FAT-TALK NATION

*The Human Costs of America's
War on Fat*

SUSAN GREENHALGH

CORNELL UNIVERSITY PRESS
ITHACA AND LONDON

First published 2015 by Cornell University Press
Printed in the United States of America

Library of Congress Cataloging-in-Publication Data

Greenhalgh, Susan, author.
   Fat-talk nation : the human costs of America's war on fat /
Susan Greenhalgh.
      pages cm
   Includes bibliographical references and index.
   ISBN 978-0-8014-5395-3 (cloth : alk. paper)
   1. Weight loss—United States. 2. Weight loss—Social aspects—
United States. I. Title.
   RC628.G743   2015
   613.2'5—dc23   2014048582

Cornell University Press strives to use environmentally responsible suppliers and materials to the fullest extent possible in the publishing of its books. Such materials include vegetable-based, low-VOC inks and acid-free papers that are recycled, totally chlorine-free, or partly composed of nonwood fibers. For further information, visit our website at www.cornellpress.cornell.edu.

Cloth printing   10 9 8 7 6 5 4 3 2 1

Contents

PREFACE

"Tiger Mom puts 7-year-old on drastic diet!"
"Chris Christie had secret weight-loss surgery."
"Good news? AMA declares obesity a disease."
"Fitness Crazed"

This is not another book about how to lose weight or become fit. In my search for a publisher, I encountered one literary agent after another who told me that on the topic of obesity, the only thing people would read is a book on how to shed pounds. My book would not sell, they said—and the headlines above, which are daily fare in our fat-phobic culture, seem to suggest as much. Yet I am reluctant to agree. From my conversations with Americans of many ages and backgrounds, I sense a hunger for new ways to think about the troubling epidemic of obesity and related disorders, which seems to grow ever more dire as a medical crisis, even as it stubbornly resists solution at the individual or societal level. I sense a longing for a way to push back against the well-worn narrative in which America is facing a "childhood obesity epidemic" so threatening to the nation that it be fought no matter the cost—an account so pervasive that it has become the cultural common sense about obesity and virtually the only way to understand the problem and how to address it.

This book responds to the yearning for fresh insight into the vexed issue of weight in America. It asks how the war on fat works; how it has recruited all of us to fight fat by lecturing, badgering, and shaming fat people into shedding pounds; and how it has come to weave itself so deeply into the fabric of our society that it has remade who we are as a nation—our culture, our relationships, our economy, our science and technology, and even our politics.

In all the talk about fat in America, there is one voice that is almost never heard: the voice of those targeted in the fight against excess pounds. How do heavy people feel being the object of such visceral hatred, verbal abuse, and outright discrimination? We do not know, and they cannot tell us without risking further abuse. *Fat-Talk Nation* gives voice to people who have been shamed into silence. It tells the human story of today's war on fat in the voices of its main objects of bodily reform: the young. Featuring 45 in-depth narratives of personal struggles with diet, weight, and "bad BMIs," it shows how the war on fat has produced a generation of young people who are obsessed with their bodies and BMIs, and whose most fundamental sense of self comes increasingly from their size. It shows that no matter whether obese, overweight, normal, or underweight, almost everyone is miserable about their bodies and almost no one is able to lose weight and keep it off. This book shows that the war on fat, which is supposed to rescue America from obesity-induced national decline, is itself damaging the bodies of the young and disrupting families and intimate relationships. The human trauma caused by the war on fat is disturbing—and it is virtually unknown. By exposing what the war has wrought, this book aims to change the conversation about weight in America today.

In telling the stories of those targeted for bodily reform, this book turns the war on fat itself into the object of inquiry. It argues that fatness today is not primarily about health; more fundamentally, it is about morality and political inclusion/exclusion or citizenship. To unpack the complex dynamics of fat politics today, I introduce a cluster of concepts—biocitizen, biomyth, fat-talk, biopedagogy, bioabuse, biocop, and fat subjectivity—and show how these biophenomena work together to produce so much hype and such deep investments in the attainment of the thin, fit body.

I draw on scholarly work in fat studies, medical anthropology, biopolitics, and medicine and public health, and I aim to contribute to the conversations in those fields. Yet because the obesity issue affects virtually all Americans, and because the stakes in how we understand and address it are so high for us as individuals and as a nation, I also aim to reach a wider general public. In particular, I aspire to reach the young people who are the primary targets of the war, as well as those charged with their upbringing, from parents and doctors to teachers and coaches. To reach that broad readership, I keep scholarly trappings to a minimum and draw only selectively on the literature. For those wanting a comprehensive review of the burgeoning writings on fat politics, the reference list contains citations to numerous helpful sources.

Many books on the cultural politics of fat reflect, at least in part, efforts by their authors to come to terms with the fat oppression they have endured throughout their lives. This book has a different and rather unlikely genesis. It was born in a classroom on the leafy campus of the University of California, Irvine, in the heart of sunny, body-obsessed southern California. As I taught my students in "The Woman and the Body" about the rise of this new "epidemic" and the launch of the national war on fat, they taught me, through their essays about their own lives and the lives of those close to them, about the dynamics of weight in their daily existence; about their struggles, mostly futile, to lose pounds and keep their weight within "healthy BMI" levels; and about the trauma they experienced as they watched their happy childhoods or promising athletic careers vanish, lost to the struggle to drop weight. I had no idea until reading their essays of the extraordinary suffering young people endure simply because their bodies carry extra pounds. Their essays left me stunned and saddened. Why are fat people berated and stigmatized while thin people are treated like health heroes, when their body weights are due more to genetics and the environment than to any bodily virtue on their part? Reading my students' essays made me see the war on fat as a problem of social (in)justice and compelled me to undertake this project to make their stories part of the national conversation about the war on fat and how we have fought it so far. It is to these young people, and especially to the roughly 600 students in "The Woman and the Body" classes of 2010 and 2011, that I dedicate this book.

Beyond sharing their powerful stories, my students have contributed to this project in countless other ways. In California, Leticia (Lety) Sanchez and Laura Stipic served both as able research assistants and as mentors on the body culture of their generation. On the other side of the country, in Cambridge, MA, my Harvard students have deepened my understanding of how the war on fat plays out in parts of the country outside southern California. Through critical engagement in the classroom and close readings of my work-in-progress, undergraduates Helen Clark, Marissa

Cominelli, Parker Davis, Amalia Duncan, Charles He, Courtney Hooton, Anne Carroll Ingersoll, and Briana Jackucewicz lent nuance to my interpretations and affirmed my sense that the life stories of my California students are quite typical. My teaching assistants at UC Irvine—Elsa Fan, Caitlin Fouratt, Cortney Hughes Rinker, Elham Mireshghi, Erin Moran, Lydia Zacher, and Ather Zia—and my teaching fellows at Harvard—Neal Akatsuka, Marty Alexander, Cynthia Browne, and Zoe Eddy—were critical interlocutors on the politics of the body in the United States today. Graduate students in my seminars "Biopolitics" and "The Body in the Age of Obesity" also stimulated new thinking. Lively discussion in class with Non Arkaraprasertkul, Sara Hendren, Melissa Lefkowitz, Jacob Moses, James Sares, Jason Silverstein, Sonya Soni, and Kimberly Sue left all of us with a deeper appreciation of the contradictions inherent in today's framing of obesity as a medical matter.

A number of professional colleagues—Esther Rothblum in fat studies, Megan Carney and Suzanne Gottschang in medical anthropology, Becca Scofield in American Studies, Sarah Gurley-Green in narrative medicine, and two reviewers for Cornell University Press—read the manuscript in full, providing invaluable feedback, as did my dear friend and SoCal insider Gary Sohl. I am indebted to Katherine Flegal and Cynthia Ogden of the CDC for insight into the science of obesity and its making. This book also benefitted immeasurably from discussions with Anne Becker and S. Bryn Austin on the still mostly uncharted connections between eating disorders and obesity, and with Arthur Kleinman on the pathways from social stigma to social death.

I was privileged to present some of my work-in-progress to members of the Science and Technology Studies Program at the University of California, San Diego; the Institute for Social, Behavioral, and Economic Research at the University of California, Santa Barbara; the Anthropology Department at the New School for Social Research; the Social Anthropology group at Harvard University; and the Research Center on Public Health and Institute for Science, Technology, and Society at Tsinghua University in Beijing. I also presented papers from this project at the annual meeting of the American Ethnological Society and the conference on BIOS: Life, Death, Politics, hosted by the Unit for Criticism and Interpretive Theory at the University of Illinois, Champaign-Urbana. For their trenchant comments and words of encouragement at these events, I owe special thanks to Miriam Ticktin and Lisa Rubin of the New School for Social Research, Hazel Clark of Parsons Institute, Val Jenness at UC Irvine, Sarah Fenstermaker of UC Santa Barbara and the University of Michigan, Paul Rabinow of UC Berkeley, Alma Gottlieb of the University of Illinois Champaign-Urbana, and Naomi Oreskes of UC San Diego and Harvard. Some of the material in chapters 1 and 4 draws on my article "Weighty Subjects: The Biopolitics of the U.S. War on Fat," *American Ethnologist* 39(3), August 2012, 471–87.

These words of appreciation would not be complete without mention of Fran Benson, my acquisitions editor at the press. Her infectious enthusiasm for the project and critical suggestions on framing and approach helped make this book everything it is now.

Part 1

THE POLITICS AND CULTURE OF FAT IN AMERICA

1

A BIOCITIZENSHIP SOCIETY TO FIGHT FAT

When I was an 8-pound baby who was a week early, it should have been a sign that being skinny would never be my destiny. In high school and college I have been bothered and ashamed by my weight. I noticed that food is my "support" and I abuse it. When I am stressed, I eat. When I am depressed, I eat. When I am angry, I eat. When I am bored, I eat, creating a vicious cycle that is spinning out of control, snuffing out the person I am inside. Looking to food to comfort my hormonal and emotional episodes is unhealthy because, if during one of my "feeding frenzies" I happen to gain weight, even just one or two pounds, I flip out and feel disgusted with myself. I can feel the disgust manifest in the pit of my stomach like it has a voice, and with every growl and every grubble, it is like a knife into my self-esteem telling me I am too fat and asking why I eat so much.

I believe my problems with my weight began when I was a little girl. My father's side of the family is very materialistic and looks-based; if you're not rich, pretty, and skinny, you are nothing. My mother is quite a large woman, and so my father's mother didn't like her and always ignored her. When my brother and I were born, my mother gained 60 pounds and my grandmother's cruel words became more vocal, to the point where as a second grader I knew my grandmother thought my mother was too fat to be with her son. Yet as the years went by and my mother didn't lose any weight, and I began to grow rounder, her hurtful needle-like words became aimed at me. I will never forget the pain and disgust I felt when I was about in fifth grade. My grandmother, father, and I were at the family restaurant Islands. I was eating a chicken tenders kid's meal, yet my grandmother thought this was too much for me. So in the middle of the meal, she looked at me and told me to "stop eating, because if you don't then one day you will look like *that*." "That" happened to be an extremely large woman in the restaurant, with my grandmother's finger pointed directly at her. I felt confused and hurt. All these thoughts swarmed in my head: I knew I was big, but was I fat? That day changed my life forever. I have not been able to look at myself the same way again.

Elise, twenty years old, Caucasian from Sherman Oaks, California;
from her personal story "A Rock Weighing My Spirit Down"

When I was ten years old, I went to the doctor's office for a routine checkup. Little did I know I was about to experience one of the most traumatic events of my life. I knew I had weight problems, but no one had ever called me fat directly. This doctor told my mom that if she did not do anything soon, I would be in danger of contracting diseases like high blood pressure, diabetes, and hypertension. I did not realize it at the time, but those words caused lasting trauma. My self-confidence was shot down. Since then I have always thought of myself as a big girl; even though I have now lost more than 35 pounds and kept it off, I still think of myself as big.

Society is very cruel toward overweight people, especially young children. When I was in elementary school, we were all playing outside during recess when this boy tore up my self-confidence. There was a game of basketball and I wanted the ball, but no one would give it to me. Finally I asked for it. The boy said to me: "Why do you want the ball? You are fat, I'm sure you can't even shoot!" I froze for a couple seconds. I could not believe that someone would say something so insensitive and rude to me. I ran to the girls' bathroom and cried for a few minutes. That day is one I will never forget. He broke me down. For years after that I felt ugly, fat, disgusting, and not good enough. I assumed that every boy was as mean and disrespectful as that one. So I began to eat. Food was delicious and it made me feel good. Slowly but surely, I gained more and more weight until I became borderline obese.

Lauren, nineteen years old, Salvadoran American from Lynnwood, California;
from her personal story "Overcoming the Abuse"

A National War on Fat: Narrative of a Nation in Decline

By all accounts, America is in the midst of an obesity epidemic of cata-strophic scale in which rising proportions of the public—now two-thirds of adults, and one-third of children and adolescents—are obese or over-weight. Between the late 1970s and 2012, the proportion of Americans who are obese rose from 15 to 34.9 percent among adults and from 5 to 16.9 percent among the young.[1] Although the rate of increase has recently slowed or stabilized in some groups, the now-heavy burden of fat, influ-ential voices maintain, continues to threaten the nation. In the dominant story told by government, public health, and media sources, the country's fatness is eroding the nation's health, emptying its coffers, and threatening its security by depriving it of fit military recruits.[2] The response has been an urgent, nationwide public health campaign, officially launched by the U.S. surgeon general in 2001, to get people—and especially the young—to eat more healthfully and be more active in an effort to achieve a "normal" body mass index (BMI).[3] Toward that end, the surgeon general's office and other government departments concerned with the public's health have repeatedly urged all sectors of American society—from parents to elected officials, to school administrators, health-care professionals, lead-ers of nonprofits, and private companies—to help reduce the burden of fat. First Lady Michelle Obama's "Let's Move!" campaign, which aims to "solve the challenge of childhood obesity within a generation," is only the latest initiative in what has been the nation's standard approach to remedy-ing the problem of growing girth for the last decade and a half.[4]

American antipathy toward fatness is nothing new. For roughly the last 150 years, being fat has been seen as a cultural, moral, and aesthetic transgression that marked one as irresponsible, immoral, and ugly—"grotesque" in the indelicate language of former Surgeon General C. Ever-ett Koop (who served 1982–1989).[5] In the last few decades, however, there has been a critical cultural shift in our concern about fatness, from "self-control" (or virtue) to "health." The now routine definition of excess weight as a disease, the rapid growth in medical research, and the prolif-eration of news on obesity and overweight mark this cultural shift.[6] As the sociologist Abigail C. Saguy argues, the biomedical frame for understand-ing obesity has become so naturalized that people do not even realize it is a conceptual frame, one among many possible frames.[7]

While weight as an attribute has been medicalized, that is, defined as a medical condition requiring diagnosis, two categories of weight—overweight and obesity—have been pathologized, treated as diseases in themselves. No longer are chunky and fat people merely "lazy"; in the current discourse they are also biologically defective; chronically ill; at risk of yet other, obesity-related diseases; and in need of ongoing medical treatment. It is this "diseasification" of higher weights, and its framing within a narrative of obesity-induced national decline, that has justified our government's intervention in the obesity "epidemic" and the use of taxpayer dollars to support these interventions. With two-thirds of American adults and one-third of children now deemed abnormal and in need of remediation, there would appear to be strong grounds for taxpayer-supported government involvement, including not just public health actions but also financial support for a mushrooming research enterprise devoted to understanding the causes and consequences of this new disease. This disease model of weight, requiring government management, has not replaced the moral model of body size but has built on it in ways that greatly intensify the already heavy pressures to be thin.[8]

Because personal health in our culture is a mega-value, equivalent to the good life itself, the medicalization of weight has had huge societal consequences. In the national anxiety that has grown up around the obesity problem—what sociologists such as Natalie Boero call a moral panic, marked by exaggerated concern about the threat to core American values[9]—these broader consequences of treating heaviness as a disease have received scant notice. But they deserve our closest attention. The shift to health as the primary grounds for concern about adipose bodies has led to a dramatic expansion of the social forces seeking to intervene. The result has been an explosion of fat-talk of all kinds. By *fat-talk* I mean communications of all sorts about weight—spoken words, written texts, visual images, and moving videos—along with the associated practices, such as dieting, exercising, and many others. Where do we hear fat-talk?

In the news there has been a veritable explosion of articles on obesity. Between the early 1990s and 2010, the number of published news reports on obesity rose from virtually none to 6,000 a year.[10] Feature articles in news, women's, and science magazines appear regularly, accompanied by cover images of fat babies holding gigantic tubs of french fries or fat children snorfing down double-scoop ice cream cones. (Such images have become less common in recent years.) In the political sphere, anti-fat legislation aimed at limiting food ads for children, requiring food labeling in restaurants, or reengineering car-centric environments is advancing at the federal, state, and municipal levels, producing noisy debates over the "nanny state's" right to tell Americans what they should eat and the ability of hefty officials to govern. The New Jersey politician Chris Christie has received more than his share of press commentary about his size.[11]

Corporate interests have been a major force behind the escalation of fat-talk. Slimming down has become a huge sector of the economy as the pharmaceutical, biotech, fitness, food, and restaurant industries have figured out how to use a rhetoric of medicine ("it's good for your health") to exploit people's fear of the disease of fat to generate some $60 billion annually in profits.[12] In our image-saturated world, the ads of corporate America, with their trim figures and seductive messages, have been powerful forces behind the growing fixation on fat. Building on an already deeply ingrained culture of thinness,[13] the new medically driven concern with weight loss has also propelled corpulence to the center of our popular culture. The new genre of Fat TV—featuring weight-loss reality shows such as *The Biggest Loser* (NBC), *Weighing In* (Food Network), and *Celebrity Fit Club* (VH1)—is only the most conspicuous of these new forms of fat culture. Finally, in everyday social life, fat-talk has become a routine way of communicating with one another as we visually size people up; comment on their body size, the fit of their clothing, the food they are eating, and so on; and judge them according to their adherence to the normative thin-body ideal. The harsh warnings of Elise's grandmother and the cruel jabs of Lauren's classmate are perfect examples of fat-talk in action. It is no exaggeration to say that fifteen years after the official launching of the war on fat, America is obsessed with fat—what it means for us, how bad it is for us, and what we must do to rid our individual and collective selves of it. We have become, in short, a fat-talk nation, in which fat-talk is ubiquitous, marking good and bad, deserving and undeserving Americans.

In this way, what started as an urgent public health call to action in the early 2000s has grown into a massive society-wide war on fat that involves virtually every sector of American society and leaves few domains of life untouched. In the late 1990s, former Surgeon General Koop, one of the most outspoken and influential warriors in the battle against tobacco, coined the term *war on obesity* to draw attention to the need for a national mobilization against fat that was every bit as forceful as the nation's war on tobacco.[14] In 2004, in the wake of 9/11, then–Surgeon General Richard Carmona described the rise in childhood obesity as "every bit as threatening to us as is the terrorist threat we face today. It is the threat from within."[15] Such metaphors are not innocent. In likening fat people, including fat children, to terrorists, Carmona was justifying an all-out war against fat individuals that entailed treating them as veritable enemies of the American people and the American way of life. The message was not only that it is un-American to be fat but also that hostility toward large people was warranted and necessary and beneficial to "us all."

In this book, I call this broad-based campaign a *war on fat*. I use the term *war* not just because some government and public health advocates routinely use that metaphor but also because that word captures the feeling of many of its targets that not just their bodies but also their persons are under perpetual attack. I use the colloquial word *fat* because that is the term many heavy people prefer, finding the official term *obesity* too objectifying.[16] And I focus on the war on fat, rather than on obesity, because this is a war not just on obesity (defined in terms of the BMI) but on every extra pound of flesh, whether the excess is on an "obese," "overweight," or "normal" body. The twenty-first-century war on fat is profoundly remaking the political, economic, social, and cultural worlds in which we live in ways that are very partially understood. Although this book deals only with the United States, weights are rising around the world, producing what the World Health Organization calls a "global pandemic of obesity"[17] and, in turn, urgent efforts by governments and transnational bodies to contain it. The problem, then, is not only an American problem; increasingly, it is a global problem. Given the centrality of America in the world, how we respond is likely to affect policymakers and ordinary people in the tens of millions around the globe. Will the warlike approach to obesity championed by the United States be a positive model for the rest of the world? That question is rarely asked in public and health forums, but it should be.

Whatever its broader consequences, the war on fat has not yet reduced the national waistline. Despite the huge investment of public and private resources to fight fat, rates of obesity have scarcely budged. Between 2003–2004 and 2011–2012, there was no significant change in obesity prevalence among youth or adults. There was, however, a substantial decline in obesity among preschool children ages two to five, a finding that appears promising but remains unexplained.[18] The reasons obesity has stopped climbing in most groups remain unclear; the slowdown could be related to basic biology—a saturation of the population that is genetically vulnerable to weight gain in our environment—and have little to do with the war on fat.[19] The response has not been to step back and rethink the nature of the adversary and the warlike approach to its eradication; the response has been to hunker down and fight even harder. For example, health officials in some areas have turned up the heat on fat kids and their parents. In late 2013, Children's Healthcare of Atlanta released a controversial video, "Rewind the Future," which was aimed at warning negligent parents by graphically depicting the future of a child, Jim, whose diet of junk food led to massive weight gain and eventually a heart attack.[20] With a growing recognition of the limits of diet and exercise, and a marked rise in obesity-related diseases, anti-fat advocates are left with few treatment options other than surgery and drugs. Weight-loss (or bariatric) surgery—which is very costly, carries substantial risks, and imposes severe dietary restrictions for the rest of the patient's life—has been extended to new patient categories, including severely obese adolescents as young as twelve.[21] Since 2012, the Food and Drug Administration (FDA) has approved four new diet drugs: Belviq, Qsymia, Contrave, and Saxenda. Like fen-phen, which was withdrawn in 1997 after evidence emerged of serious heart-valve damage, all have the potential to cause cardiovascular and other problems. And none of the drugs is very effective.[22] With large proportions of Americans labeled ill, few safe and effective cures in sight, and a growing reliance on costly and risky methods, today's approach to fat hardly seems like a promising route to creating a healthy, vibrant, revitalized America.

Why Worry about the War on Fat? Listening to Our Young People

In all the public talk about the national plague of obesity and the lazy, irresponsible fat people who are bringing the nation down, there is one voice that is rarely heard: the voice of those targeted by the war on fat. Young women such as Elise and Lauren are the main targets of the war on fat, yet the kinds of stories they tell are virtually never heard. Almost every day on the news, we hear from medical researchers and government officials announcing a new finding about the health effects of obesity or a new campaign to tax soda; we hear from corporate advertisers and spokespersons promoting weight-loss products; and we hear from anxious parents and teachers concerned about their chubby young charges. Once in a while a lone voice can be heard complaining about the cultural hatred of fat. In fall 2012, for example, the feminist blog Jezebel carried an angry article titled "It's Hard Enough to Be a Fat Kid without the Government Telling You You're an Epidemic."[23] Complaining bitterly about the common assumption that fat kids are fat because they eat too many Pizza Poppers and bowls of chocolate cereal, the author, once a fat kid and now a fat adult, argues that the anti-fat campaign amounts to an anti-people campaign that will do more harm than good. Around the same time, Jennifer Livingston, a full-bodied TV news anchor in Milwaukee, spent several minutes on the air responding to a man who had e-mailed to inform her that "obesity is one of the worst choices a person can make" and that she was a poor role model for young girls.[24] Using the occasion as a teaching moment, Livingston insisted that such attacks are not acceptable and that we need to teach our kids kindness, not cruelty. The outpouring of support she received leaves no doubt about the sea of unhappiness and pent-up exasperation that exists about the maltreatment of overweight people in our culture. Yet sympathetic outlets for such complaints are few indeed. As is usually the case with Internet critics, just as quickly as a fat-rights voice emerges, it disappears from public view, leaving no lasting cultural critique, no sustained challenge to the dominant approach to the problematic of weight as an epidemic. And if heavy adults are rarely heard, heavy children and adolescents, the campaign's major targets, are virtually inaudible.

The Critique of the Fat Acceptance Movement: Is Anyone Listening?

Underscoring the absence of a wider cultural critique of today's approach to obesity, voices such as these amount to little more than complaints about how the war on fat has affected the speaker personally. This is a far cry from a systematic critique of the anti-obesity campaign. Such an analysis does exist, but it is likely that few Americans have even heard of it. It is called the fat acceptance movement (or simply, FAM), and its main organization, the National Association to Advance Fat Acceptance, has been around for decades. Researchers and activists broadly aligned with the FAM have developed two main criticisms of the anti-obesity campaign, one focusing on the politics of the war on fat and the other on the science of obesity.

In its political critique, the movement argues that the real problem we face in this country is not obesity but rampant fat stigma and size discrimination, which, it contends, are worsened by the crisis framing of the obesity problem.[25] Drawing on a large array of statistics, FAM researchers point out that fat people face discrimination in every arena of daily life—from education to employment to medical care—with consequences that diminish their social and economic well-being, harm their romantic prospects, and compromise their health.[26] Common treatments for fatness are not only ineffective over the long run, but many lead to weight gain and, on top of that, pose serious risks to people's health. Far from diseases that should be medically treated, the FAM argues, fat and weight more generally are forms of bodily diversity. Like height, weight is a relatively immutable, biologically and genetically based part of our identities that should be accepted and respected. Instead of wasting time and money seeking to achieve an artificial standard of thinness, they argue, we should aim to be "healthy at every size."[27] Seeking to redefine weight as a legal and political matter, the movement works to end size discrimination and gain legal protection for the rights of fat people. By openly celebrating fat pride and circulating alternative images of fat people having fun, smashing bathroom scales, or enjoying the companionship of normal-size men who love fat women, the movement is challenging the erasure of fat people in our culture while constructing new, positive identities and embodied practices for the fat community.[28] The FAM offers the encouraging and inclusive messages that there is beauty in all bodies and that health can come at any size.

This alternative paradigm deserves serious consideration, yet it has had little discernible impact on the public conversation about the obesity problem. The movement does seem to have injected into some of the public health campaigns greater sensitivity about the damaging effects of stigmatizing images on heavy people.[29] Yet its larger argument that weight is not a disease but a form of bodily diversity having to do with human rights has gained little traction, despite the scientific evidence that genetics plays a very substantial role in bodily weight and that the body fights weight loss. Few members of the general public seem to be aware of the movement and its work. (And, of course, some bloggers who are aware have been dismissive of the "fat-empowerment stunts.") The FAM was born and remains loosely based in California, yet few of my University of California students had heard of it. After learning about it in class, few found it relatable. That may be because the images of its spokespeople I shared featured mostly very large, white, middle-class, middle-age women. Beyond the different demographic, though, was the bigger problem that the young adults I worked with, far from wanting to proudly claim a fat identity and demand rights on that basis, simply wanted to fit in and be normal. Perhaps because the war on fat was launched and is legitimated in the name of science, and the FAM speaks largely in the name of politics and human rights, its voices are easily ignored by mainstream obesity researchers. Some of the spokespersons for the movement may also face other problems in getting their message heard. As very large individuals themselves, they may be so stigmatized by the dominant fat-hating culture that they are accorded little credibility. Sadly, their voices may be discredited simply because they are fat.[30]

The work of the historian Amy Farrell helps us to understand why fat people are allowed so little space for self-expression in our culture. In *Fat Shame*, her pathbreaking history of fat culture in America, Farrell argues that, based on a long history of fat shaming, fatness today is such a stigmatizing attribute that it is utterly discrediting.[31] Fatness is not only a physical stigma, it is also a character stigma that allows others to treat fat people as not quite human, as not worthy of normal standards of respect. This stigma then justifies active discrimination against them that further diminishes their life chances. Mainstream culture, she argues, is reluctant to give fat people any but circumscribed acceptance—that is, they are tolerated and allowed a public voice as long as they stay within their group and accept the limits imposed by the non-fat culture. In the United States today, there are precious few public scripts that fat people can follow or positive identities that they are allowed to occupy. They can be "fat and funny," like the main characters on the CBS television program *Mike and Molly*. Or they can accept the dominant obesity narrative and present themselves as "fat and ashamed" and working desperately to lose weight—like the contestants on the NBC show *The Biggest Loser*. They can post humorous or biting comments on online sites, such as the StopHatingYourBody microblog on tumblr, where like-minded people share reactions and photos. But once they try to step outside those delimited circles—say, by criticizing their treatment in the larger culture—they are punished and shamed into silence. No wonder so few dare to demand broader inclusion in mainstream society. How do fat people feel being the object of so much verbal vitriol and moral condemnation? We can only guess, and they cannot tell us without risking further maltreatment.

Closely aligned with this political activism is a body of interdisciplinary scholarship in the emerging field of fat studies that, although perhaps not (yet) reaching the general public, is powerfully shaping the scholarly understanding of the country's so-called "obesity epidemic"[32] Through analysis of a wide range of political, cultural, and scientific materials, as well as selected interviews, this work has shown how the notion that the United States faces an "obesity epidemic" was historically constructed by particular actors, who, working as moral entrepreneurs, created a moral panic around the issue and how that "crisis" construct has persisted to become the hegemonic narrative about obesity in America, despite the problematic nature of some of the underlying science.[33] This work has also illuminated some of the harmful effects of the crisis framing, including a worsening of stigma and discrimination against fat people and a heightening of social inequalities along the lines of gender, race, and class.

Although I build on this research, in this book I tackle a different set of questions. I seek to understand not fatness or its cultural and political representations but how the war on fat—a different focus from the commonly studied public health campaign—is actually playing out on the ground and with what effects, especially on the young. The younger generation—that raised since the early 1990s—is a critical focus for this research. In her work with adult participants in weight-loss programs, Boero found that people did not see their fatness as a risk to personal health or contributor to a public health crisis, a finding that suggests that the public health narrative is having little impact on ordinary Americans.[34] That conclusion, this book will show, does not hold for younger Americans. As the first generation raised in a world obsessed with the "crisis of childhood obesity," young people's experiences with the crisis story are more piercing, penetrating, and consequential than those of many adults. As they grow into adulthood, their life experiences will increasingly shape who we are as a nation.

To understand how the war is working in daily life, I introduce a new kind of data and a new set of theoretical concepts. I draw on anthropological research on the real-life experiences of young people in one part of the country, listening intently to how they describe their worlds and lives, and making their accounts the centerpiece of my own. I also develop a repertoire of interrelated concepts that includes a robust notion of subjectivity, which remains underdeveloped in the work in fat studies, and a set of notions that show how a historically specific morality, politics, and science of weight intersect in everyday life to produce the kinds of effects noted in the existing literature as well as others that have not been brought to light. As noted in the preface, I hope to reach not only scholars and students of American society but also members of the general public, who are themselves the unwitting participants in the war on fat, with effects they may not fully appreciate. In hopes of engaging that broader readership, I have used colloquial language and placed scholarly citations and discussions in the notes at the back of the book.

Unhappy at Every Size: Young People Share Their Stories

As a university professor and researcher located for many years in the Los Angeles region (and now the Boston area), I have listened carefully to the voices of young adults who since childhood have been the main targets of the war on fat. I have listened most closely to the students in my course "The Woman and the Body" at the University of California. The majority of them were technically "overweight" or "normal." A handful would be considered "obese" or "underweight." Regardless of how they were categorized, scarcely a one was happy with his or her body. Most were acutely aware of the society-wide war on fat and that it made them feel like damaged goods. One overweight young woman, whom I call Anahid, put her feelings into these words: "When there is so much talk about obesity, you feel bad about yourself as a person. Even if you are a kind person, you feel down because the whole nation is saying that excessive weight is bad and that's it. It makes you look at yourself and think that there is something wrong with you. It is not a good feeling at all; it makes you feel like a failure and more importantly, it makes you feel as if you have failed others" [SC 92]. Virtually everyone felt oppressed by the constant pressure to achieve a certain body size and shape.

The following chapters present the in-depth accounts of the weight struggles of forty-five people—mostly in their late teens and early twenties, but some in mid- and late life—of both genders and many different ethnicities. Each account is unique, but the accounts taken together tell a larger and troubling story about the effects of the war on fat on its prime targets. That tale is not one of successful weight loss and newfound health and happiness. Instead, it is one of joyless childhoods and shrunken lives marked by the sorts of trauma described so poignantly by Elise and Lauren.

Back in the late 1990s and early 2000s, when the anti-obesity campaign was being launched, its advocates' main goal was to draw attention and resources to the nation's newly discovered rise in obesity, which they found alarming. Although figures like Koop and Carmona certainly amped up the pressure with their rhetoric of "crisis" and "war," they probably did not anticipate that, because the issue of fatness taps such deep veins in our culture and morality, a war on fat would offer so many benefits to so many parties that more and more social forces would join the fight. Yet the stories this book presents suggest that is just what happened, with the result that the campaign against fat has ballooned into something much bigger and more consequential than anyone expected—or fully understands. Young people's stories need to be heard, not only by today's promoters of the anti-obesity campaign but also by the parents, teachers, coaches, and friends who have been recruited to serve as foot soldiers in that war. They need to be read not only by those who are actively trying to shape the weight of America but by everyone who thinks heavy people are disgusting and repulsive—which includes a large portion of the American public.

Drawing on their accounts and other materials, this book tells the human story of the war on fat, a story of both hidden dynamics and untallied costs. Although I share some of the concerns of the FAM, especially about the damaging effects of weight stigma, this book extends those concerns beyond the fat population to a wide swath of Americans, documenting the effects on Americans of many weights, both genders, many ethnicities, and diverse classes. As already noted, it also provides a broad theoretical framework for understanding how the war on fat works on the ground and produces its unintended effects. By centering the voices and stories of young people, while shaping them into a larger, theoretically grounded account of the war on fat that ties it to questions of citizenship and the nation, this work seeks to change the cultural conversation about fat in this country. I will show that the war on fat affects not just obese and overweight people, though the consequences to them are harmful enough. Instead, it affects us all—as individuals and as a society—in ways that are profoundly concerning.

The Value of Auto-Ethnography

What opened my eyes to the human dimensions of the war on fat was ethnography. The classic tool of anthropology, ethnography is a mode of inquiry that relies on deep immersion in a culture and mostly qualitative methods such as interviews. The term also describes a form of writing. As both research method and text, ethnography tries to capture and reflect human subjects' own views of their lives and the larger context that shapes them. In *auto*-ethnography, the person being studied crafts his or her own description and analysis of his or her life and world.[35]

In the pages that follow, I rely primarily on auto-ethnographies— individual stories of struggles with eating, exercising, weight control, and eating disorders that were shared with me—to tell a new story about fat in America. How, readers might be thinking, can personal stories possibly challenge the truths of science? Because this book makes big claims, it is important that readers fully understand the grounds on which it is making them. Making an argument based on ethnography entails a different mode of explanation from the one used by the medical researchers who usually write about the obesity issue. The biomedical (and public health) research tries to persuade with numerical data that are presented as scientific facts based on supposedly neutral scientific objectivity. Quantified data are generally good at presenting the big picture, but they tend to reduce individuals to a few attributes and to omit the larger context in which people's lives play out. In medical research, people are treated as objects for study by scientists. Scientists speak for people, imposing their understandings of what matters and why on people's lives. Their understandings can be powerful, but what scientists think is most important may differ from what individuals consider the most important parts of their lives.

By contrast, auto-ethnography persuades with personal stories, stories that, ideally, compel assent by their very humanity—both the human content and the narrative structure of a life's unfolding. Ethnographic accounts are explicitly subjective, with the factors that shape the angle of vision (gender, age, and so forth) being not only acknowledged but often made part of the story. Scientific data are evaluated by being replicated by other researchers; ethnographic accounts can be considered sound if they feel right: if they map onto our understandings of the world, if they are believable, and if they are supported by other kinds of evidence in our culture and society.

Ethnographic data offer certain advantages over the quantified data of science. By viewing the war on fat through the eyes of its targets, auto-ethnography allows us to see how it affects individuals and their bodies and lives. In ethnography, people are not objects but rather subjects who can tell us what they consider most important. Key to understanding the human consequences of the war on fat, auto-ethnography allows us to capture selfhood or subjectivity—people's own sense of who they are—using their own voices. Rather than reducing people to a few quantifiable variables, ethnographic writing captures a wide range of the often quirky, unmeasurable things that make them human. By illuminating the causal links between individual lives and their wider historical and cultural contexts, ethnography also enables us to move beyond individual experience and trace the connections between broader structural forces and personal experience.

The main limitation of ethnography is its focus on relatively small numbers of individuals; because the "sample" is not scientifically selected, one cannot generalize to a larger population. In this book, the problem of generalizability is diminished somewhat by the number and diversity of individual cases. I gathered ethnographic accounts of 245 individuals of a great many ethnic backgrounds and from all income levels except dire poverty and vast wealth. Most of the accounts center on young people, but some feature middle-age and elderly people. Although the cases are unique, the dynamics of the weight struggles they describe are, I believe, quite general. Auto-ethnography also has limits, for the researcher cannot pursue leads or independently observe the writer in social context to verify the validity of his or her account. In using these essays as "data," we must assume that their authors told the social truth as they saw it.

The chapters that follow use the essays to answer three questions: How does the war on fat work on the ground? Is it achieving its intended goals? And what is it producing in addition to slim, fit people, if indeed it is producing those? Put another way, what are its broader social effects? The proponents of the war on fat have been so narrowly focused on fighting obesity (and uncovering its health effects) that they have not stepped back to ask about the effects of their campaign itself—on fat people or on society at large. Yet as a society we need to ask these difficult questions: Is the war on fat doing what it is supposed to do? Is it inadvertently producing some harmful effects? Do the benefits exceed the unintended costs?

Students of narrative teach that it is not enough to challenge a powerful public story; one must replace it with a better story. In the pages that follow, I seek to disrupt an exceeding powerful account of weight in America, one focused on personal blame, health, and economic costs, by telling a more compelling story that is centered on morality and political belonging, individual and societal costs, and social injustice on a very wide scale. To understand all this, we need to grasp how the war on fat works.

How the War on Fat Works, Part 1: Meet the Thin, Fit Biocitizen

How, then, does the war on fat operate, and what exactly does it do in the process of trying to make us all thin?

The Birth of the Thin, Fit, Healthist Biocitizen

To answer these questions, we need to go back some 150 years to the late nineteenth century, when fat first became a salient political and cultural issue in America. In her history of fat culture, Farrell shows how the 1860s saw a growing cultural hatred of fatness as authoritative voices began to use body size as an important marker to measure one's suitability for the privileges and power of full citizenship.[36] Fatness became a metaphor for something that threatened the United States (greed or corruption, for example). Beginning around 1900, fatness became a sign that one was inherently incapable of withstanding the pressures and pleasures of modern life, including the responsibilities and privileges of citizenship; one must be thin to be civilized. From around 1900, having the right body—a thin one—became a requirement for inclusion in the category of good Americans deemed worthy of a place in the public sphere and the rights and responsibilities of citizenship. Since at least that time, body weight in America has been a political and moral issue through and through.

Social thinkers have coined the term *biocitizenship* for this new kind of political belonging or citizenship connected to one's bodily attributes. In the United States and other Western countries, influential theorists have argued, the notion of citizen no longer means simply a subject with a legal status and set of constitutional rights and duties. Instead, a citizen is a social being whose existence is articulated in the language of social responsibilities and collective solidarity.[37] Since around 1900, one of the social responsibilities of the good (bio)citizen has been to maintain a certain kind of body—initially a thin body and, from the late twentieth century, a thin, fit body. In this book, I call this new kind of biocitizen who is the centerpiece of the war on fat the *thin, fit biocitizen*.[38] Managing our own health and ensuring a medically "normal" weight and fit body are fundamental duties of the good biocitizen today. It is important that the requirement involves active citizenship and social concern. The good biocitizen has two inter-related duties. The first is to take care of his or her own diet, exercise, and weight because it serves the individual and all others in society. As a former Health and Human Services secretary put it, "All Americans should lose ten pounds as a patriotic gesture."[39] Failing to control one's weight makes one a bad citizen because one is ignoring the interests of the common good needed for a well-ordered (that is, healthy and productive) society.

The requirements for being a good biocitizen have become ever more demanding. To be a thin, fit biocitizen today demands the constant surveillance of one's body, pursuit of rigorous diet and exercise routines, and avoidance of risky behaviors in an effort to maintain a normal BMI and a fit physique. (The BMI is a number calculated from a person's weight and height that is widely used as indicator of his or her fatness and disease risk. Technically, the BMI is an individual's body mass divided by the square of his height.) Because optimal health can never be fully achieved, its pursuit requires constant work and vigilance. There is a word for such obsessive attention to the body, and it is *healthism*. Few Americans are likely to be familiar with this term, but many enact its essence every day. Coined in 1980 by the political theorist Robert Crawford, healthism is the moralization of health which arose in the mid-1970s among middle-class Americans.[40] Stimulated by a new awareness of health hazards in the environment and by the rise of a host of new health movements—from the self-help, natural foods, holistic health, and women's health movements to the jogging, dieting, and fitness crazes—healthism defined health as a *supervalue*, one that took precedence over all other concerns.[41] Health became a metaphor for all that is good in life, and the preoccupation with personal health became a primary—often the primary—focus for the definition and achievement of well-being. Health also became a major locus of identity as people defined themselves increasingly by how well they succeeded in adopting healthful practices.

Rather than looking to larger economic, political, or environmental forces as the determinants of health outcomes, healthism situated the problem of health and disease at the level of the individual: good health was said to be the moral duty of all individuals, while bad health was attributed to individual failings. The solutions to health problems were individualized too.[42] In the 1990s and early 2000s, the war on fat absorbed this healthist strand in our culture and made it central to how the campaign was framed and carried out. Healthism is evident today in people's obsessive efforts to stay thin, fit, and healthy. It can be seen too in the overriding emphasis of the campaign to make individuals, rather than society as a whole, responsible for weight. Instead of fighting food corporations, restructuring the built environment, or tackling toxins in the environment, most public health officials have been pouring their energy into blaming and shaming individuals and urging them to "take responsibility for their health." Things are beginning to change, but the emphasis on individual responsibility for weight remains paramount.

Since the 1980s, market-oriented (or "neoliberal") values and institutions have gained supremacy, bringing a retreat of the state and a rise of the entrepreneurial individual, who exercises choice and takes responsibility for his or her own risks. Good health—especially as signaled by the thin, fit body—has become a means to prove one's self-worth in a competitive political economy. In her important book *Weighing In*, the political ecologist Julie Guthman argues that the rise of managed care in the 1980s led to a redefinition of *good citizenship* to include being a minimal consumer of state health and welfare services.[43] Under managed care, health became subject to market logics, and the unhealthy, who impose excess costs on the health-care system, were said to harm the nation. The good citizen became one who reduced health-care costs to the body politic by taking responsibility for his or her own health through lifestyle modifications. This notion that the individual should show concern for national health costs helps to explain the widespread acceptance of the notion, fostered by the war on fat, that the cost of treating obesity is a huge public burden. In the twenty-first century, the constant stream of medical news and commercials, with their stress on the growing number of health hazards we face, makes consciousness of our physical well-being increasingly unavoidable.[44] Today, health is such a positive value that it is unthinkable not to embrace it and adopt the constant self-surveillance and discipline it requires. Because body size reflects the state of one's health (or so it is claimed), what we have today is not just what Deborah Lupton, following Michel Foucault, has called "the imperative of health"[45] but also *the imperative of thinness*.

The pursuit of the perfect body is an intensely moral project. A central focus of the war on fat—a normative or "normal" BMI to which we should all aspire—functions as a moralizing discourse that divides us into two classes of American: low and high BMI, thin and fat, good and bad. Thinness is deemed a worthy, desirable, and necessary state, and thinness and fatness are associated with traits at the opposite ends of the moral spectrum, from the highly valued self-discipline and self-control, on the one hand, to the moral failings of self-indulgence and lack of self-discipline on the other.[46] The rewards to good biocitizenship are endless. Those able to achieve the proper fit, trim body are culturally celebrated and socially rewarded. Countless statistics show that they enjoy a privileged position vis-à-vis the state (including eligibility to join the armed forces; to serve on police, fire, and other forces; and to pay lower Medicare and Medicaid premiums), the health-care establishment (where they receive better treatment), and employers (who pay and promote them more generously).[47] Seeing themselves pictured positively in advertisements, the entertainment and news media, and public health announcements, they enjoy the pride that comes from being valued as good Americans. Bad citizens— all those unable to reach a normal BMI, but especially fat people—suffer cultural degradation, social exclusion, and rampant fat discrimination in almost every domain of life. They are excluded from some areas of state service and employment, stigmatized by the health-care establishment,

and discriminated against by employers. Moreover, weight bias is growing worse, increasing according to one measure by two-thirds over the last
decade.[48] This evidence—which is based on abundant studies, virtually all
with similar findings—lends empirical weight to Farrell's contention that
fat stigma today is so severe that fat people are often treated as not quite
human. Not only is it acceptable to abuse them, but they are seen to *deserve*
such treatment because they are deviant and bad people who harm the rest
of us. Fatness today is a mark of shame so discrediting and life-diminishing
that people will go to extraordinary extremes to eliminate it.

Creating a Biocitizenship Society to Fight Fat: Self and Others in Our Social World in Charge

The most straightforward goal of the war on fat is to restore the nation
to physical and economic health by transforming obese and overweight
Americans into thin, fit, proper biocitizens. Because treatments for fatness
have very limited effectiveness, a more realistic goal is to prevent those
who are not yet fat from becoming fat. That means focusing most attention
on children and adolescents. The labeling of obesity as an "epidemic" or
even a "terrorist threat from within"—both suggesting that fatness is out
of control, dangerous, and a public enemy—and use of the military metaphor for the anti-fat campaign present the elimination of fatness as an urgent task and justify extreme and discriminatory measures in the name of
vanquishing the threats and restoring the nation's health.

Because health is such a huge—one might even say primal—value, all
legitimate social institutions are obligated to promote the project. And,
indeed, the creators of the war on fat have mobilized every major sector of American society to join the fight against fat. One can be forgiven
for thinking that one of the most important tasks of the U.S. government
today is to combat fat. In addition to the White House, which is home to
the Let's Move! campaign, no fewer than nine federal agencies under the
Department of Health and Human Services (DHHS) work on obesity issues.[49] But government efforts are just the beginning of what was and still
is envisioned as a society-wide battle against a formidable foe. In its Call to
Action, the Surgeon General's Office mapped out a strategy involving efforts by families and communities, schools, the health-care establishment,

media and communications networks, and worksites.[50] And they have responded. Schools have become major actors in the anti-obesity campaign, developing fitness tests that track children's weight status, introducing healthier food in cafeterias, reducing junk food in vending machines, creating weight report cards, and much more. In medicine, physicians and bariatric surgeons have been tackling obesity in the clinic and operating room, while researchers have been energetically studying the biology of obesity and its health consequences. Corporations in many industries have been producing and marketing an ever-widening array of anti-fat products—from apps that track food and movement to gelatinous globs that fill the stomach, curbing appetite[51]—while instituting programs to improve the weight and health of their own employees. And the list goes on. The scale of the endeavor is simply phenomenal.

The most important agent in this transformation, however, remains the individual: you and me. We have already seen that the biocitizen is charged with taking care of his or her own diet, exercise, and weight. Yet it is not enough to take care of oneself. As the sociologist Christine Halse argues, a good biocitizen's social responsibilities include taking care of the nation's welfare by helping others in one's social world—family, friends, co-workers, even perfect strangers—lose weight and become good biocitizens.[52] If heavy weights are bringing the nation down, then it is our civic and moral duty as good citizens to help people who are heavy and (apparently) unhealthy to lose the weight and get fit. The good biocitizen, thus, has two duties to society: care of the self and care for others. In the chapters that follow we will meet big sisters looking out for younger brothers and sisters, aunts berating nieces and nephews, coaches ridiculing "lazy" athletes, and strangers commenting on the food choices of a neighboring diner. Far from just being catty or cruel, each of these concerned people is following the cultural mandate to help others make healthy choices and get thin bodies. And in the process, each is feeling morally superior about his or her own choices and body.

This busy biocitizen is the key to understanding how the war on fat works and what it does. It works by creating virtuous biocitizens and demanding that they not only maintain medically normal weight themselves but also coax others into dieting and exercising to reach a normal weight. Put another way, the war on fat makes self and society primarily responsible for creating the thin, fit bodies it sees as ideal. The result is a whole society preoccupied, even obsessed, with weight and weight control: a *biocitizenship society*. This is precisely the kind of society we live in now. This notion of the doubly duty-bound biocitizen has never been applied to America's (or any country's) fight against fat, but we will see that it closely fits what is happening in American society today.

How the War on Fat Works, Part 2: Fat-Talk, Fat Discourse, Fat Science

The most important tool available to the virtuous biocitizen for persuading "bad," "unhealthy" citizens to become good ones is fat-talk. In her landmark study of body culture in the 1990s, *Fat Talk: What Girls and Their Parents Say about Dieting*, the anthropologist Mimi Nichter uses the term *fat talk* to refer to a pervasive speech performance in which teenage girls verbalized the inadequacies of their body shapes, typically by declaring: "I'm so fat!"[53] This book employs the hyphenated term *fat-talk* more broadly to refer to everyday conversations about weight—conversations of all sorts, not just declarations of fatness—that circulate in popular culture through conversation, the media, the Internet, and so on, as well as in written texts, visual images, and moving videos. Far from "mere talk," fat communications of these sorts are often accompanied by concrete practices that may be backed by legal or moral force. For example, a physician's demand that a patient go on a diet is accompanied by the entering of the patient's BMI score and diagnosis on his or her chart, practices given weight by the physician's legal authority to diagnose and treat disease. The list of such nonverbal practices accompanying weight talk is endless: the teacher assigns exercise as homework, the parent empties the kitchen of sweets, and the classmate excludes the chunky child from the playgroup. Fat-talk and the material and cultural practices associated with it have powerful yet often invisible effects.

Fat-Talk Is Everyday Talk, and It Is Contagious

As noted before, the society-wide campaign to eradicate fat has produced a veritable epidemic of fat-talk. Comments and conversations about weight, diet, exercise, and related topics are ubiquitous in virtually every domain of social life. Increasingly, fat-talk seems to be a social norm, a common language with which people strike up friendships, argue, and generally engage one another. Nothing can illustrate this better than a real-life example. So let me introduce Carrie (a pseudonym), an eighteen-year-old from Long Beach, California. Once Carrie began reflecting on how often she teases people about their weight, she realized to her surprise that it was almost all the time.

> I always seem to pick on people and their weight. I never purposefully chose to pick on people's weight to be cruel or hurtful. It was just a friendly way of starting a conversation or pok[ing] fun at someone. When I realized this, I started considering how many times I did this and to how many people. It was practically to everyone in my [residential] suite and I did it frequently.
>
> Shortly after the beginning of this quarter, I ate lunch with a group of my hallmates. I sat next to this boy from my hall, we'll call him Sam, and he's a really quiet guy. I didn't know how to start a conversation with him, so I waited a while and noticed that he had gotten a Pizookie. Then he got another one. And that's how I began my conversation with him. I started joking around with him and pretending to be all shocked that he had two Pizookies instead of just one, the little fatty. Now, every time I see him I always throw a fat joke at him, especially if he's eating something. Recently, he's been getting back at me by also making fun of my weight. He'll joke around by stumbling towards me and saying that I'm so big that I have my own gravitational field. Even though I know I'm pretty skinny and it's a joke, though, I sort of take it into account when I start eating. [SC 255]

All this warm and fuzzy teasing about weight and food has real effects, though, causing people to become weight conscious and diet- and exercise-obsessed. In 2007, research published in the prestigious *New England Journal of Medicine* suggested that weight is socially contagious and spreads through social networks; if your close friends, sibling, or spouse becomes obese, you have a higher chance of becoming obese yourself. The weight of neighbors had much less effect, ruling out the impact of shared environments.[54] Why weight levels spread is the subject of much debate.[55] The authors suggest that people adopt the weight norms of their close friends. This is certainly true, but there may be biological mechanisms of infectiousness as well.[56] Another important vehicle by which obesity (and thinness) spread through social networks is fat-talk. Let's listen to Carrie again.

> Sam is not the only friend I tease about weight. Since I've commented on my friends' weight, though, it seems they've decided to start commenting on mine, too. They're joking, but I always keep [their remarks] in the back of my head. I thought my weight was perfectly fine when I came into school, then freaked out when I gained 10 pounds. I thought I was getting fat—[and] I still do. Every time I go to eat I get a little worried about whether the food I'm about to eat is going to [make] me fatter. Perhaps some part of this standardized ideal for skinniness has rubbed off on me. It seems to be normal for girls here to be super skinny while eating super healthy: no soda, just water and always a salad. So when I see myself eating a bunch of junk with soda, I feel a little [self-]conscious. I never cared about what I wore or how I ate until I came to this college filled with skinny girls. [SC 255]

Carrie suggests that, through fat-talk, first weight- and diet-consciousness and later weight-obsession become contagious, spreading from person to person within a tight network of friends.

Fat Discourse

While everyday fat-talk such as that of Carrie and her friends is important, it is but the conversational component of *fat discourse*. By *discourse*, I mean a complex, internally structured, historically specific body of knowledge that structures how weight and weight-related behavior can be talked about and that does things or produces effects, many of them unintended.[57] Fatness has always been framed within a larger discourse, but that discourse has shifted. In the Middle Ages, for example, fleshiness was a symbol of physical vigor and prosperity, while gluttony was deemed a religious sin.[58] In the nineteenth century, corpulence was an aesthetic transgression. Today, with the medicalization of weight, the discourse on fat is increasingly a scientifically based discourse aimed at optimizing a biological dimension of human existence. In this discourse, the science does critically important political work.

Based on the science of weight, today's fat discourse establishes weight-based categories based on the BMI. In this classification scheme, a BMI of 18.5–24.9 is "normal," 25–29.9 is "overweight," and 30 and higher is "obese," while under 18.5 is "underweight." The BMI discourse, then, is not only *normalizing*, specifying an ideal or norm and urging all to normalize their status, it is also *subjectifying*, setting out weight-based identity categories into which people are supposed to fit themselves. Although slender bodies have long been a cultural obsession, now overweight and obese people—the main targets of the fat discourse—are no longer considered simply unattractive (and morally flawed), they are also understood as "abnormal" or "defective" in some essential, biological sense. Because they are flawed, they are in need of remediation. Because fat discourse is a biomedical discourse, the abnormal categories are deemed diseases, chronic in nature, that must be treated according to the best medical practice, which primarily means diet and exercise.[59] It is now a physician's professional duty to measure weight regularly and diagnose and treat weight-based "disease" in all of his or her patients, adult and pediatric.[60] Thus, fat discourse identifies the fat targets to be normalized and instructs them to follow diet, exercise, and other regimens to reach normal weight and become biologically normal subjects or persons. This is what I mean by political work.

Essential Biomyths

As a bodily or biological discourse, fat discourse makes scientific experts (doctors, public health specialists, physical education teachers, and so on) the authorities on body weight and its management. Drawing on the still enormous cultural authority of the biological sciences and biomedicine among the general public, these body experts speak in the name of the truth and few challenge their authority.

The research and clinical communities face a problem, however: although they have designated overweight and obesity diseases, they have no reliable way to successfully treat these diseases and make their patients "normal" or "well." The absence of effective treatments was emphasized in the mid-1990s, when the rise in obesity first came to light. For example, the authors of the 1994 *Journal of the American Medical Association* (*JAMA*) study revealing the striking increase in heavy weights since the 1970s described them as problems "for which no efficacious, practical, and long-lasting preventive or therapeutic solution has yet been identified."[61] But once the anti-obesity campaign was labeled a national war, requiring hope not discouragement, concerns about the lack of good treatments were greatly downplayed; indeed, by the 2000s public figures had shifted the focus to children and were announcing that obesity is "completely preventable" (Richard Carmona) and that the problem of childhood obesity "can be solved" (Michelle Obama)[62]—this, despite major advances in finding effective ways to treat or prevent obesity.

Given the significant role of genetic and environmental factors in obesity, it is not surprising that the field of bioscience has not yet found a cure for fatness. Indeed, the specialist literature suggests that, for most individuals, there are few if any safe and reliable ways to achieve long-term weight loss. A major review of studies of the outcomes of calorie-restricting diets shows that diets often work in the short run, producing short-term weight losses of 5–10 percent of body weight, but the vast majority of dieters regain the weight.[63] And somewhere between one-third and two-thirds regain *more* weight than they lost. Moreover, the longer the period of time measured, the greater the amount of weight they regain. Surprisingly, even those who remain on reduced-calorie diets regain the weight after a period of time. And weight gain, including the notorious weight cycling (the repeated loss and regain of weight), results in health problems of its own. In short, diets promote neither lasting weight loss nor health benefits. For its part, exercise has substantial health and fitness benefits, and it appears to help with the maintenance of weight loss. It rarely, however, leads to weight loss. As noted earlier, diet pills have been associated with serious health problems and are minimally effective in any case. Surgical solutions—lap-band and other bariatric surgeries—are expensive, pose serious health risks, and have unknown long-term outcomes.[64] For a physician seeking to help his or her patient lose weight, this is a discouraging situation.

Yet many if not most in the medical and public health fields deeply believe that obesity constitutes a genuine public health crisis and poses a serious threat to the health of affected individuals. They have responded in two ways. The first has been to acknowledge that individual treatment rarely works and, instead, to encourage prevention by promoting societal-level interventions in what is known as the obesogenic environment. Prominent advocates of this approach include former New York City Mayor Michael Bloomberg (who served 2002–2013), whose many efforts to combat obesity include banning the use of trans fats in restaurants; tightening nutritional standards and eliminating junk in the city-run schools, senior centers, hospitals, and so forth; adding bike lanes to the city's streets; boosting public awareness through high-profile ad campaigns; and a (failed) effort to ban supersized sugary drinks.[65] In public health, the obesity researcher Kelly Brownell, who founded the Yale University Rudd Center for Food Policy and Obesity, advocated a wide range of measures aimed at redesigning our toxic environment.[66] Such programs, and those aimed at preventing childhood obesity, hold considerable promise, but evidence of their effectiveness remains limited.[67]

The second approach, which continues to hold out hope that heavy individuals can lose weight and keep it off (or that excessive weight gain can be prevented in children), has promoted what might be called "best-guess" medical practices and hoped for the best. Best-guess medical practices are those that physicians believe, based on some experience, may work to lower weights, primarily the well-known dyad, low-calorie diets and increased physical activity. Given that obesity had not previously been treated as a full-fledged disease in a large number of patients, in the late 1990s scattered information about what might work was all that was available. In recommending this approach, the Expert Committee of the American Academy of Pediatrics, which created an early set of guidelines for diagnosing and treating overweight in children, acknowledged that the guidelines did not represent evidence-based medicine but rather a pragmatic accommodation to a perceived urgent need:

> Obesity in children and adolescents represents one of the most frustrating and difficult diseases to treat. The management recommendations presented here represent an important attempt to provide those who care for children with practical directions on how to assess and treat overweight children. Many of the approaches also apply to obesity prevention. Because so few studies of this problem have been performed, the approaches to evaluation and therapy presented here rarely are evidence-based. Nonetheless, they represent the consensus of a group of professionals who treat obese children and adolescents.[68]

Since then, the number of clinical guidelines for the treatment of pediatric obesity has grown, and the recommendations have become increasingly evidence-based.[69] Yet the emphasis has continued to be on the limitations of the recommendations, especially regarding obesity prevention and treatment in primary-care settings. For adults, although a cure remains elusive, new drugs and devices have been introduced that, doctors emphasize, can produce modest weight loss that improves patients' lives.

A similar pragmatism underlies the official advocacy of the BMI as the core measure of fatness and health risk. The pediatric guidelines, as well as similar recommendations for treatment of adult obesity, urge use of the BMI despite its well-known limitations (described next) because it is easy to calculate and because there is international support for its use.[70]

This best-guess approach to individual weight management means that the war on fat has come to embed many assumptions that the scientific community itself considers dubious or controversial yet embraces as pragmatic compromises in the interests of "doing something about the urgent problem of obesity." These assumptions then get endlessly reproduced in clinics, in schools, in the news, in advertisements for diet and exercise products, in the popular media, and in everyday conversations—appearing everywhere as credible and true because they come wrapped in a cloak of science and because they are repeated over and over. I call these working assumptions about the body, weight, and health that guide many professional interventions as well as ordinary people's behavior *biomyths*—myths because they are part of cultural common sense and persist despite their contested status in the scientific community.

Fundamental to the story this book tells are six core biomyths:

1. Weight is under individual control; virtually everyone can lose weight and keep it off through diet and exercise. Weight-loss treatments work; if they don't, it's due to lack of willpower on the part of the dieter.
2. Parents (or other caregivers) can control, or at least significantly influence, the weight of young people.
3. The BMI is a good, reliable measure of fat and health risk.
4. Obesity and overweight are not only risk factors for other diseases; they are also diseases in themselves.
5. "Normal" weight signifies good health; "abnormal" weight is invariably associated with disease.
6. Obesity and overweight cause a host of other diseases, many of them very serious and even life-threatening.

Unfortunately, none of these is quite true. Or perhaps I should say that each has many detractors, for the science of weight is rife with controversy and contention. Let us take them one by one, drawing on the work of critical obesity researchers, including some affiliated with the FAM.[71] The influence on weight of biology, genetics, and the environment (social, built, and natural) means that individuals actually have limited control over their weight. The research we have just reviewed suggests that, although some people are genetically fortunate and can achieve and maintain "normal" weights, most people cannot and common treatments to lower weight do so by only a small amount and only in the short run (in contrast to bio-myth 1). The medical community is aware of the difficulty of achieving sustained weight loss, but in the political economy of hope[72] on which the war on fat runs, which is imbued with faith in the promise of science and technology to find solutions, it does not emphasize this to patients or the public. If people have limited control over their own weight, then the in-fluence of their caregivers is even smaller (biomyth 2). To be sure, parents can restrict the food coming into the household and teach their youngsters healthy eating and exercise habits, but beyond that, their influence is fairly circumscribed.

The limitations of the BMI are widely appreciated in the biomedical and public health communities, where it is considered a useful, although not especially good, measure of obesity. Indeed, the BMI was originally created for surveillance and screening, not as a tool for individual diag-nosis. Nevertheless, it is widely used in that way today. Assuming the ex-istence of a "standard body," the BMI fails to allow for variations in body composition (muscle, bone, fat), or regular differences along lines of gen-der and race/ethnicity. At best, the BMI may account for 60–75 percent of the variation in body fat content in adults.[73] And it cannot account for the character and placement of fat deposition in the body, which have well-known impacts on health outcomes (biomyth 3).[74]

Is obesity (and overweight) a disease in itself, as claimed by biomyth 4? Growing numbers of organizations—including, in June 2013, the Ameri-can Medical Association (AMA)—have declared obesity a disease, yet the controversy remains far from settled. Indeed, the membership of the AMA voted to label it a disease over the objections of its own expert committee, which argued that obesity should not be deemed a disease because the BMI, the measure used to define it, is simplistic and flawed and because there are no specific symptoms that are always associated with it.[75] Because there are no specific symptoms linked to the different BMI categories, weight status by itself cannot correlate with the health state (biomyth 5). Instead, there is great diversity in the connection between BMI and metabolic health. In the United States today, fully one-third of obese people are metabolically healthy, while one-quarter of normal-weight people suffer from metabolic abnormalities.[76] The everyday association of BMI with health is highly problematic.

The last biomyth may appear to be the strongest and least mythlike of the six, but it too is problematic. In both adults and children, obesity is statistically associated with a host of serious diseases. According to the Centers for Disease Control (CDC), children who are obese are more likely to have risk factors for cardiovascular disease (high cholesterol and high blood pressure), and to have prediabetes, bone and joint problems, and breathing difficulties. In the long term, they face the risk of adult obesity and so are more at risk for adult health problems such as heart disease, type 2 diabetes, stroke, several types of cancer, and osteoarthritis. Yet these well-known associations, many emphasize, are mostly ones of *correlation* rather than *causation*. The science shows that it is not obesity per se that causes these diseases but, instead, a complex array of metabolic changes in the body that are set in motion by significant weight gain. These happen because adipose tissue (where excess fat is stored), previously thought of as an inert mass, turns out to be metabolically active; when it increases and is out of balance with other organ systems, it precipitates a cascade of changes likely to worsen health.[77] "[Obesity] is the middleman," writes the cardiologist Carl J. Lavie, "that can exacerbate existing conditions and contribute to premature death by aggravating chronic disease."[78] Responding to the argument of the FAM and others that some people are fat *and healthy*, the biologists Michael Power and Jay Schulkin suggest that obese people can indeed be metabolically healthy in the short to mid-term. Over the long term, though, the excess fat tissue on their bodies is likely to catch up with them and lead to ill health.[79]

Further complicating matters is what is known as the "obesity paradox," the finding that for people diagnosed with serious diseases—from cardiovascular disease to arthritis, kidney disease, diabetes, and cancer— being overweight or mildly obese is actually protective, with heavier people living longer than thinner ones.[80] Lavie, author of *The Obesity Paradox*, resolves the puzzle this way. When we're young and healthy, becoming obese will certainly cause problems in a matter of years. With age, though, the balance is likely to tip in favor of extra weight. Ideal weight from the vantage point of health and mortality cannot be specified in general terms but, rather, is likely to vary with age, sex, genetics, cardiometabolic fitness, and the existence of preexisting diseases.[81] Lavie and others argue forcefully for the need to decenter weight and BMI in discussions of health and to focus instead on metabolic fitness, including cardiorespiratory health.

Although these everyday premises are deeply problematic, the discussion of controversial issues tends to be confined to the specialist literature. Rarely does it reach the general public (although Lavie's book might change that). For some ten years now, Paul Campos, Glenn Gaesser, Eric Oliver, and other critics aligned with the FAM have tried to publicize such problems, but their voices have been marginalized or simply ignored by the medical community.[82] Public consciousness of these problems tends to be low except when, once in a while, a controversial new finding that challenges one of these biomyths is picked up by the popular science press. When a controversy does erupt into the mainstream news, however, it is not easy for the lay reader to sort out who is right and who is wrong.

For example, in early 2013 an article published in *JAMA* used new data to confirm the long-standing finding that BMIs in the overweight and low-obesity range are associated with *lower* mortality levels than normal BMIs—findings that might weaken the claim that overweight as well as obese individuals face elevated health risks.[83] These findings, reached by scientists at the CDC, were quickly reproduced on the health pages of the *New York Times* and elsewhere, gaining wide attention.[84] But they provoked immediate controversy, with a handful of influential obesity researchers arguing that the research was marred by methodological flaws that invalidated the findings.[85] In a National Public Radio interview, a prominent nutritionist at Harvard's School of Public Health called the study "a pile of rubbish . . . [that] no one should waste their time reading" and convened an expert symposium to discredit it. A few months later, *Nature*, the top science journal in Great Britain, took the unusual step of publicly chastising him in an editorial for using such dismissive, black-and-white language as "rubbish" when gray is the true color of science.[86] Clearly, the health consequences of obesity are bitterly contested in the scientific community itself. Indeed, a review of some key episodes in the history of obesity science that have been charted by fat studies scholars (and a few participants in that history) reveals that the field has been riven by bitter disputes over fundamental issues for decades.[87] But the general public is not privy to these debates. And when the controversies do come to light, the public, lacking insider data, ends up confused and troubled, and, needing some information on which to act, often simply falls back on the conventional wisdom embodied in the familiar biomyths.

Although influential public figures are increasingly working to alter the obesogenic environment, the emphasis on individual responsibility for weight persists in doctors' offices, schools, social media, and popular culture. The dominant biocitizenship approach to obesity thus continues much as it has for the last fifteen years. The building of the anti-obesity campaign on such problematic foundations raises troubling ethical issues as heavyset people are being labeled diseased and insistently urged to lose weight through techniques that either do not work for most people or that work at serious risk to their health. Heavy people are, in effect, asked to do the impossible and then socially punished for failing. Questions of medical ethics and social justice need to be pointedly raised.

Biopedagogical and Bioabusive Fat-Talk: Making Weight-Centric Identities

These complex dynamics of the war on fat help us understand its powerful yet largely neglected social effects. The first and perhaps most important is on personhood or subjectivity. By *subjectivity* (or *selfhood* or *personal identity*, terms I use interchangeably), I mean all the things that make us unique humans or subjects with agency—our views, our feelings, our beliefs, our hopes. Our subjectivities shape how we act in the world—what behaviors we adopt, how we treat each other, and so on. People have multiple and shifting selves—familial, professional or work-related, bodily, and so forth. Research has shown that people's sense of self is shaped through dialogue-type interaction with social (including scientific and political) discourses in their environment.[88] For example, the discourse on religion in my church may turn me into a devout believer and churchgoer. The discourse on weight may turn me into a shameful "fatso" and anxious dieter. This book shows how people acquire weight-based subjectivities, especially that of a fat subject, and how that identity is becoming the pre-dominant one in many people's lives.

To understand how self-identified fat persons are being created, we need to take a close look at the social discourses that circulate around fatness and how individuals interact with them. One such discourse is that of the BMI, which, we have seen, sets out weight-based identity labels that people are encouraged to take as their own. But discourses circulating more widely in society play important roles too, especially in transporting those scientific discourses into individuals' lives. In my California research, I identified two kinds of fat-talk, with different effects on identity formation. In the first, *biopedagogical fat-talk*, the discourse on weight serves to inform people of their weight status ("too fat," "too skinny," etc.) and instruct them on what practices they must adopt to achieve a normative body weight.[89] Biopeda-gogical fat-talk is routinely dispensed by the authorities in young people's lives: physicians, health and physical education teachers, coaches, and so forth. But it is also offered by family and friends, often on a daily basis in the form of unsolicited commentary on the size of our bellies, the fat content of our snacks, and other such matters. Biopedagogical fat-talk can be criti-cal ("If you don't stop eating, you'll look like that fat person") or it can be complimentary ("Wow, you've lost weight; you look fantastic!"). Because weight is such a sensitive topic, both negative and positive pedagogical fat-talk can have big effects on the person being addressed. Complimentary fat-talk—positive feedback on our bodies or weight-loss efforts—may seem benign, or at least innocuous, but we will see that an approving nod can be just as powerful as an insult in triggering extreme reactions.

The second type of fat-talk is *fat abuse*, delivered through *biobullying* of various sorts. "You should not be buying that donut!" or even "You're so fat, you can't even run a block!" are common examples.[90] It's important to remember that both kinds of fat-talk are actively encouraged by the war on fat, in which our duties as virtuous biocitizens include trying to transform fat people into good biocitizens by educating them about the whys and hows of losing weight. If those educational efforts don't work, then we should up the pressure and try coaxing them. If that still does not work, then it's quite okay to shame, ridicule, or humiliate them—any kind of bullying that motivates them to lose weight is justified as being for their own good and for the good of the country.

Everyone knows that abusing people is wrong, yet when it comes to weight, we do it all the time. Fat abuse is utterly ubiquitous in America today. In the conventional media and on social media, derogatory comments about heavy people are routine. In everyday life, many people issue abusive remarks about the overweight and obese seemingly without a second thought. From a large literature, we know that heavy-weight young people are targets of often cruel verbal abuse, and that the heavier the child, the greater the abuse.[91] When we think of biobullying, we usually imagine mean kids in the hallways or on the playground at school. Yet recent research on stigma has shown that not just peers but also teachers and even parents can be fat-abusive toward youngsters.[92] This is saddening, but it is not surprising because we are all encouraged to be biocops who engage in biopolicing, constantly monitoring everyone else's weight, and "helping" those who are not good biocitizens become them by offering pointed pedagogical and abusive comments. Public health research suggests that stigmatizing comments rarely, if ever, motivate people to lose weight, yet the belief that they do persists in our culture.[93]

Although some readers may find it troubling or offensive, I use the language of bioabuse and biocop for parents who use sharp words and methods to get their kids to lose weight. Such terms violate our cherished image of the warm-hearted parent, yet from the viewpoint of at least some on the receiving end, those terms feel exactly right. And in seeking to help youngsters they care for lose weight, parents are really little different from the teachers, coaches, and other child authorities—all of them are trapped in the biomyths that encourage such treatment of fat kids. And so I use these terms in full knowledge that they may provoke discomfort and debate.

This book shows how the two kinds of fat-talk work together to turn obese and overweight people into *fat subjects*. A fat subject is different from an obese person. An obese person is someone with a BMI of 30 or higher. A fat subject is someone who, regardless of his or her weight, identifies as fat, organizes his or her life around that fatness, and acquires the attributes of a typical "fat person." There is not much public discourse about "normality" (except as the medical ideal), but normal-weight people are vulnerable to fat-talk too. Subject to constant warnings about the dangers of weight gain and the health consequences of fatness, they see their health as always in jeopardy because they are at risk of becoming fat and acquiring weight-related diseases. These people become *potential* or *at-risk fat subjects*, who maintain a constant vigilance over their bodies and anxiously engage in prophylactic dieting and exercising to avoid that fate. Very thin people are subject to a variant of fat-talk that I call *skinny-talk*— suggestions that they are unhealthily skinny. People so teased often start seeing themselves as abnormally "underweight" or, in the colloquial, *skinny persons*, and begin eating more in an effort to become "normal" and stop the abuse. The auto-ethnographic accounts presented here will show how the pervasive fat-talk in the worlds of our young people is turning virtually all of them into fat-subjects of some sort, producing a cascade of other effects unlikely to be deemed desirable by the war's makers.

A Look Ahead

This book has ten chapters divided into four parts. We begin in southern California (SoCal) where, as everyone knows, the bodies are beautiful and the body pressures are intense. All the same, in chapter 2 I argue that SoCal is a microcosm of the United States, a place whose denizens have the same dreams as other Americans (getting a good body to get a good life) but face tougher standards and pressures. In chapter 2, I map out how the anti-obesity campaign, a pet project of former Governor Arnold Schwarzenegger, has been carried out in California and with what effects on its young targets. If those with whom I worked are any indication, the campaign has been a smashing success, helping to transform young Californians into virtuous biocitizens who mostly know their BMIs, believe the biomyths, and are obsessed with their weight and health. The chapter moves on to describe my research project before briefly mapping out the social dynamics of the fight against fat (differences by ethnicity, income, gender, and place), essential background for the chapters that follow.

In part 2, I delve into the core issue of selfhood, showing how the weight classes of the BMI have been internalized in such a way that people of all sizes increasingly define themselves by their weight. In chapter 3 I focus on people labeled "obese," in chapter 4 on "overweight" selves, in chapter 5 on those labeled "underweight," and in chapter 6 on those labeled "normal." This part of the book documents how the war on fat has turned almost everyone into a fat subject of some sort, producing a society in which virtually everyone is obsessed with his or her weight, few are able to lose (or gain) pounds, and no one is happy with his or her body or life.

The national narrative underlying the war on fat worries about the health and economic costs of obesity to the country, but the costs of the war on fat itself are rarely mentioned in public communications, let alone systematically tallied up. In part 3, I hone in on some of the unmeasured costs of the war borne by the youth who are its main targets. In chapter 7, I reveal how the war on fat, by exerting intense pressure on young people to achieve the thin, fit body, has put their physical and mental health at risk. In chapter 8, I show how the fight against fat has frayed some of our most fundamental bonds. Struggles over weight have pulled mothers and daughters apart, set sibling against sibling, forced heavy kids out of their families, and fostered fat abuse in intimate relationships that destroys its victims and their marriages.

Despite the human costs of the war on fat, from a societal point of view it might still be worthwhile if the war works to reduce obesity. In chapter 9, I ask whether the core strategy in the war—good biocitizens working to persuade, coax, and badger heavy people to shed pounds—can help the very fat, who face seriously elevated health risks. The answer, unfortunately, is no. In virtually every case, the biocitizen program has backfired, doing more damage than good. It has failed because it is unable to address some of the most the powerful forces underlying obesity today: poverty, genetics, and psychosocial distress. In chapter 9, I expose some of the real-life limits on today's war on fat.

In chapter 10, the conclusion, I argue that the war on fat, by giving two-thirds of American adults and one-third of American children a life-diminishing diagnosis of "overweight and unhealthy" while lacking the means to effectively treat the disease and make them well, constitutes a serious ethical violation on the part of medicine and a grave injustice to society. Concerns with social suffering and social justice call for winding down the war on fat and bringing it to an end. In the chapter's last section, I map out a set of strategies with which to jumpstart that process, offering them not as concrete proposals but as springboards for discussion and debate.

2

CREATING THIN, FIT BODIES

The View from SoCal

In SoCal the whole society pushes beauty.
Celebrity body culture is almost impossible to achieve, yet we all try.
Guys also fall victim to wanting that perfect body.
COMMENTS OF YOUNG SOUTHERN CALIFORNIANS DESCRIBING
THEIR SOCIAL WORLD, 2011

SoCal: The (Fantasy) Land of Perfect Bodies

I am not a native Californian, but for seventeen years (from 1994 to 2011)
I lived and worked in Orange County (OC), the wealthy coastal jewel in
the crown of the southern California mega-region (SoCal for short) that is
home to 23 million people—fully 60.9 percent of Californians and some
7.4 percent of all Americans.[1] As every consumer of American popular
culture knows, SoCal, with its hyped-up Hollywood celebrity culture and
its laid-back OC beach culture, is the epicenter of the cult of the perfect
body. For women and girls, and increasingly for men and boys as well, the
thin, toned, "beautiful" or "ripped" body (depending on one's gender) is
a central measure of human value and core currency of social success. In
the photos of glossy promotional magazines such as *OC Riviera* and *Image
Magazine*, those of us fortunate enough to inhabit this sun-drenched cor-
ner of the United States live in large, beautifully appointed homes over-
looking the Pacific; work in law, banking, or investment firms; work out

at expensive sports clubs; and shop and dine at world-famous malls such as South Coast Plaza. We inhabit the apparently effortless product of all that outdoor living in the California sunshine: slender, toned, healthy bodies that are the envy of the nation and the model for much of the world. In SoCal, the images say, perfect bodies bring perfect lives.

Where the Weather Is Fine . . . and the Body
Pressures Are Intense

The connection between fabulous bodies and fabulous lives can, of course, be found all over the country. Countless statistics show that Americans with trim, lean bodies are advantaged in every way imaginable. But in SoCal, the cult of the body is more extreme. Not only are the body ideals more exacting—for women the ideal is slender, big breasted, tall, toned, and tanned, and for men it is tall, buff, lean, and tanned—but also the pressures to reach those ideals are more intense. Everywhere in the United States, young people are exposed to the bright media images of successful thin Americans and, at the same time, to the dark public health messages about a national epidemic of obesity warning them to avoid getting fat at any cost. These inducements and blandishments blanket southern California too. In SoCal, though, the pressures to be thin and fit—and to avoid being fat and unfit—are heightened by the regional culture. According to my native informants, three aspects of the area's storied culture intensify the demands for perfect bodies: the beach and the weather (of course), Hollywood (ditto), and the enormous wealth of the region.

Immortalized by the Beach Boys in their 1963 hit, "Surfin USA" ("San Onofre and Sunset, Redondo Beach, LA, everybody's gone surfin', surfin' USA"), the iconic southern California beach and the warm, sunny weather create cultural expectations that people will have "perfect, bikini-ready (or, for guys, tank-top-ready) beach bodies" all year round.[2] The beach environment, combined with the year-round warm weather, means that people are expected to show skin, to wear skimpy, revealing clothing that displays their tight abs, rippling muscles, flat stomachs, and deep cleavage. According to another informant, "SoCal weather is beach weather; you're considered 'weird' if you are not showing your legs, arms, and skin." The materialistic values of the area breed a "show-off culture" in which pridefully displaying one's possessions—the car, the house, the expensive toys, and the three-T body (tanned, toned, and tight)—is expected. As one young woman put it, "Every girl in SoCal wants to have a skinny figure, nice abs, and decent boobs so she can proudly strut around in a bikini." The demands are similar for guys, with an extra emphasis on athleticism: "Men want that perfect chiseled body [that] they can show off at the beach. They are always at the gym lifting heavy weights to get more buff."

The presence and centripetal force of Hollywood in the region, with its seductive images of glitz, glamor, and the good life, provide a constant reminder of the enormous rewards that come to those with beautiful bodies. "In SoCal," one informant explained, "body image matters a lot. Because we live so close to Hollywood, the culture is to copy that perfect body by any means." LA is of course a culture of celebrities, and these gorgeous people, including the many reality TV stars, are everywhere—on the small screen, on the big screen, on magazines covers, on the Internet, on social media sites, and even on the streets in certain upscale areas of the city. For those who grew up here, the celebrities' presence, whether physical or virtual, was "in my face daily," as one Angelena put it. Of the 255 young California women I surveyed in 2011, fully four-fifths said they grew up comparing their bodies to those of their celebrity idols. The message they took away was that both to get and to be seen as deserving of the good life, all women need to look like celebs. The physical proximity of Hollywood and its stars—one can almost reach out and touch them—makes their lives seem attainable, leaving young people not just dreaming but concretely aspiring to have celebrity bodies and the lives that go with them.

Finally there is the general affluence of the area, where median household income in the three largest counties ranges from 1.07 to 1.44 times the national average.[3] Especially along the coast, there are lots of people with lots of money to buy the means to create beautiful bodies—fresh organic foodstuffs, gym memberships, personal trainers, botox injections, and cosmetic surgery. One informant put it succinctly: "SoCal culture is one of looking beautiful and having nice things. It's a purely consumerist culture that emphasizes that all you need is money." And lots of money supports what another called a "health-crazed culture: a culture of health consciousness [that] values yoga, exercise, vegetarianism, and organic food." All these beautiful wealthy people, who can be seen everywhere, both set the body standard for all and lead people, even those without much money, to believe that such perfect bodies are within their reach.

Although body consciousness and the desire for a slim, toned body are widespread among young people around the country, the pressure to achieve the ideal is especially intense here. The unforgiving character of the bodily expectations is reflected in comments such as these: "Living in LA is hard. There is lots of pressure and a constant need to feel skinny. It's hard to be born and raised in a city where's it's all about your looks." And men are hardly immune: "Guys are obsessed, too, they try to build their bodies up to look their biggest and baddest. They want to be like the guys from [the reality TV program] *Jersey Shore*."

For the majority of women, the dominant body ideal is simply unattainable. It is equally impossible to escape, leaving people feeling flawed and unable to measure up. "The area's culture makes me feel I am too fat, while all the diet commercials make me want to lose my 'weight problem,'" one lamented. In a climate in which every tiny imperfection is blown up, the feelings of inadequacy, of not being part of mainstream American society, were especially painful for women of color, who could never achieve flawless white skin—or tall, skinny bodies. One Mexican American woman wrote, "The skinny-body-obsessed culture of LA made me think I was not good enough or not part of this society and needed to change." A Middle Easterner wrote, "Growing up and living in LA has completely shaped me and greatly lowered my self-esteem. Everyone looks like models and I can't live up."

One could say, perhaps, that southern Californians have the same dreams as other Americans (getting the good body to get the good life) but that the standards are tougher and the pressures to have perfect bodies are more intense. And so the anxieties about being fat and flabby are deeper. The very extremeness of the body obsession in the area allows us to see with special clarity how the culture of the thin, trim body works and what effects, intended and otherwise, it is producing. SoCal is by no means typical, but it is a microcosm of all the forces that play out in American society around the slender, trim body. And lest we forget Tinseltown, SoCal is also important because it represents the cultural cutting edge that, through the power of the Hollywood media, exports its dreams of perfect bodies and perfect lives to the rest of the world. To an important extent, Hollywood culture is America's culture.

The SoCal Body Politics Project

From 1995 to 2011, I taught a large course at the University of California, Irvine (UC Irvine)—located in the very heart of the OC—on the culture and politics of the gendered, raced, classed, and sexed body in the United States today. In ways I did not expect, "The Woman and the Body" became a space for intense conversations about the politics of the trim, toned body in SoCal, where some 78 percent of the students I taught grew up. The course also served as a virtual ethnographic fieldsite and a springboard for further fieldwork in southern California more generally. In 2005, I added a segment on the rise of the "obesity epidemic" and the war on fat, which by then was sweeping through SoCal like a tsunami.

Because young people are the prime target for the anti-obesity campaign, the class provided a rare opportunity for learning about how the campaign was working and what kinds of effects it was having on its main targets. Given the opprobrium heaped on heavy people in our society, among young people deemed "too fat" the subject of weight evokes feelings of intense shame and personal failure, feelings too humiliating to share with anyone. Even the methods of anthropologists (interviews, hanging out with our informants), which are designed to gain in-depth understandings of social life, are not very effective at eliciting feelings of this sort. In 2010, I offered students extra credit for writing a three- to five-page ethnographic essay on how issues of diet, weight, and the body mass index (BMI) play out in the life of a person they know well. The prompt urged them to "provide a richly detailed account: describe how the person felt, what she or he said and did, how it affected others, [and so on]." (The full prompt can be found in the book's appendix.) Assigning these essays as a pedagogical tool, I was not prepared for what I received. Full of tales of California childhoods dominated—and often devastated—by battles over weight, the essays were eye-opening, disturbing, and, in cases, heartbreaking to read.

For several years, I had been troubled by the growing drumbeat of alarmist news about the "crisis of childhood obesity" that was "undermining America's future" and the moralistic tenor of the public health campaign against obesity. That is why I added the segment on the obesity epidemic—to help students see that there were other ways to think about the obesity question. Yet up to that point, I had not taken up obesity as a topic for research. My students' essays put a human face on the war on fat. And that face had tears rolling down its cheeks. As a person of slender build, I had never fully grasped the sheer intensity and unremitting nature of the bullying, abuse, and downright torment heavy kids endure simply because they have bigger bodies. The essays made clear that the campaign against obesity was imposing a heaping dose of blame and shame, which the students had internalized in endless—and largely futile—efforts to lose weight. Reading their stories of suffering made me see that a real social injustice was being perpetrated in the name of public health. And when I put myself in the picture, I saw that the social injustice was two-fold, for even as heavier people are unfairly punished for something they mostly cannot control, slender people are unfairly rewarded for having bodies that are a product more of nature (genes, environment) than of their own "hard work." Why, I wondered, had no one talked about how people who are naturally slender come across as health heroes—responsible, disciplined, virtuous biocitizens who take care of the nation by taking care of themselves? These troubling questions needed to be aired.

The essays my students wrote were so poignant, I felt they had entrusted me with some deeply private and often painful secrets, secrets they nonetheless felt relieved to divulge because it meant they were no longer alone with their fears. Because I had unknowingly encouraged them to unearth those troubling accounts, I felt an obligation to get their voices out, to ensure that their stories were more widely heard. It was, then, my concern about the social injustice being perpetrated by the war on fat, coupled with a more personal sense of obligation to my students, that led me in summer 2010 to undertake the SoCal Body Politics Project. I taught the class at UC Irvine once more, in 2011, during which I took the opportunity to offer the extra-credit essay one more time and to gather other, more systematic class-wide information on the politics of weight in the worlds these young people inhabit.

This book draws on four sources of information: the ethnographic essays, targeted interviews, survey questionnaires, and informal conversations and experiences. The first and most important source is the ethnographic essays gathered in 2010 and 2011. The majority (three-quarters) wrote auto-ethnographies about their own experiences; the rest wrote about siblings, parents, other relatives, or close friends. I received permission to use 222 of them (of the 264 essays for which permission was sought and the 236 whose authors responded). A few essays described the bodily concerns of more than one person; this brought the number of individuals whose experiences were documented to 234. Because one important ethnic group in California—Latinos—was underrepresented, I also conducted in-depth interviews with eleven additional students, bringing the number of individual accounts to 245. To gain more systematic information on the young people's body practices; the influence of their parents, doctors, and teachers; and the wider culture of weight in the southern California region, I also distributed questionnaires in class on these topics. This book draws on three such questionnaires: beginning-of-term surveys from 2010 and 2011 (distributed before students knew anything about the course, a total of 601 surveys) and an end-of-term questionnaire from 2011 asking about a few factual matters that were unlikely to be affected by the subject matter of the class (303 surveys). Finally, the book draws on countless informal conversations, encounters, and observations gained simply by my living in southern California for seventeen years.

360 Million Excess Pounds: The War on Fat Comes to California

Southern Californians have long been obsessed with having healthy, fit bodies, but this preoccupation has been greatly intensified by the public health campaign against fat. We have witnessed the massive efforts taken by key agencies of the federal government to mobilize all Americans and all major institutions of American society to fight fat, especially among children and young people. It is at the state and local levels, however, that the war on fat connects up to individual bodies and lives. With the financial and technical support of the Centers for Disease Control and Prevention (CDC), states are encouraged to develop programs to combat obesity at the level of the individual, family, school, and community.[4] In 2013, twenty-five states had such CDC-funded programs. For its part, California, home to 38 million people (in 2012)—some 12.1 percent of the American population—responded with alacrity. A close look at the state's efforts makes clear that the creation of thin, fit biocitizens is not just a theory but a political reality in California—and around the country.

The key figure in California's response is former bodybuilder, action hero, and governor, Arnold Schwarzenegger. During his seven-plus years in Sacramento (November 2003 to January 2011), Schwarzenegger made fighting the obesity epidemic a personal cause. Before the governor became involved, obesity prevention efforts had been occurring on an ad hoc basis. Building on his star power, in 2005 Schwarzenegger launched a series of innovative anti-obesity initiatives that he hoped would help make the state a leader in tackling the problems of an overweight and underactive population and transform it into the healthiest state in the nation.[5]

The Vision: A Model State Full of Good Biocitizens

In 2005, the governor released his "Vision for California—10 Steps toward Healthy Living," challenging the state to make California a national model for healthy lifestyles. To serve as a call to action, at the same time he convened the Summit on Health, Nutrition, and Obesity. In 2006 the Department of Health Services issued the *California Obesity Prevention Plan: A Vision for Tomorrow, Strategic Actions for Today* (or *COPP*) to guide a statewide response to the state's growing obesity epidemic. Maintaining that all sectors of society have roles and responsibilities to play in improving nutrition, increasing physical activity, and combating obesity in California, the plan identifies action recommendations for every sector. A close look at this plan reveals the incredible effort undertaken by the state government to mobilize virtually the entire society to fight fat.

In its crisis framing of the obesity problem and in its proposed solutions, the California anti-obesity plan mirrors the approach developed in the national campaign and used around the country. In the last decade, the document states, California residents have gained 360 million pounds of excess weight, leaving a third of children, a quarter of teens, and over half of adults overweight or obese. While noting that the epidemic affects everyone, it points out that obesity affects those of lower-income and minority backgrounds the most. Imposing severe costs on the public—an estimated $28 billion in added health care costs and lost work productivity—heavy people are a burden on the state and the taxpayer; they are, the report implies, either irresponsible and/or poorly educated citizens whose understandings and behaviors must be changed. Because fat children are likely to become fat adults, children must be the key target for change.[6] The state's response is "a call to action for all Californians" to become what I have called trim, fit biocitizens who are responsible to self, family, state, and nation. The state government is taking the lead in tackling this threat posed by obesity, but it is up to every Californian, every organization, and every sector of society to promote this critical cause.[7]

The Plan: Instill New Norms, Remake the Environment

California's approach to creating good biocitizens has two main prongs. The first is a massive public education campaign to change social norms so that the "new normal" is eating healthful food and living an active lifestyle. Drawing on California's proud reputation as the healthy and fit state, the document frames this lifestyle as "California living."[8] To ensure that citizens are sufficiently concerned about their weight and its health implications, citizens must come to view their sense of self in terms of their weight. The goal is to have all Californians know their BMI, grasp its profound significance to themselves and society, constantly monitor it, and act responsibly on that knowledge to keep it within normal range. The BMI is also a key tool of the state and its agents in their fight against fat. As the central tool for assessment, surveillance, and monitoring of bodies, and for the study of the health consequences of obesity, the BMI has been introduced and its use routinized in clinics, schools, homes, and other sites throughout the state where bodies are shaped. Health-care givers are supposed to treat it as a vital sign and document it in the patient's medical record. Health and physical education teachers are required to assess BMI as part of a mandatory physical fitness test (PFT) given every California fifth-, seventh-, and ninth-grader.[9] And parents need to monitor their kids' weight and BMI to make sure they stay within the bounds of "normality."[10] Like virtually every other government program to combat fat, California's thus embeds and authoritatively propagates the notion that the BMI is a reliable tool in the assessment and management of fat and its health effects.

The second prong is a campaign to alter the state's environment to support healthy choices in food and activity. The *COPP* charges all sectors of society—from government and business to agriculture, education, land-use planning and development, architecture, transportation, retail, public safety, health care, and the media—to work together to create healthful environments.[11] Parents are made responsible for ensuring that family members choose nutritious foods, limit caloric intake, eat at least one healthy meal a day together, restrain TV viewing and computer gaming, and participate in physical activity as a family every day. Teachers and school administrators are duty-bound to ensure that children receive quality physical education, institute healthy food and beverage standards, and provide nutritious breakfasts and lunches. Doctors and health-care insurers are asked to rely on prevention (rather than treatment) of obesity, especially in children, and to implement standards of care sensitive to culture, age, and abilities. California's obesity prevention plan thus maps out a program for creating a model biocitizenship society in which three idealized figures—the good, responsible parent; the good, health-focused teacher; and the good, weight-conscious doctor—each has a fundamental role to play in creating a new generation of healthy, fit, trim California biocitizens.

Starting in 2005, the governor introduced a series of innovative policies that made California a leader in child obesity prevention.[12] At a second high-level summit in 2010, this one attended by President Bill Clinton, the governor reiterated his commitment to the cause. Based on new figures suggesting that the costs of overweight and obesity had risen to $41 billion by 2006, and that the fraction of Californians at unhealthy weights had grown, the state updated the *COPP* and created new initiatives to meet the challenges.[13]

The state's campaign to combat fat has clearly intensified the pressures on southern Californians to optimize their diets, physical activities, and weight. It has done so by pathologizing heavy weights, that is, treating them as chronic illnesses that must be medically attended to; by tasking parents, teachers, and doctors with constantly monitoring and managing kids' weight; and by making body weight a matter of governmental concern and action. As a result of the state's involvement in the issue, concerns about childhood weight have become more structured, more institutionalized, more medicalized, and perpetuated by ever more sectors of society. Fears of the obesity epidemic and the war on fat were huge parts of the world in which the young people I studied grew up. If the "average" person I worked with was twenty years old in 2010, then he or she was four when the federal government discovered the rising epidemic of obesity; six when California introduced standardized fitness tests with BMI assessments; eleven when the surgeon general announced the national war on obesity; and fifteen when California started systematically introducing anti-obesity reforms in schools, clinics, and workplaces around the state. Through these initiatives of the federal and state governments, as well as the broader cultural forces they have helped to spark, the war on fat has profoundly shaped the lives of California's young people. Although the details may vary, the same is happening in states around the country.

Producing Virtuous Biocitizens

California's obesity prevention plan maps out a picture of an ideal biocitizenship society. To what extent does social reality conform to this ideal? The SoCal study provides some striking answers.

A Biocitizenship Society Par Excellence: Weight Preoccupation and BMI Knowledge

In a biocitizenship society, weight is a core measure of health and good citizenship, central to one's identity, social value, and political deservingness. In such a society, weight consciousness is sure to be high. And, indeed, in the SoCal surveys, almost 60 percent of women and 30 percent of men said they were concerned about their weight "almost all" or "much of the time" (the exact figures can be found in table A.1 in the appendix). Another 35–40 percent (of both genders) were concerned occasionally. Weight dissatisfaction was fairly high. Over 50 percent of women and 30 percent of men said they felt "way too heavy" or "somewhat too heavy." Women were far more concerned than men about being too heavy; men were far more worried than women about being too thin. Some 20 percent of men felt "way too thin" or "somewhat too thin"; only about 5 percent of women considered themselves too thin.

If a good biocitizen is dedicated to keeping his or her weight within normal range, he or she must know his or her BMI score and where it fits on the scale from "underweight" to "obese." Among the young people I worked with, an astonishing 92 percent knew their BMIs. Most had learned their scores much earlier—in middle school (roughly 40 percent) or high school (35 percent). These percentages differed little by gender (see table A.2 for the details). The school fitness tests described earlier were major incubators of weight and BMI consciousness. Over half the students (roughly 55 percent) indicated that they learned their BMI from an instructor (see table A.2). In most cases, the source of the information was a health or physical education teacher who was carrying out a school fitness test. In a small minority of cases, it was a coach or fitness professional.

Physicians: Weight Warnings in the Examining Room

With obesity and overweight deemed chronic diseases, the medical field has a major role in the war on fat. In the survey, roughly 20 percent of young people said they first learned their BMI from a doctor, usually during a regular physical check-up (table A.2). Roughly the same proportion reported that they had been told by a doctor that their weight or BMI was something to worry about and work on (table A.3). Differences according to gender were small.

Learning Weight Consciousness and Good Biocitizenship in the Home

Like parents around the nation, many California parents are intensely concerned about their kids' weight. Beyond any pressures they may feel from the family doctor or school nurse, there are compelling reasons for them to worry. Not only are the child's health and social life believed to be deeply affected by his or her body size but parents themselves are judged by the size of their kids' bodies, with the parents of fat kids deemed "bad parents" or "bad mothers" for producing obese kids. So deeply entrenched is the assumption (biomyth 2) that parents can control their children's weight that in recent years some parents in other states have had their severely obese children seized and sent to social services for "better upbringing."[14] Among the California young people in the study, as many as three-fifths had been scolded by their parents for being the wrong weight (see table A.4). Here there was a large gender difference, with over 60 percent of young women but under 40 percent of young men reporting being reprimanded for unacceptable body weight. In other words, the daughters' weight was monitored more closely than the sons'.

Youngsters also learn body ideas and practices from listening to and observing their parents. Hoping to understand the extent of an intergenerational transmission of weight concern, I asked my students whether their moms and dads had been concerned about their own weight when the young people were growing up. Two-thirds said their moms had been very concerned about their weight (see table A.4). There was a huge gender difference, with dads much less preoccupied than moms. These proportions differed little between SoCal parents and parents from other places, mostly northern California (or NorCal). As anticipated, kids tended to model their body ideals and weight behavior on those of their same-sex parents. The proportions of moms and daughters, and of fathers and sons, very concerned about their weight were remarkably close (68 percent of moms and 57 percent of daughters compared to 31 percent of dads and 30 percent of sons).

Diet and Exercise: Healthism in Action

A good biocitizen is one who lives a healthist life, eating nutritiously, dieting when necessary, and exercising regularly to keep his weight "normal" and his body toned or buff. In early 2011, 40 percent of the women and almost 30 percent of the men I studied had been dieting the previous fall, in the sense of limiting their food intake because of weight concerns. These numbers may sound low, but only people who considered themselves too heavy were likely to be dieting. The numbers of women and men who felt too heavy and who were dieting were quite close, suggesting that the great majority who thought they were too big were trying to lose weight. The exact numbers and the types of diets followed can be found in table A.5. Lifetime dieting was almost twice as prevalent as dieting at a particular point in time. Fully two-thirds of women and nearly one-half of men reported having been on a weight-loss diet at some point in their life (table A.5).

Exercise is performed both for weight control (whether it works or not) and to achieve toned or fit muscular bodies. Not surprisingly, given the definition of "real manhood" as the possession of chiseled, muscular bodies, men were particularly avid exercisers. Almost 40 percent said they had exercised three or more times a week during the previous fall; another 25 percent had worked out once or twice a week. Exercise was common among women, too, but somewhat less so (see table A.6). Judged by their body practices, these young people are generally extremely virtuous biocitizens, with women more focused on dieting and men on working out.

Believing in the Core Tenets of Biocitizenship Culture

Finally, a good biocitizen is one who accepts the dominant public health discourse on obesity and works to spread its ideas throughout society. Perhaps the most fundamental tenet underlying the war on fat is the notion that everyone can achieve a normal weight through diet and exercise (biomyth 1). In a survey, I asked students if they agreed with this statement: "Weight can be safely and effectively controlled by virtually everyone; achieving normal weight is a matter of personal willpower." This is a very strong version of biomyth 1. Even so, fully 55 percent of respondents agreed with it. Another one-sixth said they were not sure, but over one-quarter disagreed. Men were more certain about their ability to manage their weight than women; almost two-thirds of the men but only one-half of the women agreed that weight is under personal control (see table A.7, panel A). Men may be more accepting of this biomyth about control because they have less experience trying (and then failing) to lose weight.

A well-indoctrinated biocitizen also accepts the BMI as a valid, scientifically sound measure of body fat, weight, and health risk. I presented my students with a strong version of the BMI biomyth (biomyth 3), asking whether they agreed with this statement: "The BMI is a reliable, scientifically sound measure of body fat that applies to everyone, regardless of body shape, ethnicity, and so on." Over one-quarter had great trust in the BMI, while another 30 percent were not sure about its scientific merit. Just over 40 percent were skeptical about its reliability or wide applicability. Again, the men were more trusting of the science than were the women (table A.7, panel B).

Another core idea in the war on fat is that, in a biocitizenship society, everyone has the responsibility to educate, coax, and, if necessary, badger others to diet and exercise so as to achieve a healthy, thin, toned body. Do young people in southern California believe they have these responsibilities to biopedagogize and biobully their fellow Americans? To a surprising extent, yes. I asked my students whether they agreed with this statement: "If family members or friends are overweight, it is our responsibility to let them know we've noticed, and to provide suggestions for diet, exercise, and other techniques they can use to lose the extra pounds." Over two-fifths agreed, while another one-quarter were not quite sure (see table A.7, panel C). One-third disagreed. One-half of men agreed that we are duty-bound to persuade others to become thin, fit biocitizens. Perhaps more attuned to the sensitivity of weight issues, only 40 percent of women agreed with the statement.

The survey evidence thus suggests that the war on fat is in full gear in southern California. Doctors, teachers, and parents are dutifully instilling health and weight consciousness in their charges. Young people know their BMIs, live reasonably healthist lives, and by and large believe in the core tenets of the war on fat. That's the big picture. For a more nuanced and complex story, we turn to the individual auto-ethnographies.

The Ethnographic Essays

After being offered extra credit for writing about how issues of diet, weight, and the BMI play out in everyday life, roughly half the class (48 percent of 274 students in 2010 and 332 students in 2011) wrote essays that ranged from three to twelve pages in length.

Topics of Their Own Choosing

The students had complete freedom in choosing their topics, framing their stories, and deciding which incidents to relate. Because the essays were not graded (all students who turned one in received extra credit) and I did not specify any particular content, there was no incentive to frame the essays any particular way or to "tell me what I wanted to hear." (Indeed, as far as they knew, I might not even read the assignments.) A substantial proportion of the essayists did not follow the prompt's instructions very diligently, instead just writing what came to mind on the topic.[15]

The course certainly had some effect on their decisions about what to write, though it is difficult to specify exactly what it was. The extra-credit essay was assigned early in the section on the obesity epidemic, but it was not due until we had completed that section and a section on eating disorders. The three class sessions devoted to the obesity epidemic mapped out two approaches to the issue (public health and fat acceptance) and introduced the notions of medicalization of weight, fat abuse, and the limitations of the BMI, among others. Based on a close reading of the essays, I believe that those ideas were the ones that empowered many to write about their experiences. Before the class sessions, heavy students did not have a story to tell; instead, internalizing the dominant view, they saw themselves as lazy, irresponsible, and deserving of ridicule because they had not succeeded in losing weight. By suggesting that this account was problematic and that weight ridicule might constitute abuse, the class unleashed long-buried feelings and memories, making those emotions and experiences understandable. Although the students were just beginning to question what they had always known to be true, the class made them see that it was legitimate to feel bad about being bullied, enabling them to tell a story they had not been able to articulate before. The class material was very general, however. There was nothing in the readings or lectures on how the issues of weight and weight management play out in the lives of real people. Figuring this out was their assignment, and each student did it in his or her own way. It is therefore of some interest to see what was on their minds as they were listening to the lectures and doing the readings on obesity.

In my initial sorting, I divided the essays into five clusters by general theme or topic. When the essays from the two years were combined, the largest number of essays (57 percent) dealt with what I call everyday weight struggles. These featured people who were, by and large, overweight or normal but, facing overwhelming pressures to be skinnier, were obsessed with losing weight. A substantial number of essays in this group focused on the pressures on athletes in certain sports (such as gymnastics, dancing, and wrestling) to achieve extreme body types. The second-largest cluster (22 percent of the essays) dealt with eating disorders, primarily bulimia and anorexia—topics that were not mentioned in the prompt. Smaller numbers of essays focused on people at the extremes of the weight continuum, those who felt "too fat" (7 percent) or "too skinny" (7 percent), both of whom were desperate to achieve a more normal weight. A final 8 percent of the essays centered on other topics, including fat-talk, medical misdiagnoses, and spousal fat abuse.

For the cultural analyst, these essays by those targeted by the fat-talk for bodily reform provide extraordinary insight into how the broader war on fat has shaped their practices, identities, and relationships over the first twenty years of their lives—a relatively long time frame in this field of research. Just as a diarist can write about shameful things he or she would not be comfortable telling anyone in person, the auto-ethnographer can write about feelings he or she would be too embarrassed to openly admit or talk about in an interview. As we will see, these young people are incredibly keen observers—and, in many cases, also analyzers—of the micro-politics of weight in their social worlds.

Finding a Voice, Discovering a New Self, Contributing to Public Understanding

For many of the young authors, writing the essay provided a positive, even therapeutic and empowering experience. Writing about difficult issues that may have never risen to consciousness before helped them organize their thoughts and feelings and make sense of them, often for the first time in their lives. Through writing, some were able to acknowledge for the first time a difficult truth—that they suffered from an eating disorder, for example, or that intimate partners were fat-abusive toward them—and come to terms with it. Acknowledging such problems is often a first step in the process of healing.

Perhaps just as important, writing about these matters enabled these young people to find their voice. In a society in which fat seems to be the last socially acceptable grounds for prejudice, heavy and, especially, fat individuals are some of the most stigmatized and silenced people in America today. As we have seen, there is a growing push-back against the excesses of the fat-is-bad mantra in the expert literature and within the fat acceptance movement, yet rarely does this critique spill over into the domain of popular culture, where fat people are supposed to feel shamed into extreme dieting and exercising, not complain about fat abuse. Shows like *The Biggest Loser* provide the script—and there are few others. For these young people, the essay provided a vehicle through which they could express feelings that had lain buried, unheard, often for years. Here is how some expressed their gratitude for the opportunity to articulate and share some painful feelings.

> Before I start, I would like to mention that this is my story and it is something I have never really talked about to others. It wasn't until this project that I really took a look and faced a reality that I never wanted to face. [SC 150]

> As I re-read this paper, I'm not too sure if this is the essay that you wanted, Professor. But even if it is not, I can honestly be thankful that I got the chance to write about this issue that has plagued my entire life. Thank you

for giving me an opportunity to be able to express my feelings about this matter. [SC 17]

Realizing the extraordinary power of these essays as personal testimony and cultural evidence, I sought approval from the university's institutional review board to use them and then requested permission from each student to use his or her essay in my research. As noted earlier, of the 264 students I contacted, 10.6 percent did not respond.[16] It is not clear why. They may not have received the e-mail because it was summer and many were involved in other activities or had graduated. Or they may have felt uncomfortable and simply not replied despite a second, reminder e-mail. Of those who responded, 94.6 percent gave me permission to use their essay. Far from reluctant, the vast majority were thrilled to be included in the research. In part, they were excited that I had sought them out and was interested in their stories. Those who had felt unheard for years were grateful to have someone bear witness to their suffering. My reading of and caring about their stories was a form of affirmation, a signal that they and their struggles mattered to me. One student, whom I call Tiffany, wrote:

> The essay is personal to me, but I'm happy to share it with you. Writing about my feelings and problems was a good way to expose how I was feeling to someone else other than myself. For me, it was a difficult paper to write, but I feel it helped me to figure out a bit of my "problem." Thank you for reading my story; it's good to know that someone did listen to me. [SC 150]

Many replied that they were honored to be asked to have their essays included and hopeful that their accounts might help reframe the public debate about obesity by exposing the struggles and suffering so many endure in the name of health. Here are some typical responses:

> I would be more than happy to assist you in any way that I can. Thank you for the opportunity to be a part of something that can help the community. [SC 150]

> I am ok with my essay being part of your research! I will be happy if my little participation can [help] change the situation of [the] obesity epidemic. [SC 17]

Five percent of the students I contacted asked that I not use their essay because their stories were about friends or family members, and they did not want them to be embarrassed by public exposure of shameful secrets. In one unusual case, an author gave me permission to use all of her essay except the part about a family member who had expressed disgust at the author's weight in an exceptionally disturbing way. I had hoped to use precisely that part because it revealed so forcefully the lengths to which family members sometimes go in their efforts to force kids to lose weight. I replied that I understood fully and respected her decision. Five months later she wrote to me again saying she had had a change of heart. She had done a lot of soul-searching since graduation and realized that what was driving her to consider a certain set of careers, all in the health field, was a desire to make a difference in the world and to help others. She wrote:

> I realized that your research could potentially make a very large and posi-
> tive contribution to society (you know, since obesity is such an "epidemic")
> and that if I allow you to use my paper I would, in turn, also be making a
> small but important contribution to society's understanding of obesity. It
> would be nice to let people know what it feels like to be looked down upon
> and criticized for being "too fat." My negative story should be used for pos-
> itivity [in] research that could help people. [SC 220, e-mail, October 2, 2011]

We agreed that she would conceal her and her family's identity by alter-ing certain identifying (but substantively unimportant) information. This powerful account can now be found in these pages.

Preserving the Authors' Voices

I selected for inclusion and analysis the essays that were most compelling or affecting and that addressed the core issues treated in this book. These forty-five essays are not, of course, representative cases, but the stories are ordinary ones, typical of the accounts I collected.[17] Most of the stories are auto-ethnographies, but about 10 percent are accounts of friends or family members. Although these secondhand accounts are unable to reflect their subjects' feelings as fully or accurately as the firsthand ones, this subset of essays is extraordinarily valuable because it draws our attention to kinds of experiences that are so painful they are unlikely to have ever come to light unless they were written up by a caring friend or family member.

Because I want to honor what the young people have to say—their stories, in their own words and with their own emphases—rather than present excerpts, I include the complete essays or substantial portions of them. I have preserved them in their original language, correcting only spelling and grammatical errors. In a few places, to clarify the meaning, I have changed a word or two or slightly reworked the text. My alterations are in brackets. For the longer essays, I have also added subheadings to structure the text. Because of space limitations, I have omitted portions of text that do not deal with weight. Whenever possible I have retained the original titles chosen by the authors. When the essays lacked a title, I created one, often using quotations from the essay itself. In the following chapters, for each case I include a brief introduction to the central figure (ethnicity, hometown, and so on) and then, following the essay, present a short analysis highlighting what it adds to our understanding. I bring the findings from all the essays together in the conclusion of each chapter and in chapter 10.

The Social Dynamics of the War on Fat: Ethnicity, Income, Gender, and Place

Social differences of ethnicity, income (or class), gender, and place shape how the war on fat plays out in individual lives. To understand this broader social structuring of the war on fat, I asked the authors of the essays to provide basic information about their subject's ethnic background, family economic level, and home city. (The subject's gender was clear from the essay itself; I did not ask about sexual orientation.) The essays do not and cannot bring out the full influence of these social attributes on the body politics of the young people I worked with. That is because the authors did not emphasize (or perhaps even see) the role of ethnicity and other factors in their struggles. Moreover, I had a small and nonrandom selection of essays to draw on. Although the full range of effects must remain invisible, the influence of these social factors is quite evident and can be teased out, in part by comparing essays centering on people of different social backgrounds. And although the findings can't be generalized to the population as a whole, they can be used to generate hypotheses that can be tested with larger-scale data sets in the future.

Hyphenated Americans: A Portrait of America's
Ethnically Diverse Future

America is fast becoming a minority-majority country, and SoCal is on the
leading edge of this trend. In 2010, people of color made up 46.5 percent
of Americans under eighteen. The figure was 73 percent for California.[18]
In the Los Angeles–Long Beach–Santa Ana metro area, the demographic
core of SoCal, nonwhites made up an astonishing 79 percent of the youth
population.[19] Given the demographic trends—by 2018, minorities will
make up the majority of all young Americans—SoCal is especially important, providing a glimpse into the nation's future.[20]

SoCal is home to people from all over the world, making it a fascinating
place to study and live. Many southern Californians are the first, second,
or third generation of families who immigrated to the United States. That
diversity is reflected in the ethnic backgrounds of the subjects of the ethnographic essays. The breakdown of the subjects by ethnic background
and country of origin can be seen in table 2.1. Although the proportions of
whites and blacks in our study group are similar to those for the region as
a whole, among the young people we will meet Asians are overrepresented
while Latinos are underrepresented.[21] Following local use, here I generally
refer to members of these ethnic groups as, say, Asian rather than the more
cumbersome Asian American. That is, the term *Asian* signifies not where
the subjects were born but simply their families' cultural background.

Ethnicity is an issue for the anti-obesity campaign because aggregate
data show that blacks and Hispanics are more likely to be overweight and
obese than whites. These findings hold both for adults and for young people
under twenty.[22] Obesity researchers have drawn on common stereotypes
about these minority groups to attribute their higher weights to ignorance
of healthy practices and cultural differences in weight-related ideals and
behaviors. For example, in mid-2013 the feature article on the CDC webpage labeled adult obesity facts was titled "Compared with Whites, Blacks
Had 51% Higher and Hispanics Had 21% Higher Obesity Rates."[23] The
article cited three possible explanations for the disparities. The first two—
racial differences in behaviors that contribute to weight gain and differences in attitudes and norms regarding body weight—located their higher
weights in cultural attributes of the groups. The third—differences in access to healthful food and safe places for physical activity—acknowledged

TABLE 2.1 Ethnic Backgrounds of Essay and Interview Subjects (%)

Caucasian		18.4
African American		2.9
Hispanic/Latino		11.8
Mexican	6.9	
Other (mostly Salvadoran and Guatemalan)	4.9	
Middle Eastern		8.2
South Asian		4.5
East Asian		24.5
Chinese	15.9	
Korean	6.5	
Japanese	2.0	
Southeast Asian		24.1
Vietnamese	12.7	
Filipino	8.6	
Other (mostly Thai and Cambodian)	2.9	
Two or more races/ethnicities		5.3
N.A.		0.4
Total		100.1

Notes: Sample includes 234 essay subjects and 11 interview subjects. N.A., not available.
Source: Information provided by essay authors

the possible role of environmental factors beyond the groups' control. Although recent years have brought greater acknowledgment of the role of structural factors in minority obesity, the emphasis on overcoming "cultural barriers" to healthy weight persists in governmental and other anti-obesity programs.[24]

Social scientists have seen racism and classism in such apparently neutral scientific interpretations. Under a veneer of scientific legitimacy, they argue, research like that of this CDC article blames childhood obesity on poor minorities, and especially African American and Latina mothers, whose "poor feeding practices" and "failure to recognize overweight" are said to endanger their offspring.[25] Social science research emphasizes the crucial role of the media in perpetuating racist stereotypes about obesity. In their study of American news reporting on weight during 1995–2005, the sociologists Abigail Saguy and Kyerstin Gruys find that many articles in such highly regarded publications as the *New York Times* blame ethnic communities for contributing to higher rates of obesity.[26] Ethnic minorities (at least blacks and Hispanics) are depicted as backward or ignorant, reinforcing the social stereotype of minorities and the poor as lazy, irresponsible, out of control, and hence unworthy of full inclusion in the political community.

For many years, public health studies of obesity focused almost exclusively on these three broad groupings. But other ethnic groups—in particular, Asians—make up a growing segment of the population, especially in high-immigrant areas. In 2012, Asians were 5.1 percent of the U.S. population but 13.9 percent of the California population.[27] Starting in 2014, the CDC began publishing findings for what it calls "non-Hispanic Asians" based on new data from 2011–2012. These data show that Asians, both adult and youth, have much lower levels of overweight and obesity than any other major racial/ethnic group (for example, among Asian youth, 19.5 percent were overweight or obese compared to 31.8 percent for youth of all groups).[28] Although at a given BMI level, Asians (at least adults) may have more body fat and different risk profiles for morbidity and mortality, these differences in weight (or BMI) remain striking.[29] In recent years, a lively online discussion has developed about "why Asians are so skinny" and what body practices everyone else can learn from this supposedly fortunate group. Echoing the model-minority stereotype, what has emerged in the online discussions is an image of the "good Asian," whose "healthy behaviors" are contributing to the nation's health, in sharp contrast to the "bad black and Hispanic," whose "laziness and ignorance" are worsening the obesity epidemic. The great ethnic diversity of people featured in the student essays provides an opportunity for us to hear the voices of cultural groups whose weight struggles have remained largely hidden. We can also read the stories of some blacks and Hispanics, and of many more East and Southeast Asians, to see whether the figures of the "good Asian" and the "bad black and Hispanic" fit the social facts.

Cultural differences shape bodies and body practices in many ways, ways that are little studied and poorly understood. Several connections between ethnicity and body politics emerge clearly in the essays. One is cultural differences in body ideals for women, a subject that has been studied in some groups. Existing research suggests that, relative to whites, Latinas tend to prefer "curvier" bodies while blacks like "thicker" bodies.[30] The SoCal essays support these broad generalizations but show that "cultural preferences" such as these are anything but uniformly shared by all members of a given ethnic group. Rather, preferences for "ethnic" bodies tend to be stronger in the older generation and among more recent immigrants. Young, acculturated Latinas, for example, face such a heavy dose of peer and media pressure dictating the necessity of having skinny bodies that they often abandon their parents' ideals and apply the skinny-body norm to themselves. Among certain East and Southeast Asian groups, the essays reveal, body norms are far more stringent than the scientific norm of the anti-obesity campaign.

Ethnic differences in parent-child relations also shape the way the war on fat plays out in different communities. Cultural norms regarding parent-child communications are especially important, given the centrality of fat-talk in negotiations over weight. The essays suggest that in Caucasian families weight is considered so sensitive a subject that there is a strong norm discouraging parents from openly scolding youngsters for being heavy; parents are expected to use more subtle tactics to get their kids to change their ways. In many Asian families, by contrast, it is perfectly acceptable—indeed, it is even normal and expected—for parents and adult relatives, all of whom care deeply about their sons and daughters, to openly criticize, berate, and humiliate them about their weight (and other matters, such as grades). Readers unfamiliar with these common cultural dynamics may be shocked at the level of fat shaming or bioabuse meted out to children by parents who believe they are helping the youngsters lose weight. Especially because so many Asians populate these pages, it's important for readers to understand the cultural logics of a parenting style that may be unfamiliar.

Research in Asian American studies reveals a distinctive style of parenting that is rooted in Confucian values of respect for authority yet reflects immigrant adaptation to American culture.[31] As the sociologist Min Zhou explains, in Chinese American families (which make up the majority of Asian Americans) a modified version of Confucian values stressing filial piety (unconditional obedience to parents and suppression of a child's self-interest), hard work, discipline, and education serve as normative behavioral standards for socializing the young.[32] In a cultural context in which the interests of the collective outweigh those of the individual, divergence from these expectations brings shame on the whole family and so is negatively sanctioned by both the family and the ethnic community, where bragging about high-achieving children is commonplace. In the American context, parental expectations regarding education, hard work, and other issues are often hard to enforce because children born or raised in the United States belong to two ethnic worlds and develop strong desires to become more "American." Despite the strains, Zhou suggests, many children live up to their parents' expectations, in good part because of their involvement in a well-organized ethnic community that reinforces Asian values and penalizes those who don't conform.

In 2011, Amy Chua threw a bomb into these relatively calm academic discussions with her memoir *Battle Hymn of the Tiger Mother*.[33] In this account of bringing up her two daughters, Chua describes the stern, demanding, and emotionally unsupportive "tiger parenting" techniques that, she claimed, enabled her to raise highly successful children. Her book drew fierce criticism both for its stereotypic depictions of "Chinese parenting" as invariably harsh and demanding, and for exalting a style of parenting that, testimonials of Asian Americans suggest, can leave children traumatized. The book spurred a new wave of research, which finds that among Asian Americans "tiger parenting" exists but is not common; parenting styles vary greatly, with many parents incorporating Euro-American practices; and "tiger parenting" produces poor outcomes, both academically and psychosocially.[34]

How do Asian American parents deal with the issue of child weight and with what effects? To my knowledge, this question has not been explored by ethnic studies scholars. The essays leave no doubt that children's body size is now an important measure of family and community success—and another source of intergenerational strain. The uber-thin body ideals that Asian parents establish for their youngsters suggest that Asians have applied their overall high expectations for their kids to the issue of body size. Yet achieving a thin body is for many youngsters an impossible quest. Do parents turn to tiger tactics in frustration? What are the effects on their children and on family relationships? The essays provide a rare window on the dynamics of biocitizenship in this rapidly growing segment of American society.

Families of Privilege and Privation: The Role of Income or Socioeconomic Class

Southern California is a region of great riches and great economic gaps. According to the latest census, in 2007–2011 the median household income in the largest counties of the region ranged from about 145 percent of the U.S. average (for Orange and Ventura counties) to 106 percent (for Los Angeles and San Bernardino counties).[35] Southern California is also home to vast differences in economic prosperity and insecurity, with areas of great wealth existing in close proximity to areas of extreme poverty. Far from the glittering malls and velvety beaches of the coastal communities lie tiny Imperial County (population 176,000), with household incomes only 75 percent of the national median, and Kern County (population 856,000), with incomes at 91 percent the U.S. average. The same is true within counties. In Orange County, for example, the wealthy (mostly white) coastal enclave of Newport Beach, with a median household income of $108,946 lies but 13 miles from the working-class (mostly Latino) city of Santa Ana, with a median income of $54,399. The wealth gap in Los Angeles County is even vaster, with exclusive enclaves such as the (mostly Asian and white) San Marino ($154,318) having four times the average household income of poor Latino and black cities such as Compton ($43,311).[36] As these data suggest, income and ethnicity are tightly bound up together.

This regional picture of overall prosperity concealing big disparities is reflected in the economic backgrounds of the people my students wrote about. Of the subjects of their essays, 13 percent came from financially struggling families while 50 percent came from middle-income households. A relatively high proportion—22 percent—came from financially privileged backgrounds. The other 12 percent fell between these major categories. (For the definitions of these categories, and exact percentages in each, see table 2.2.) A close reading of the essays reveals very few people at the extreme ends of the economic distribution. That may well be because of the provenance of the sample. Very poor kids are unlikely to be able to afford college (and especially the University of California), while very wealthy ones are likely to attend private colleges rather than a state university. Still, there is a fairly wide distribution, with ample numbers of subjects representing every economic group except the extremely poor and the ultra-rich.

Economic advantage and disadvantage affect body weights and practices in countless ways, yet, with a few exceptions, those influences are hard to detect in the essays. Some of the writers commented on the effects of economic distress (they never called it "poverty") in terms like this: "My boyfriend grew up in rough circumstances," or "Both my

TABLE 2.2 Family Economic Well-Being of Essay Subjects (%)

Financially struggling[a]	12.8
Financially struggling[a] to middle class[b]	6.8
Middle class[b]	50.4
Middle class[b] to well-to-do[c]	5.1
Well-to-do or financially privileged[c]	21.8
Other, N.A.	3.0
Total	99.9

Notes: Sample includes 234 essay subjects; it does not include the 11 interview subjects. The information was provided by essay authors via email. The categories are based on my understanding of what "struggling," "middle class," and "well-to-do" mean to people in the southern California region. N.A., not available.
[a] *Financially struggling:* Main breadwinner probably has blue-collar type of job, main breadwinner may not have stable or steady work, family probably lives in a rental apartment, and family does not always have enough money to buy the things it wants.
[b] *Middle class:* Main breadwinner has steady work and makes a pretty good income; main breadwinner may own a small business, be a middle manager, or have a professional job; family probably owns its home; and there is money for some extras, but the family has a habit of economizing.
[c] *Well-to-do or financially privileged:* Main breadwinner has stable job and earns lots of money; main breadwinner may work in the professions, law, or business; family owns a home and lives in an especially nice or expensive home; and there is ample money to buy nice things.

parents had to work so I grew up on fast food." Young people from well-to-do families almost never drew attention to their economic privilege, instead taking their ability to afford the good things in life for granted. A second reason the influence of class remains hard to see is that many other forces were interacting with family economics to shape weight practices, making it difficult to isolate the effect of poverty (or wealth) from the effects of these other forces. For these reasons, many of the class dynamics of weight and biocitizenship attainment remain out of sight.

Yet one can see the impact of family economic well-being in many, often subtle (but occasionally glaring) ways. The essays starkly illuminate the advantages the financially privileged enjoy in pursuing the goal of biocitizenship. Members of such families have the education to understand the complex rules of healthist living; the money to buy the things that bring thin, fit bodies (healthful food, gym memberships, and trainers—and cosmetic surgery when those fail to work); and the time to pursue the goals of health and good looks. With the necessities of life easily secured, they have the luxury to worry about achieving the cultural ideal of the thin, fit body.

Families in difficult economic circumstances not only have little education, money, or time but tend to live in unsafe, amenity-poor neighborhoods that make it difficult for kids to eat well and get enough exercise. Members of these families are more worried about making ends meet than whether their bodies are trim, buff, and of the scientifically recommended weight. A theme that runs through many essays is the emotional stress that family economic hardships (or travail of any kind) put on young people. Kids often deal with the stress by eating more—especially more sweet, salty, and fatty foods, which are the easiest to find, the cheapest to buy, and the most intrinsically rewarding to eat. And so the cycle of poverty and obesity continues.

Thin Girls and Buff Boys: Fat-Phobia Evens Out—a Bit

As a long line of feminists has emphasized, an obsession with diets, weights, and perfectly proportioned bodies has long been a female affliction.[37] Today's war on fat, however, is an equal opportunity campaign that expects boys as well as girls to become fit, trim biocitizens. In young men, the campaign seems to have found a newly vulnerable target. We have seen that in SoCal, young men are almost as obsessed with their bodies as are women, though with different emphases (muscles for men, slenderness for women). Far from being specific to California, these divergent emphases are central features of American consumer culture today.

In *Body Panic*, the media specialists Shari L. Dworkin and Faye Linda Wachs trace recent shifts in idealized male and female bodies in health and fitness magazines.[38] Such magazines are perfect for our purposes because our ideas about bodies are so heavily shaped by the images in consumer culture (such as those shown in these magazines) and because body ideals are increasingly promoted in the name of "health" rather than "beauty." The authors find a striking change in gendered ideals in recent years. While both males and females must be free of excess fat, increasingly the ideal female form is slender, firm, curvy, and lacking in strong musculature, whereas the ideal male is muscular, with a cut form and bulging upper-body muscles. Women are small, tight, and toned, while men are big, hard, and cut—exactly the body ideals I found in southern California.[39] The images, articles, and other content in these magazines not only help define the cultural ideals to which we all strive, they also teach a morality of the body in name of "health." The morality for men is that size makes the man and only he who succeeds is a valued American. By making men (and women) feel inadequate because so few can ever reach the ideals, the health and fitness magazines also keep readers obsessively focused on body routines. This is a superb illustration of how popular cultural forms (which include the ads of corporate America) work together with the public health campaign to promote weight consciousness and fat hatred.

With both genders preoccupied with achieving perfect biocitizen bodies, the worlds of young people of both genders are full of fat-talk. Are boys and girls subject to equal amounts of it? Does all the talk about weight invade boys' identities as much as it does girls'? The limited research of cultural anthropologists suggests that, compared to teenage girls, boys in this country are less closely monitored and criticized for their weight—in other words, they are subject to less fat-talk. That is because boys' identity and self-worth are tied more to their abilities and achievements than to their looks and because social acceptance by others is less critical to their identity formation.[40] The surveys I conducted support this finding, showing that boys are less likely to be scolded by parents and doctors for their weight (tables A.3 and A.4). The essays, however, make clear that in SoCal fat boys are mercilessly—and probably increasingly—teased about their weight. One researcher working elsewhere found that boys were relatively immune to the feelings of personal failure that girls endured. Another found that boys were hurt by the harsh critiques but, following codes of masculinity, had to "play it cool" and hide the pain.[41] Which view is correct in California today? We find out later in the book.

So far we've talked about masculinity (and femininity) as though it had no ethnicity, but in reality gender and race/ethnicity are deeply intertwined. In their discussion of the cultural construction of male ideals, Dworkin and Wachs describe how hegemonic masculinity—invariably pictured as white, tanned, athletic, and strong—is marked as different from and superior to the subordinated masculinities of racial minorities and lower socioeconomic classes. The "superiority" of the white, musclebound male is achieved in part by rendering the "inferior" males invisible, that is, by omitting any images of them in magazines that purport to show "healthy American men." How do nonwhite men react to this erasure from the public imagery of what it means to be a real man? California is a splendid place to be posing these questions because the ideal of the white muscled male is absolutely hegemonic—what more iconic image of ideal American manhood is there than the blonde, white surfer boy?—and because there are so many men of nonwhite, subordinated groups in local society to talk to.

Of the essays I gathered, 82 percent focused on women and 18 percent dealt with men. (This proportion is similar to the ratio of women to men enrolled in the class.) Because the experiences of men suffering weight abuse are so poorly documented and understood, I found the essays on men particularly fascinating. They also hold special interest because, just as women are expected—and even taught—to emote about their weight concerns, men are culturally forbidden from expressing feelings of being "hurt." Yet, perhaps because this was a personal essay written for an understanding female professor, some men were willing to share those and other feelings. In other cases, sisters or girlfriends who knew the men well enough to be able to decode their feelings told their stories. Both sorts of essays were very touching. For these reasons, I have tried to include as many of the essays about men as possible. In the end, some 29 percent of the essays featured in this book center on men.

SoCal, NorCal: Everywhere You Go, It's the Body State

The great majority of the essay subjects (roughly three-quarters) were raised in the ten counties of southern California. One-third were from Los Angeles County (which includes the City of Los Angeles) and one-fifth were from Orange County. Fifteen percent of my subjects came from northern California (primarily the Bay Area and the Silicon Valley), and another 6 percent came from other states or countries. The details can be found in table 2.3.[42]

Although northern Californians, especially those from the San Francisco Bay Area, tend to look down their noses at their southerly brethren for their superficial body obsessions, when one examines the body ideals and practices of people raised in the two Californias, the differences are not that great; almost everyone is pretty obsessed with having a trim, fit body. There are probably two reasons for this. One is that the bodily pressures on young people living in southern California are so extreme that even more "enlightened" northerners, once they move to SoCal (to go to school, for example), feel they must comply with the local body norms to fit in and be socially accepted. Another reason for the lack of north-south difference is

TABLE 2.3 Home County, State, or Country of Essay and Interview Subjects (%)

SoCal		73.9
San Luis Obispo and Kern counties	1.6	
Santa Barbara County	0.8	
Ventura County	2.0	
Los Angeles County (includes city of Los Angeles)	32.7	
Orange County	20.0	
Riverside County	5.3	
San Bernardino County	2.0	
San Diego County (includes city of San Diego)	6.5	
Imperial County	0.8	
Two or more counties, due to moves	2.0	
SoCal and other area(s)		4.1
SoCal and other state(s)	0.8	
SoCal and other country(ies)	3.3	
NorCal		14.7
San Francisco Bay Area	7.3	
Silicon Valley	4.5	
Other	2.9	
Other state or country		5.7
Other state	3.7	
Other country	2.0	
N.A.		1.6
Total		100.0

Notes: Sample includes the subjects of the essays (234) and interview informants (11). Location listed is where the subject grew up and/or where most of the events described took place. Information was provided by essay authors via email. N.A., not available; NorCal, northern California; SoCal, southern California.

that diet, exercise, and other body practices are now undertaken mostly in the name of "health" rather than superficialities like "attractiveness." Northern Californians may not be willing to admit to vanity, but they will proudly assert their attachment to "health."

More important than the part of the state the subject hailed from is the community he or she grew up in. As suggested before, in wealthy communities (such as San Diego County's Rancho Santa Fe, OC's Newport Coast, or LA's Beverly Hills), one finds more exacting body standards and expectations, greater pressures to comply and, in turn, more extreme body practices (weight-loss drugs, cocaine, surgery, and so forth). In poorer communities such as Calexico in Imperial County or Santa Ana in Orange

County, one generally finds the opposite; standards are more forgiving, pressures are less severe, and healthist body practices are more minimalist, in good part because family incomes and the environment provide little support for sustained diets and exercise routines. The authors of the essays certainly did not analyze the role of these community factors, but when they had a noticeable impact on weight, the authors brought that out in their essays. My subjects came from a large number of communities all over California (and the country and the world). Although it's impossible to say how each home town shaped its residents' body practices, to help contextualize the stories, in the introductions to the essays I identify where the subject lived during the incidents described in the essay. Those familiar with California's diverse communities should be able to make some important connections.

The University Setting: Boot Camp for Weight Obsession

Finally, a few words about the university setting, which all participants in my study had in common. Weight and other body anxieties are not created in college, but they are certainly heightened there. As the journalist Courtney E. Martin puts it in *Perfect Girls, Starving Daughters*, college is a boot camp for body obsession.[43] The essays presented here suggest that young people living and eating together tend to become hypersensitive about their appearance and weight, which are usually the first things people judge them on. Young people thrown together soon begin to silently compare their bodies, ranking one another by the criteria of pride and shame set out by the rules of biocitizenship. As Carrie's earlier comments show, in such close quarters, fat-talk and the weight preoccupation that follows become contagious, spreading from one anxious person to another. And with college comes the "Freshman 15." Although some claim to have debunked the reality of this risk of weight gain, for many of my students, and especially freshmen who dined at the all-you-can-eat commons, it was only too real. The extraordinary ethnic diversity of the Irvine campus added to their weight worries, as people compared themselves to those of other ethnicities, finding their own bodies inevitably wanting. Neglecting biological differences, for most it was the skinniest girls (Asian) and the buffest guys (Caucasian) who set the standard for all. College years are also the conventional mate-hunting time, making both girls and guys hypersensitive about meeting the codes of femininity and masculinity and making their parents hyperconcerned about their ability to find an appropriate partner. These and other aspects of the university experience, documented in great detail, certainly affected my informants' body ideas and practices.

Yet, in this project, the effect of the college setting is not as great as one might expect. UC Irvine is a commuter campus, with just under 50 percent of all students (but 80 percent of freshmen) living in dorms or other college-owned, operated, or affiliated housing.[44] Moreover, many of the essays about the young people themselves focus on life experiences that unfolded when they were in elementary, middle, or high school. Still other essays (roughly one-quarter) deal with a relative or friend, none based at UC Irvine. My ballpark estimate is that roughly 40 percent of the essays deal, at least in part, with young people in their college years. For these, the influence of the college setting is important.

Part 2

My BMI, My Self

3

"Obese"

Being raised to see beauty as being skinny, I saw myself as ugly for having
gained so much more weight than most girls I knew. In high school, my
weight definitely made me feel that I was uglier than all my friends, which
led me to think negatively of myself and have low confidence. It was hard
for me to communicate effectively with boys or prettier girls, since I felt that
I was too ugly to speak to them. This led me to have few if any male friends.
Overall, I felt that I was inferior to everyone and that I would disgust people
because I was fat.

AMY, FROM HER ESSAY "WEIGHT-OBSESSED CULTURE" [SC 26]

Over the last two decades, I've argued, the war on fat has been quietly
remaking American society by fostering the formation of new, medicalized identities based on the body mass index (BMI). Through a whole series of verbal and nonverbal cues, individuals have been urged to take
their BMI classification as the measure of their health, adopting their new
weight-centric identities (obese, overweight, etc.) as their own and acting
according to the medical and cultural expectations for that "condition."
Because health is a super-value in our culture, I have suggested, increasingly this new weight-based identity is becoming one of the core identities
of Americans everywhere. If these arguments are correct, this amounts to
a striking transformation of American society and selfhood. To my knowledge, no one has systematically investigated whether people see themselves
as "normal," "underweight," and so on.[1] The essays I have gathered can
help answer these questions. In this and the following three chapters, I use
them to understand self-making and selfhood among young Californians.
I start with the identity "obese," whose incumbents are the main target of
society's war on fat.

To be fat in America is to be "ugly," "disgusting," "inferior," and "unworthy" of friendship or romance. Kids like Amy learn this early. Through an endless stream of fat-talk and other anti-fat communications in their social worlds, they learn that fatness is evidence of a biological flaw, moral turpitude, and civic irresponsibility. To be fat is to be a personal and moral failure. The public health campaign seeks through both derogatory labeling and directed fat-talk to educate them and, if that doesn't work, then shame them into becoming virtuous biocitizens who will diet and exercise their way down to normality. In the biocitizenship society in which we now live, everybody, from intimates to strangers, has both the right and the responsibility to shame and discipline fat people into becoming good biocitizens. In a world full of such fat-talk, people targeted for discipline and abuse have few conceptual, narrative, or visual resources with which to construct alternative identities, reject the demeaning comments, or critique the hurtful jabs of which they are victim.

In the official discourse of the war on fat, the labeling and fat-talk are deemed positive and constructive. Rarely do we ask if the fat-talk and other measures aimed at the obese are actually working in the intended ways. Nor do we ask what happens to people—the great majority, according to the science—whose biologies refuse to cooperate. By looking at how obese (and near-obese) young southern Californians see themselves and their lives, this chapter tackles those questions. In part because extra pounds accumulate with age, very few youngsters, at least on California college campuses, are truly obese (that is, have a BMI of 30 or higher). (A 5′ 6″ person is "obese" at a weight of 186 pounds or more.) Of the 234 subjects featured in the essays, only seventeen (7.2 percent) were fat.[2] Surprisingly, the great majority of those were of East or Southeast Asian descent, a finding that flies in the face of the stereotype of "the thin Asian."

In these chapters, I ask three sets of questions. The first concerns the workings of our biocitizenship society. What kinds of cultural pressures do very heavy youngsters encounter? What categories of people act as responsible biocitizens who try to induce heavy people to lose weight? Is their fat-talk biopedagogical, bioabusive, or both? Who, if anyone, supports them? Second, how do heavy young people react? Do they internalize the fat identity and reorganize their sense of self around their fatness? What cluster of emotions, social behaviors, and bodily practices goes with being a "fat person"? Who becomes a fat subject and who, if anyone, resists that identity? And third, what are the larger consequences of accepting a fat identity for young people's health and lives? Is the war on fat helping these prime targets lose weight and become socially valued biocitizens?

The essays show that obese people exhibit an array of responses to these pressures. While all those we will meet accept their fatness as fundamental to their identity, not everyone accepts that fat is bad or tries to become a good biocitizen. A first group follows the dominant cultural script, internalizing the fat-person identity and struggling to follow the bioscript of dieting and exercising to become thin, fit, socially valued biocitizens. A second group, finding the fat-is-bad story impossible to abide, finds some relief by creating alternative social identities that allow them to claim a positive selfhood in public, even though in private they continue to feel like shameful "fat persons." A third group, finding the bad-person story intolerable and the diet-and-exercise solution ineffective, ends up rejecting the dominant narrative and claiming that "fat is good and so am I."

Fat and Unworthy (Ugly, Undeserving, Bad): The Classic "Fat Person"

Let's begin with what we might call the classic fat person. For working purposes, I define a *classic fat person*, or subject, as a very heavy individual who internalizes the dominant construction of obesity as a shameful condition, identifies as being fat, feels bad about him- or herself, and tries to lose weight. Other attributes may emerge from the essays, but these are the most fundamental. Amy, whose bleak words of self-loathing open this chapter, is an example of such a person. In this section, we meet two young people who have suffered enormously from being labeled "fat" their entire lives. Seeing no way out, they simply endure, hoping for something to happen that will relieve their misery.

Stuck in a Fat Body: Kim's Story

Kim is a nineteen-year-old Thai American from an upper-middle-class family in San Francisco. An early developer, Kim was subject to some of the most vicious biobullying documented by my young informants. Unable to challenge her tormenters and unable to lose weight, she simply removes herself from the world that has caused her so much pain.

Not all Asians are skinny. I should know. I am a 19-year-old Thai female and I am fat. Medically speaking, my BMI tells me that I am on the border-line between overweight and obese. On a good day I am just overweight. On a bad day, I am obese.

Big Breasts and Hips Bring Bioabuse from a Tender Age

I was a skinny child [who] hit puberty in the fifth grade. When I was in sixth grade, my classmates [figured] out that I had started my period because I kept leaving class to go to the bathroom for "personal lady reasons." I was teased by male friends. They asked me: "Can you fly?" I wasn't sure what they meant so they clarified: "Do you have wings?" They were referring to whether I wore pads with wings.

A couple months later, a rumor started about me. A popular boy from school that I had a crush on came up to talk to me for the first time. He told me that he heard some girls spreading rumors about me and how I "stuff." I didn't even know what that meant. I asked him to explain it to me. He said "using tissue," and I still didn't [understand]. I asked him if he thought the rumor was true. He said, "No, why would you stuff? Only guys do that to make their penis look bigger." When he said that, I [realized] that the girls were starting rumors that I was "stuffing my bra."

In middle school it got worse. Ever since I hit puberty, my boobs grew. But I also gained weight everywhere, so I thought [my body] was [well] propor-tioned. For example, I have always had a big butt and huge thighs. One time, a friend's friend looked at me and told me that my boobs were "too big" and that I was "very unproportional." I thought she was complimenting me so I smiled at her and said thank you. She shot me a dirty look. For some reason [I could not fathom], this girl was criticizing my body.

My school was like the movie "Mean Girls." There was a clique of popu-lar girls. They always had the best clothes and got the best-looking guys. Ev-erybody wanted to be their friend so they could be popular like them. These girls were skinny Asian girls with no boobs and a couple of skinny white girls with small boobs. A friend came up to me during PE this one time and [said]: "Those girls over there are talking about you and I don't like that." She pointed over to the popular girls who were all sitting or lying on each other in their "sisterly, little perfect clique" while playing with each others' hair and talking about me as if they didn't have a care in the world. I was really sad be-cause there was no way I could confront those girls who had the entire school wrapped around their fingers.

It got [even] worse after that. I began hearing rumors that I was sexually active. People I [didn't even know] would walk by me just so they could taunt me and call me a slut to my face. [They would then] walk over to the popular girls so they could tell them what they did to me and then continue talking about me. Everywhere I walked in school, I would hear whispers or even yells calling me a slut. The worst point was when strangers actually started throwing their trash at me. They would [hurl] their crumpled hamburger wrappers and empty soda bottles at me. It got so bad that I would just stop walking around [the school campus].

A Mother's "Encouragement" Feels Anything But

The verbal abuse didn't stop there. When I was in high school my mom started commenting on how I'm so short. (By the way, we are the same height.) After [learning from the doctor] that there was nothing I could do to change my height, my mom started picking on my weight. She would tell me that I eat too much. I need to eat more vegetables. My shoulders are wide. My neck is so short and fat. The list goes on and on.

When I got into college, I moved out of the house because I didn't want to commute. When I would come home for the weekend, my mom would start to up the ante. She would not only call me fat, but she would tell me that I was so fat I will have a heart attack. She even went so far as to mock me by tensing her left arm, grabbing her chest, falling on the floor, and thrashing her body because "That's what you will look like when you have a heart attack because you're so fat." This happened every time I went home, without fail. Eventually I just stopped going home altogether.

My mom missed me and called to ask why I haven't been coming home. I told her it's because I was tired of [hearing] her call me fat all the time, and she responded with "But you are!" I hung up on her. There was no way I was listening to her shit anymore. When I started going home again, every time she called me fat or commented on my weight, I would walk away. Soon she learned not to do it anymore. I know that she's my mom and that she cares about me, but what she thought of as "encouragement" I thought of as bullying. Anyway, her bullying stopped when she realized how much it was hurting me. Now she still encourages me to work out because I am a lazy hermit (she didn't call me that, I am just admitting that I am). She also tries to encourage me to eat more healthily. I hope she learns that criticizing me in a mean-spirited manner and doing the "heart attack" thing won't help me change. Although I want my parents' approval, the stress gets to me, and I am actually diagnosed with depression and anxiety.

When the Bioscript Fails

I'm pretty sure I should lose weight, but when I try it [almost] never works. When it does work, I end up gaining the weight back in a couple of months anyway. I believe that people have a set weight. Even though some people are able to control their weight, those people need to realize that not everyone is as lucky as they are, and stop teasing and looking down upon overweight people. I have always been jealous of anorexics for having so much self-control and being able to achieve a thin body. What has stopped me from being anorexic has been my love of food. What has stopped me from being bulimic is the grossness. I hate the taste of throw-up. So for now I am stuck in this fat body, at least until I can save up enough money for liposuction or therapy [to help me accept my body the way it is].

Kim: Forced into Hiding

Kids can be cruel, and we will encounter a lot of cruelty in these pages, but what Kim endured was more than cruel—it was vicious ejection from the community that went beyond the verbal to the physical: literally throwing trash at her as if to force her to get out of sight. And she did; the ridicule and rejection were so extreme that the only way Kim could survive was to hide in the far peripheries of the school campus. The terrible abuse continued at home, where Kim's mom, desperate for her to fit in and be popular, opted for harsh critique, going to the extremes of acting out a fat-induced heart attack to impress on her daughter the seriousness of her (apparently wilfully chosen) condition. Revealing the power of a common biomyth—that body weight is under individual control—Kim's mom mercilessly criticized her bodily flaws even though Kim had inherited her height, and apparently also shape, from her mother.

What did Kim do to deserve such inhumane treatment? Perhaps her fatness, accentuated by her shortness (under 5 feet), was so beyond the bounds of the culturally acceptable that her body was considered what one of my SoCal informants called "visual pollution." In a place where "we are used to, and feel we deserve to, see beauty and hard work on the body everywhere; fatness is simply unforgivable," it may have been not just Kim's fatness but also her failure to adopt the norms of a good biocitizen—diligent exercise and diet—that justified the treatment. Whatever her tormenters' rationale, this horrific abuse tells us more about our fat-bashing culture than it does about Kim herself.

From an early age, Kim has had a "fat" identity thrust upon her. Not surprisingly, she has made that identity central to her sense of self.

What has that identity entailed? Although Kim does not talk about feelings of being defective or unattractive, it seems clear she feels that way because she has tried to lose weight many times. She also feels emotionally traumatized, depressed, and anxious. Inhabiting social worlds that reject her, lacking social support of any kind (that she mentions), and unable to defend herself from her abusers, Kim feels her only option is to physically escape and dream of a time when she can afford a surgical solution to correct her bodily flaws. Kim's plight serves as a powerful metaphor for the place of heavy people in SoCal society—there may well be none.

I Wish I Believed in Myself: Jessica's Dream

Jessica is a twenty-two-year-old Chinese American whose middle class OC family is full of weight-preoccupied biocitizens. Although the fat-talk directed at her has been more encouraging than abusive, it has slowly eroded her sense of herself as a good person to the point that she looks in the mirror and sees a "fat, ugly, abnormal" person.

In My Own Skin
I want to be pretty, I want to be thin
No matter how hard I try, I just can't fit in
I go on diets, I go to the gym
I count calories, Just to be slim
I take diet pills, Eat Kellogg's meal bars
Drink Slim fast, To look like TV stars
I want to be pretty, I want to be thin
So I can feel better, In my own skin

I wrote this poem five years ago. I have never thought of myself as a pretty, cute, or good-looking person. As shallow as this may sound, my main reasoning would be due to my weight. I am currently 5'6" and weigh in at 189 pounds [BMI of 30.5]. I never talk about how much I weigh to anyone, whether they are family, friends, or strangers. The thoughts that constantly play over and over in my head deal with weight. I keep telling myself, "if I am able to lose weight, I will look better," "if I am able to lose weight, people will like me better." I can't explain why I choose to believe that my identity is based solely on my appearance. I do not judge others this way and my friends do not judge me this way. Every single day I struggle with my weight and I do my best to hide it from everyone else.

Wii Fit Says I Am "Obese"

Weight loss is very popular right now. There are a lot of media that have come out with weight-loss videos or games. I got sucked into Nintendo's Wii Fit. On this game, before you are able to do any of the exercises or active games, you have to weigh yourself. The game gives you your weight in pounds [and tells you where] you stand on the BMI index. According to the Wii Fit game, I am obese [so] my character becomes obese as well. This is horrifying to look at. It makes me feel awful about myself.

Every time I look in the mirror, the only thing I see is how overweight my body is. I think about the muffin-top stomach fat that pools over my jeans and how my underarms flap away when my arms move. I currently count calories whenever I can and keep a food journal to review my previous meals. I no longer have enough confidence to wear skirts and always cover my upper body with some sort of jacket or sweater. I am always on a diet and force myself to go to the gym. I try my best to not eat over 1,500 calories a day and try to leave out carbohydrates as much as possible.

Shopping Traumas

I feel the most insecure and self-conscious about my body when I go shopping for clothes. I am afraid to see the size of pants I will have to pick up as well as how they will look on me when I try them on. I didn't start worrying about my weight until I went shopping with my friends one day freshman year. Everything was going great and I was very happy until we walked into Forever 21. All the girls had clothes they favored and went to try on, including me. I was the only one who didn't fit into the clothes she tried on. I chose the largest sizes Forever 21 offered. I felt naked when I looked in the mirror. Why didn't they fit me? My only answer was that I was too fat. I wasn't normal like all of my friends. I was overweight and because I was overweight I was ugly.

I will not allow myself to ever be put in that situation again. If I go shopping with my friends, I will not grab clothes to try on because my logic is that I am too fat to fit in them anyway, so why even try? As I stand in front of clothes that I think are cute but won't fit me, I begin to break down. I don't want my friends to see me cry so I excuse myself to grab some fresh air. The more clothing stores I walk out of, the more depressed I am when I get home.

I am not my only critic. My family heavily criticizes me for my weight as well. My father constantly will remind me not to eat too much because I am too fat. My mother will always remind me about how beautiful I was five years ago when I was 125 pounds. She will e-mail me pictures with captions that say, "Jessica, you are so beautiful here. Make sure you take care of your body." My mother is also constantly saying that she is on a diet. She too is trying to lose weight. My oldest brother is a health nut. Even though he does not do it to lose weight, he is always watching what he eats and reading the newest books on fitness. My sister-in-law and second older brother both have a gym pass and talk daily about wanting to lose weight.

I was not always like this. In high school, I could care less about how much I weighed and who thought I was too fat or too skinny. Besides the fact that I was not fat in high school, I ate what I wanted when I wanted. My main goal was to get through high school and find happiness in myself. [Since then] my personal weight issues have affected me emotionally and psychologically. I no longer like to go to the beach unless I am fully clothed. I haven't even purchased a bathing suit in six years. With the society that I live in right now, I am too afraid of what will come of my future if I am overweight or considered ugly. I wish I could be happy again. I wish I did not care about what others say or believe about me. I wish I believed in myself.

Jessica: Fearing the Future as a Fat Adult

In Jessica, we have a young woman who, subjected to the pervasive familial and cultural pressures to be thin, has in the short space of five years come to see herself as fat and fat as her most fundamental identity. In her telling, what sparked this dramatic transformation was a shopping trip with friends. Her essay elaborates on a common theme in the ethnographies, the normalizing role of women's clothing; how the size range available defines bodily normality and how today's cute clothes flatter thin and toned, but not thick and fleshy, bodies. With its standardized, tiny sizes, contemporary fashion is for many a form of tyranny. The unavailability of extra-large sizes in popular clothing outlets not only makes it difficult for fat girls to find the in-styles but also excludes them from the social life of shopping, one of the most important social activities of young women. For Jessica, the discovery that she could not be clothed was so traumatizing, it led her to reorganize her sense of self, leaving her with a fragile identity that she has spent the rest of her young life trying to protect.

Jessica's essay brings out the role of fat-culture media, such as the popular Wii Fit game, which has spread biocitizen culture by normalizing the use of weight as a basis for identity and promoting weight loss as an important cultural project. For Jessica, and no doubt many other players, having to view her "obese" character as other gamers see it made her feel terrible. These and countless other popular fat-cultural forms have taught her to evaluate her worth in terms of weight and to see her large body as an assortment of unacceptable parts to be given disparaging labels and made the target for weight-control efforts. Her family of dedicated biocitizens only heightens the pressure on her to conform.

Subject to such relentless pressures, Jessica has come to see herself first and foremost in terms of her fatness. That new identity has profoundly changed her life. From someone who cared nothing about her weight, Jessica has become obsessed with her extra pounds and has taken up the weight-loss practices expected of a heavy person. They have had little effect, however, leading to emotional distress, social withdrawal, and deep fears for her future in a society that treats fat people as legitimate objects of stigma and discrimination.

Creating Counter-Identities: Re-Imagining the Person in the Fat Body

Some young people, after years of suffering, find the fat identity so intolerable that they create an alternative public identity that gives them self-respect in social settings, even though they may continue to feel like degraded fat persons inside. Those we meet here—Mai Ly, Sajeda, and Caroline—are highly creative in refashioning their external selves. Although the new identity is largely imagined and probably ephemeral, it makes them feel happier and more in control of their lives and selves. In the last case, Caroline's, the new identity seems to be changing her most fundamental sense of self for the better. Whether the new identity will endure remains to be seen.

Tough Girl Outside, Sad Girl Inside: Mai Ly's Secret Life as an Obese Person

Mai Ly is a heavy twenty-one-year-old Vietnamese American from a financially struggling family in Oakland. Enduring fat-abuse her whole young life, Mai Ly has developed an exterior persona as an aggressive, take-charge girl who loves her body. Inside, however, she is dying to be thin and lives with a welter of insecurities about preserving her social ties in a world in which fatness is legitimate grounds for social abandonment.

According to the BMI chart, I am obese, standing at 5'6" and [weighing] about 235 pounds [BMI of 37.9]. My whole life, I was always a bit chubbier than the rest of the little girls. My best friends were always the smallest of the small, even though they ate enormous portions at least six times a day. I, however, was not that lucky. Everything I ate seemed to make me gain weight like crazy, even if it was healthy food in small portions. It was really hard for me to take jokes [about] "fat people" when my friends sometimes made fun of them because I always considered myself one, even though all my friends didn't think that way. Nonetheless, there was always that certain group of people that needed to pick on me. For those people to get me going, they always directed their putdowns [at] how big I was because they had no other bad thing to say about me. It was the most obvious, I suppose.

"Tough Big Girl" Yearns to Be Skinny

From there on, I became known as this "tough girl" among my group of friends. I felt like I needed to be known in this way so that people would be scared to make jokes about my body. My friends think that I don't worry about my body and how I look compared to them because that's how I present myself: loving my body the way it is. However, it is hard holding on to that image because truly I have many insecurities.

Sometimes I see girls going on extreme diets and doing so many different things to maintain their beauty that I don't seem to do. I don't show or say it at all, but it makes me jealous. I compare myself to my friends enough times to say that sometimes I wish I were them, which is sad, I know, but it's true in a sense. Every time I look at myself in the mirror, I feel like if I were as skinny as they are, I could take over the world. I know myself as being one of the most aggressive people [in my circle of friends]. I take the initiative and make things happen, but I feel like my image of being overweight holds me back because people judge me before they take me seriously. I guess it's a good thing, though, because it makes me try ten times harder to get the respect I deserve.

Negotiating Fatness in Daily Life

For me, the two hardest parts of being overweight are dealing with my family and dealing with my boyfriend. From my family, I always get told that I should lose weight. They say that it is unhealthy and that it is not how to live my life. [The worst] is my mother. She finds so many ways to make me feel like I am a bad person. Every chance she gets, she tells me that I will never find love because of my weight. It's funny because, even after I told her how I have a boyfriend now (not my first), she continues to tell me how it will never last. It is hard to deal with and I know I should listen at times, but I sometimes feel happy the way I am. I mean, I would love to lose weight and be skinny, but being told to lose weight doesn't speed the process.

With my boyfriend, it's more of a big insecurity within myself. I feel like I am lucky to find such a sweet and very good looking guy, but I am always scared that he will find another girl who is more compatible with him in a body image sense. I get jealous when he talks to girls that I think look better than I do because they are skinnier, but he tells me every day that I don't need to worry. Sometimes it's hard not to worry, though. My dad mentions it too. He met my boyfriend once and said that he was a pretty skinny guy and that if I wanted to keep him then I would have to lose weight. Lately I feel like my jealousy is hurting our relationship, so now I have to try my best to control how I feel unless I want to lose him.

Other difficult issues I have to face are [eating and] shopping with my friends. My roommates find it weird sometimes that I buy food and go directly [to] my room to watch TV sitcoms. When I finish, I come out to hang out with them. I mean, I'm not that embarrassed to eat with them but sometimes I guess I feel like I am being watched when I eat. I love to shop, but I usually can't shop with other people. All my friends are really skinny, so they have no issue in finding clothes that look cute on them. I, on the other hand, am limited in clothes choice. I mean, I can still find things to buy in the shops they go to, but it's not the same sometimes. An example would be H&M. Clothes there only go up to a size large or a size 13/14, but I am a size 16 or extra-large. It's hard sometimes, but I tend to deal with it okay.

My friends are really supportive, which is why I forget [for] the most part how big I am compared to them. Many of them actually tell me they are jealous of me for being so comfortable and proud of how I look, but it kills me sometimes to think that it isn't always true. I claim that I am a big shot, and that I love myself in all ways possible, but there is always part of me that wishes so much to be thin.

Mai Ly: A Brave Façade

Mai Ly's bold strategy for warding off fat-abuse—creating a public identity as an assertive, even aggressive person—is quite common in the essays, though it is more common among boys, who become bullies or join gangs to scare off the would-be biobullies. In Mai Ly's case, the strategy worked to scare off abusers among her peers, but it didn't silence her biocitizen parents, who resorted to both educational and abusive fat-talk to convey their concerns. Nor did it deal with her self-deprecation, internalized after so many years of parental and peer reproach. Despite her brave declaration that she "loves herself," deep down, her greatest wish is that she could be thin like her friends, indeed, that she could stop being herself and become them. Like Jessica, Mai Ly finds her life dominated by struggles to maintain a social life and feel good about herself in a biocitizenship society that equates fatness with badness. Beneath the brave tough-girl-who-loves-her-body exterior, Mai Ly is a fat subject who struggles to cherish herself.

It Was I Who Was Never Good Enough: Sajeda's Story

A Pakistani American, twenty-one-year-old Sajeda grew up in northern Orange County, where her immigrant family moved from poorer to richer cities as they recovered their pre-immigration status as economically privileged. Despite her many academic achievements, Sajeda is unable to view herself as accomplished because of her heavy weight. Faced with an intolerable identity, she comes up with a highly creative way to produce that perfect self.

"Too Thin and Sure to Die": The Prognosis at Age Four

I was born and raised in Lahore, Pakistan. I came from a wealthy home; my father invested in several stocks and worked as an investment banker. I had an amazing childhood with British-based private schooling and lots of play dates and museum visits.

I was four years old when my family noticed something was off in my eating habits. I was an active child, loud and energetic. I was on the thinner side but never unhealthy. I refused to eat certain foods and eventually I completely stopped eating the healthy foods my parents preferred. The combination of my eating habits and body size led my parents to believe that I was too thin and weak. I felt confused, rejected, alone. I was the one member in my family who was thin; the rest had some extra weight. I wanted to be like them. [One night] at a family dinner, my aunt, a pediatrician, pulled me aside. At just four years of age, I was told I was too thin, too weak, and, in [her] extreme words, "*tum mar jao gi*"—"you will die." These words still haunt me today. This incident was the beginning of a long battle [with] weight cycling.

I sat in my aunt's clinic, nervous, cold, and naked. She walked in with a folder in her hand, which held my calculations. She told me I was underweight. My mom sat there in disappointment, as though it were my fault. I looked at her for confirmation that I would be alright. I saw fear in her eyes. She smiled at me and hugged me. My aunt handed my mom a piece of paper—my prescription—which would change my life forever. Inside the white bag [my mom picked up at the pharmacy] I saw a syringe with needles. I stayed quiet, assuming that was not my medicine, and that it was for my mom's diabetes. I went home and my mom asked me to take off my pants. I was confused but took the shot anyway. I was pleased to know that I would soon be normal, not sick anymore, and that I would look like my sisters.

A Traumatic Move to the United States: Finding Comfort in Hot Cheetos

Soon afterwards, the stock market in Pakistan crashed, and the stocks my father had invested in followed [the market down]. Our family was faced with a [wrenching] decision. We sold our mansion and moved to America. That was my downfall. My brothers and sisters stayed behind in Pakistan with other family. My parents thought that the "land of opportunity" would allow for better education and work. It offered that and more.

I [often] compared myself to a ticking time bomb. I had the appetite and now I was exposed to richer foods, a food-obsessed society, and culture shock. Food was my savior, my hobby, my obsession. My father worked as a night auditor and my mother was forced to work for the first time. I was often alone. I had no parental supervision and felt extremely [lonely]. I found friends in my neighbors and food. I would easily eat a box of pizza, a gallon of ice cream, and the largest bag of Hot Cheetos. My red fingers—from the Cheetos—became my signature mark.

The weight gain was steady and surprising. My parents assumed that I wouldn't spiral out of control [because] I was just a kid and a previously thin one. They let me eat myself to sleep every night. I couldn't figure out why I was eating. In junior high school, my eating habits caught up with me. People started to tease and taunt me for my weight. That was an all-time low. My grades dropped, I ate more, and felt worse about myself. My parents noticed their mistake. It was not [simply] the hormone therapy; rather, it was the combination of the toxic environment, my depressed state, and my newfound home in America [where I was alone much of the time].

The Fat Pretty Girl

In ninth grade, my vibrant personality and humor made me approachable. I gained my confidence back, I felt good, and [I] found a place in life. Still, something was not right: at this point, it was easy for me to eat two foot-longs in one sitting. I was overweight and then obese before I [realized that] something had to be done.

In high school I had many friends, all of whom told me repeatedly how pretty my face was. I was the fat pretty girl. They loved my features, my big eyes, long brown hair, and clear skin. They didn't, however, like my fat. I used [their criticism] as motivation, and in tenth grade, I managed to lose 60 pounds. I had gained my life [and] confidence back. I loved my life and felt accepted. I exercised obsessively, about 8 hours in the pool over the weekend and 4 hours during the week. By eleventh grade, I was at my prime. In my yearbook, I was voted the most likely to become a model. I loved the attention. I was popular and associated my happiness with my thinness. [At that point I] was 5'9" and weighed 180 pounds.

After high school graduation and a long-term relationship ended, I spiraled [out of control] again. My eating habits became worse and I gained the weight back. [Now,] three years [later], I weigh more than ever before. I thought I had achieved a lot; I transferred to the University of California, earned a scholarship, and managed to get a 4.0 GPA. It was not enough. It is horrible to admit that, despite all my accomplishments, I have not been able to view myself as an accomplished person. I have constantly criticized myself for being overweight. I am 5'9" tall and I weigh 235 pounds. I am obese according to the BMI [34.7] and, unfortunately, I feel that way.

Physical Perfection at Last—through Photo-Editing

I have a sick obsession and it's called photo-editing. I constantly edit my photos in order to make myself feel better. I have photo-shopped nearly all my pictures to perfection. If there is a mark on my face, it's gone; a bulge on my arm—gone. The most shocking detail would be that I upload these pictures to my Facebook, where I have more than 700 friends, all people I know or have met. I don't show my body in my pictures because obviously I am not comfortable with it. I continue to lead this double life, and people continue to comment on my pictures, despite knowing that I am not like my pictures.

My fight for perfection has remained [a constant] in my life. I have always wanted to be accepted and loved [by] friends [and] family. Had my parents or I known that that hormonal therapy would haunt me my whole life, they would never have opted for it. I know that in the bottom of their hearts they hold themselves accountable. I don't blame anyone but myself for my weight issues, [though,] because at the end of the day it was me that was never good enough.

Sajeda: Rejiggering a Public Identity for 700 Friends

In Sajeda's story, we have one of the more extreme cases of alternate corporeal realities, one in which a young woman, yearning to recover her former identity as a fashion-model beauty, simply photo-shops her image to match her fantasy. Although deep down she identifies as a shameful fat person, the power of the prettified images, combined with her friends' silent complicity in accepting them, allow her to hold raggedly onto the myth that the image may be—or may sometime become—the reality.

Sajeda's essay provides rare insight into how a youngster's weight can so easily balloon out of control, without anyone so much as noticing. Like many immigrant parents, Sajeda's are forced to work, leaving their child home by herself for long stretches of time. Lonely after the trauma of splitting the family, and facing profound culture shock, she finds comfort in the rich junk food that is widely available in this country. Her narrative about the inappropriate hormone shots causing her to gain weight is a little puzzling. It is not clear what kind of hormone she was given or for how long, so it is difficult to evaluate the story's merit. Nevertheless, what's important is that this is how she and her parents narrate her weight problem—as a result of a bad medical decision whose effects they could not have anticipated. The overall picture is one of steady weight gain as a product of life events over which neither the young girl nor her parents had much control. Since emerging from childhood, the teenage Sajeda has been going through a pattern of weight cycling in which her weight rises with every stressful event but falls only with obsessive exercise, for which she has no time. Yet buying into the biomyth that weight is under individual control and the morality that heavy weight makes one a bad person, Sajeda accepts the blame for a character stain so ugly that it blots out all her other accomplishments. Sajeda's story provides a troubling illustration of how our biocitizen culture blames the victim, making the victim feel her shameful status is her own fault.

Not a Bloated Lump of Fat: Caroline as "Hourglass"

Caroline is a twenty-one-year-old Vietnamese American from a relatively well-off family in the Silicon Valley city of San Jose. In this bittersweet account, she documents how her well-meaning mother, by constantly upbraiding her about her weight, destroyed her self-esteem, and how a new friend has helped rebuild it by changing the story about her body.

One Big Dieting Cycle: My Life So Far

For as long as I can remember, I have been on a diet. It wasn't self-enforced, however; [rather] I was placed on the diet by my mother. This has been the case since I was at least 10, maybe even before that. Since I am 18 now, over a half of my life so far has been one big cycle to try to put me on a diet. Since I moved out [of the house to go to] college, whenever I do end up seeing her the reaction tends to be: "Oh, you look good." "Oh, you look hot." "I missed you. I love you. Your face is messed up." The general emphasis on my beauty and attractiveness is something I wish [would stop].

It might have started when I visited Vietnam when I was younger, and my aunts, uncles, and cousins my age chided me for being bigger and heavier [than most Vietnamese girls]. My childhood memories are littered with family members making fun of and talking about my weight, while my peers spoke nothing about it and reassured me that I wasn't a bloated lump of fat. [Facing a constant barrage of] comments such as: "You're so fat I wouldn't want to be seen with you," or "You're so fat I wouldn't walk down the street with you," I was [incredibly] insecure while I was growing up.

While my mother would tell me to dress to emphasize my girlish shape and figure, and at the same time tell me that I was morbidly obese, I had contradictory messages as to whether I should hide my body or show off the fatty assets I had. I ended up going through a phase of always wearing baggy and non-form-fitting clothes to hide my shape, my fat, and myself. I didn't want to be seen, I just wanted to be passed by. My self-esteem was pretty much shattered to the point where I am not quite sure how it got repaired. While my self-esteem still constantly fluctuates, it has gotten a lot better in the last two years.

Crucial Turning Points

It wasn't until I met my best friend during freshman year [in college] that I realized that my body was actually beautiful. I was never peeved about my mind, my mind was just fine: I was a writer and a thinker and I loved to critically analyze situations and ideas. When I met Valerie I learned a lot of things. One of the first things I learned and accepted about myself is that I do have a bigger body frame than a lot of other people. However, I have assets that many people wish for but don't have. In particular, I have the sought-after hourglass figure that seems to be highly attractive in many ways. It was probably this pivotal point that brought me to realize that I was in fact not an obese blob, but just an average teenager going through a [difficult] time of life.

[Another turning point in my understanding came during a difficult conversation with my mom], when I realized how she actually viewed me and my self-esteem. I was a junior in high school and we were having a rather decent night until she brought up the subject of my weight. I did not want to hear anything about it, so I [told her] that the constant belittling was bringing down my self-esteem. [Of all the unexpected reactions,] she actually laughed! Then she continued, saying, "Low self-esteem? How can you say you have low self-esteem when you are in a program that lets you take college and high school courses [at the same time]! How many of your friends can say that they do that?" It was at that time that I realized that she did not know what she was doing [i.e., how her comments on my weight affected me]. I resumed my blank stare and mumbled replies to her need to establish the fact that I needed to be on a diet until I was over and done with my weight "problem." I wasn't going to change to be the ideal doll that she wanted me to be, and she wasn't going to stop [berating me] until I looked better. She did lay off a bit after that day.

Now I am somewhere around 5'5" to 5'6" and weigh anywhere from 160 to 165 pounds [BMI of 26.6]. My measurements are around 42/35/42 and I am fine with that. Sure, there are moments of insecurity where I think I could lose a few pounds, but then I have other things I could be doing as well. I smile more often now, I dress with a mixture of more feminine and not, and I do as I please more or less. I love my parents, I love my mom dearly, but most importantly of all, I love myself. After all those years of thinking little of myself and thinking I was not going to be as beautiful as I should have been, I never would have imagined that I could [actually] love myself. But as cliched as it sounds, beauty does come from the inside. If you can't love yourself, how can anyone else love you?

Caroline: Rescued by a Friend

Caroline's account shows how emotionally insensitive relatives—outright biobullies in the home country and a concerned but clueless parent at home—can crush a young girl's sense of herself as a good, worthy human being by relentlessly stressing appearance as the measure of feminine value and berating the youngster for her weight and looks. Despite her strong positive identity as a writer and thinker, throughout her adolescence Caroline has considered herself a big disappointment because she was not going to be as beautiful as her mom had hoped she would be. She was, in short, a fat girl, and that identity seemed to override everything else.

Caroline's story to this point is fairly typical. What is unusual here is how a weight-savvy friend restored her shattered self-esteem by creating a compelling alternative narrative about what counts at beautiful. Whether the hourglass figure is indeed considered appealing is not the point; what is important is that this idea has captured Caroline's imagination and allowed her to shed the fat-girl identity. Although Caroline's emotional turnaround remains tentative, she is finally able to reject the view of herself as an "obese blob," giving her the emotional space to cultivate her many other talents and begin creating new identities around those.

Embracing the Fat Self

Not all very heavy young people feel compelled to excise "fat" from their identities. In some cases, they are able to reject the fat-is-bad notion of the dominant culture and tell a different story about themselves, one in which they are fat *and* like themselves. In claiming fat as a positive identity, they are casting aside the whole biocitizenship narrative about their lives—including, for better or perhaps for worse, its prescriptions for healthful change. Such cases are extremely rare. In the 245 accounts I gathered, only two young people claimed a positive fat identity. Here we meet one of them.

Fat Is Who I Am: Jonathan's Story, as Relayed by a Friend

Jonathan is a twenty-year-old Vietnamese American who grew up in a middle-class family in the San Gabriel Valley city of El Monte. Subject to intense parental pressure to lose weight, and trying but failing to do so, Jonathan defies everyone and claims fatness as fundamental to who he is.

In high school I met [my] friend Jonathan. It was my sophomore year and I was enrolled in woodshop class. Jonathan was in my class and sat next to me on the first day of school. We started to talk and in time became close friends. Jonathan was my age and he was really fat while I was really skinny. We used to hang out a lot during lunch break and between classes. He had a funny personality that went along great with the way he looked. He knew he was sort of fat, but to me it seemed like he didn't care. Jonathan would get picked on by some of the Mexicans in our school because he was overweight. It seemed like it didn't faze him. He was still the normal guy I knew, aside from the fact that there was almost always verbal abuse directed at him. A lot of students at the school liked him. He was known for being funny and doing stupid things during class.

One day I talked to him about how it feels [to be] treated badly and insulted all the time. Jonathan told me about how difficult it was for him to get a girl, since he is sort of fat. He wished he could turn all the fat he has into muscle so he could get a girl easily. He told me [the fat-abuse] gets really annoying, especially since he hears it at home as well. His parents were really strict and were always encouraging him to lose weight and exercise more. His parents thought that if he were thinner he would do better in school because no one would pick on him and no one would look at him with disgust. He told me he had been trying to work out more often and do more cardio, but there wasn't much result from it. Since there wasn't much result, he didn't really care anymore, and developed an attitude every time his parents mentioned his weight or something associated with it.

In another conversation, he told me that his parents had forced him to go on a diet. He had to run at least 5 miles a week and had to watch exactly what he ate. He started to look at the calories in the food he was eating. Before he was forced onto a diet, he was able to just live freely, never checking calories. Giving up all the ice cream, chips, junk food, candy, and other goodies was one of the hardest things he had had to do in his [entire] life.

After a month, Jonathan lost some weight and his parents were proud of him. He was also proud of himself, and celebrated by eating what he ate before the diet. After that, he began to gain a little more weight because his parents became less strict on him about his weight. [As a result,] he gained the weight back twice as fast as he had lost it. The parents were disappointed in him. [They] were afraid that being overweight would cause many types of sicknesses and would be unhealthy for him. [But Jonathan] gave up on the diet and didn't care anymore. He said there was nothing he could do. He wanted to stay at the weight he was at because it was pretty impossible for him to get really skinny like me.

Even though Jonathan was pressured into losing his weight, he did not succumb to it. After long thinking, he told me he was happy being overweight. All this time he was trying to be someone else. People were forcing him to be someone else that he wasn't. He wanted to be accepted for who he is and not what he would become by losing that weight. He told me he loved the way he was and didn't care if people didn't like him. I still talk to Jonathan every now and then. He tells me that people in college are more accepting of him and his weight isn't much of a big deal in his life now.

Fat and Loving It Now: Jonathan's Transformation

Jonathan presents a seemingly typical case of a boy whose parents were virtuous biocitizens, who forced him onto strict diet and exercise programs because of concerns about the social and health consequences of his excess weight. The diet not only led to greater weight gain, it deprived him of life's greatest pleasures. At that point, the typicality ends. Jonathan decided that the diet's failure meant that being fat was simply part of his identity, a part he fully embraced. This new understanding empowered him to declare that people needed to accept him for who he really is and stop asking him to be some other, skinnier kid. What enabled Jonathan to reject the dominant biomyths, which make heaviness bad and everyone able to achieve normal weight, seems to have been his secure place in a social world in which many people liked him for his funny persona—the kind, as we have seen, most often expected of large people. Being cherished by a core of close friends seems to have allowed this young man to create a fat-positive identity strong enough to resist the pressure of all the biocitizens in his world. Such stories are very rare indeed.

How Heavy Kids Become Fat Persons

These ethnographies illuminate a social world of fatness that, to heavy children, must seem heartless and hellish. That world left a grievous mark on their selves and lives.

Growing Up Heavy in a World Full of Weight-Obsessed Biocitizens

While all the youngsters I worked with inhabited worlds full of fat-talk, the fat-talk targeted at really large kids such as these is virtually all abusive, aimed at shaming them into losing weight. These six young people, who were heavy from a young age, grew up with parents who fully embraced the biocitizenship narrative that fat kids all become unhealthy, unhappy adults and that, as parents, they are responsible for intervening early and firmly. Carriers of the dominant biomyths, their parents were the first and most important influences on their growing understanding of themselves as "fat and bad." Every one of these youngsters described emotionally disconnected parents who acted as harsh biocops, berating them for being too heavy, warning them of the social and bodily costs of heaviness, and in some cases forcing them to undertake rigorous diet and exercise programs. When their child failed to lose weight, rather than consider the possibility that genetic or other unchangeable forces might be keeping their kids large, desperate parents sometimes turned to hard persuasive tactics, telling frightening stories—even acting out a fat-induced heart attack—in an effort to scare their youngsters into taking action. More distant relatives only intensified the shaming with comments, such as those of Jessica's kin, who "wouldn't be seen walking down the street with her." In all these families, weight was deemed a critical part of the young girl's or boy's identity, and all relatives were culturally authorized to publicly (and, of course, privately) criticize the child's body.

At school, close friends often provided crucial emotional support, but they could not protect their fat friends from the verbal assaults of the mean kids. These fat youngsters faced biobullying from a multitude of cruel peers, from the "Mexican" boys who taunted Jonathan to the mean-girl clique of "popular Asian and white girls" who took pleasure in tormenting the big-chested Kim. With the exception of Jonathan, all were shut out of the popular social group because of their weight.

The wider culture these kids inhabited reinforced the message that being fat is abnormal and even freakish, and that fat kids must change themselves if they are to be accepted. Jessica and Mai Ly describe the normalizing—and exclusionary—role of contemporary fashion. Jessica's account of Wii Fit, one of the popular weight-loss games that have proliferated in recent years, shows how such media end up not helping people lose weight but reinforcing their identity as a "fat person who needs to be reformed." These are just two of the countless cultural forces that reinforce the dominant message about fat.

Developing a Fat Personhood

Subject to this unrelenting fat-abuse from key members of their social world, all six young people started identifying as a fat person at a young age. Slowly but surely, fat person became the predominant identity. Based on these and other essays, in SoCal, at least, a fat person appears to have four identifying characteristics. First, he or she sees him or herself as "bad": biologically flawed, socially unacceptable, morally irresponsible or unworthy, and/or aesthetically unappealing ("ugly"). Despite her academic accomplishments, for example, Sajeda felt like a failure because of her weight. Mai Ly confessed that she despised her body and self so much that she wished she could take on the identity of her thinner friends.

Second, the fat person engages in the mandated bodily practices—dieting and exercising—in an effort to lose that degrading weight. In most cases, the fat child was forced onto those weight-loss programs by parents, often in early childhood. Whether because the restrictions were too oner-ous for the young child, the child's growing body refused to cooperate, or the child was simply biologically programmed to be heavy, the diets invari-ably failed. Two of the young people gained back *more* weight than they had lost on the diet, ending up feeling like even greater failures than ever. And the more they pursued the impossible quest, and the more they failed, the more central fatness became to their identities.

A third attribute, common to all six young people, is social withdrawal. Faced with incessant ridicule and social rejection, the fat person retreats socially to avoid people's rude and insensitive judgment. Jessica and Caro-line hid their "disgusting" bodies in baggy clothing; Jessica and Mai Ly stopped shopping for clothes with their friends; Mai Ly ate in private; Kim physically withdrew from her family. For these kids, social isolation was preferable to constant derision and ostracism. Fourth and finally, taking on the despised "fat" identity invariably brought emotional suffering, in-cluding depression, low self-esteem, and pervasive insecurities about the person's place in the world.

Although all six became self-identified "fat youngsters," as they emerged from childhood into late adolescence and early adulthood, their identities began to slightly diverge. Although some continued to see themselves as fat and bad (Kim and Jessica), others sought to rework their public identity (Mai Ly, Sajeda, and Caroline), while another managed to reject the fat identity altogether (Jonathan). Why did some avoid (or partially avoid) this despised identity while the others continued to suffer from it? The most dramatic escape from fathood was Jonathan's, and for him his gender was crucial. While a boy can be socially accepted as "fat and funny," for a girl fat is always discrediting, regardless of other appealing attributes she may have. Because weight is less central to a boy's identity, Jonathan was able to love himself as he was. Among the girls, the most positive route taken was to create a substitute identity to claim in public. The social support of peers seems to have been crucial in the ability to do that. The two young women who were still stuck in fat personhood (Kim and Jessica) lacked the active social support of friends. Unable to defend themselves or con-front their abusers, they saw no way out of their plight. Two who cobbled together more positive public identities (Caroline and Sajeda) did so with the creative input of close girlfriends. The third (Mai Ly) also reported that her friends were "really supportive" and did not consider her fat.

Producing Thin, Fit Biocitizens?

Finally, did the biobullying and social-marginalizing tactics transform these heavy youngsters into thin, fit biocitizens? The answer is no. Even though all six young people tried following the standard bioscript, all failed to lose weight and keep it off. Not only didn't they become virtuous biocitizens, the high-pressure approach used by their families and classmates was counterproductive, turning the majority of them (all but Kim and Jessica) into bad ("irresponsible") biocitizens who simply gave up on the diet and exercise program.

How could the biocitizen program produce an effect just the opposite of the one intended? In its extreme version, the narrative tells heavy youngsters that they are very bad people indeed. When the bioabuse starts early, is protracted, and comes from many sources, it can be so damaging as to crush their sense of themselves as good, worthy people. To recover a positive sense of self—a need more urgent even than losing weight or gaining parental approval—young people either developed alternative identities that allowed them to continue their prior routine and avoid dieting, or they decided that their "real self" is in fact a fat self and that the enforced dieting was an effort by others to eliminate the "real them." The biocitizen program was counterproductive because it paid no attention to the most fundamental emotional needs of its main targets.

It is not just technically obese people who take on fat identities. Next, we will see that those who are only overweight on the BMI scale also come to see themselves as "fat."

4

"Overweight"

I know that I need to lose weight. [What] is telling me this is the number
on the scale, where I stand with BMI, and the size label on the clothing
that I buy: 2, 4, 6, 8, 10, and 0. Why are we constantly being forced to gauge
ourselves to [size] 0? The math is simple; if you're a size 8 you are 8 sizes
bigger than 0. I can [also] be told that I'm underweight, normal, overweight,
[or] obese, and just in case I forget there's a simple chart that will tell me
where I stand. So out of four different weight categories, I have a three out of
four chance of not being normal, and who doesn't want to be normal, right?
I personally feel normal and I seem normal, but I am definitely not normal
according to [the] BMI. Overall my 8 is too far from 0 and my height and
weight fall within the not-normal, so I definitely need to lose weight.

PIA, FROM HER ESSAY "I KNOW THAT I NEED TO LOSE WEIGHT" [SC 22]

We turn now to the second target of the campaign, the "overweight," who
have BMIs in the 25–29.9 range. (A 5′6″ person weighing 155 to 185 pounds
is "overweight.") This category includes a large portion of the general
public: one-third of adults and one-sixth of children and teens.[1] Among
the young adults I worked with, perhaps 30–35 percent fell in the "overweight" category.[2] How is the war on fat affecting these people?

Conventional wisdom holds that the anti-obesity campaign is helpfully
responding to the rise in the numbers of such hefty Americans by getting
them to adopt healthier behaviors that enable them to lose weight, improving their health and social life. The essays of overweight Californians suggest that the commonsense view may have things backward. Remember
the difference between being technically obese according to the BMI scale
and being a self-identified fat subject. What the auto-ethnographies suggest is that the war on fat is itself *producing* a large and growing number of
"abnormal" persons by turning young people who are only slightly overweight on the BMI chart into self-identified fat subjects. In other words,

the war on fat is creating a new kind of fat problem by expanding the number of weight-obsessed, self-identified fat subjects, who may appear normal in size but who suffer the emotional, social, and other costs associated with being labeled fat in our society. Pia's plaintive words, which open this chapter, illustrate this dynamic perfectly.

An increase in self-identified fat persons is cause for concern because of the problem of *iatrogenic injury*, harm caused by medical labeling or interventions. Although these self-identified fat subjects are not technically obese, fatness is so stigmatizing in our society that those who think of themselves as fat will suffer distress and will go to any length to get rid of the fatness. In their desperate efforts to lower their weights, these overweight fat subjects may end up endangering their emotional, mental, and in some cases even physical health.

It's easy to understand how extremely heavy young people who are subject to abusive fat-talk might come to see themselves as fat. But how could the merely overweight also start thinking and acting like fat subjects? The essays I gathered reveal two main pathways to fat personhood. Both are rooted in the normal workings of our biocitizenship society. In the first pathway, what precipitates the change in self-perception is an increase in weight teasing, abuse, and other sorts of fat-talk directed at the chunky person. In this *fat-talk pathway*, the process of acquiring a fat identity generally unfolds in three steps. A fat subject is born when an above-average-weight young person, often in late grade school or middle school, becomes subject to a growing din of derogatory fat-talk telling him or her that his or her weight is excessive and that weight is the identity that matters most to social acceptance. In the second step, his or her growing self-consciousness about weight gradually develops into a weight obsession as efforts to lose weight fail. Third, as struggles with weight come to dominate his or her life, he or she gradually adopts a fat selfhood and the constellation of emotions, social behaviors, and bodily practices that go with it.

In the second pathway, a *diagnostic pathway*, a diagnosis of "overweight and unhealthy" by a medical professional sparks the change in identity. Instead of a gradual, phased process, the change of identity tends to be instantaneous when the doctor delivers the bad news, and the accompanying parent, now worried about the child's health, immediately rearranges the child's environment and diet and exercise routines to facilitate treatment.

It takes little time for the youngster to pick up the message that there is something terribly wrong with him or her that urgently needs to be made right. In this moment, a new fat person is born.

In this chapter, I explore these dynamics, posing a series of questions similar to those I asked about the obese cases. First, what kind of social and conversational worlds do overweight young people inhabit? How do the two kinds of fat-talk work to shape self-making? Second, what kind of inner life do overweight young people experience? Do all of them become fat subjects, or do some resist that identity, and, if so, why? Finally, what are the larger consequences of becoming a fat subject for young people's health and lives? Does their health get better, as the promoters of the war on fat hope, or is the answer more complicated?

In the chapter's first section, we meet two young people who, though only slightly overweight, experience so much demeaning fat-talk that they come to feel and act like fat people. In the second section, we meet two people who are also subject to degrading fat-talk but who struggle hard to resist internalizing the fat identity that is thrust on them. In the last section, we explore the diagnostic pathway to fat personhood. We meet three youngsters, all strong, healthy athletes, who were diagnosed as "overweight and unhealthy" by medical professionals who considered only their BMI scores, neglecting the muscular composition of their bodies and the overall health of their patients. In their stories, we will see how the limitations of the BMI can create real havoc in people's lives.

From Carefree Childhood to Burdened Adulthood: Embracing (or Resisting) Fat Personhood

We begin with two slightly overweight young women who, targeted by fat-talk their whole young lives, start to see themselves as fat persons and develop all the characteristics that typically go with that identity. The first, April, is subject primarily to pedagogical fat-talk; the second, Tiffany, is the target of abusive fat-talk. So intolerable is the fat-person identity that, in their zeal to shed it, both take drastic measures which endanger their health. While April and Tiffany internalize the fat-person identity, our third writer, Binh, tries valiantly to resist that identity and hold onto other definitions of who he is.

Weight—a Ghost Haunting Me My Entire Life: April's Story

April is a twenty-year-old African American from a family of lower-middle-class background who grew up in the San Fernando Valley of Los Angeles. In her auto-ethnography, she documents a series of life-changing incidents through which she gradually picked up and internalized society's biopedagogical message that, for girls and women, a thin body is the ultimate source of happiness and sexual power.

Biobullies in School

Weight has affected me [since] I was in elementary school. I realized at the time that relationships between the little boys and the little girls were a trend. When I saw that all my friends had "crushes" and "boyfriends," I almost felt obligated to get a little boy to like me—but was never successful. That's when I learned that body image played a large [role] in attracting the opposite sex.

The two most popular girls in school were one of my best friends and my cousin. My best friend was extremely slender and athletic; she was a White girl with long brown hair, and the boys simply adored her nature. My cousin, although chubbier than my friend and Black, experienced early puberty and sported a B-sized chest and curvy hips—rather large for a 9-year-old—and the boys couldn't keep their eyes off her. Where was I in this system of body image, though? I was chubby and flat-chested, with no sensual appeal and a tomboy dressing style—I was nowhere but at the very bottom. Realizing this, I became incredibly depressed and often found myself feeling alone. Despite this, I didn't diet in the beginning. I didn't know what dieting was or that there was a way to not be "ugly." I thought I was simply born that way. However, I did know that chubbiness and no breasts were considered ugly, and slim and having breasts were beautiful. Society's standard punched me in the face, and it hurt.

Growing up and going to middle school, I began to learn more about dieting. My best friend at the time was very big, and I remember her always talking about avoiding certain foods [because] she wanted to lose weight. I always thought she was beautiful; she had large breasts, light skin, beautiful hazel eyes, and a funny personality. However, that image was destroyed when a boy called her a "fat, ugly piece of shit" right in front of me. My friend ran away in tears. It was the first time I realized that weight was a huge issue, even for curvaceous girls.

The Warnings of a Concerned Brother

It wasn't long after that that I started getting the critiques from my family. While my mother [and] father never spoke about my weight, my brother did. He constantly told me that I ate too much and that I was going to be a fat girl and that men would throw things at me. I became scared and started dieting. My dieting consisted of starving myself. I would eat a bowl of cereal at 7:00 a.m., then refuse to eat again until I got home about 4:00 p.m. and had dinner. I continued to do this every day and eventually I started to get pounding food headaches [that made me cry] because the pain hurt so much. When dinner came around, I would often binge on two large plates because I was so hungry. As a result, my metabolism dropped and I actually ended up gaining weight.

Ultimately, though, I felt fat. I remember looking in the mirror, gripping the excess fat on my stomach in my hands and imagining ripping it from my body. I imagined blowing all the fat from my nose into a trash can and immediately becoming slender and beautiful. All these fantasies haunted me like a ghost, and my confidence continued to drop as the years drifted into high school.

In high school I hit puberty when I was 14 and started to develop breasts and curves. I entered a dance class and became very active. I dropped from 140 at 5'3" to 130. As if my new body [had] triggered a reaction, boys started asking me out. I never felt more accepted in life than I did at that moment. My pride grew, but I still felt fat. I continued to diet and dance, dropping to 120 pounds at 5'4" by the time I was 15.

A Vacation I Will Never Forget

My family and I went to Jamaica that summer, and there I went through an experience I will never forget. During a boat cruise, one of the Jamaican hosts took me under deck and sexually assaulted me by forcing me to touch his privates. He was supposed to be giving me a foot massage. It was a traumatizing experience that I ended up crying to my brother about. He told me that "when you're pretty, a lot of guys are going to come on to you like that and you're going to have to deal with much bigger things later." While I didn't particularly enjoy being abused, I learned that a beautiful body really did have power over men. In addition, the reaction from my parents—who joked about the massage being my first experience as a woman—told me that seducing men was good, and the only way to do that was to be beautiful. And to be beautiful was to be thin.

High school provided a much more violent experience. One of my best friends at the time started to become jealous that I was getting attention and popularity in the dance team. So she started to spread rumors. I was called weird, dyke, and White all at once by people who were once my friends. This caused serious depression and I began to turn to food for comfort. I went from 120 to 135 and fluctuated up to 140 pounds. I was lonely and felt more fat than ever. I often told myself that I would kill myself if I [exceeded] 140, and starved myself every time I got close.

From Self-Starvation to Binging and Purging:
Weight Loss at Any Cost

When I graduated from high school food became a pleasure. Since I no longer danced, I gained more weight—I was 146–150 by the time I [left for college]. During freshman year, adjusting to a new lifestyle, I [rose to] 156 pounds by winter quarter—I was fat [BMI 26.8, hardly obese]. At the end of winter quarter, I began to starve myself to lose the weight. I ate once a day at 5:00 p.m. for dinner, usually about a 300-calorie meal. I became very weak, sleeping most of the time when I made it home from school so I would not have to think about the hunger. On the fourth day I didn't eat anything. That night the ambulance was called when I fainted in Starbuck's, where I had attempted to get food when I realized I was dizzy and on the verge of it. (I had fainted several times in high school from lack of eating.) My blood sugar was at a dangerously low level and it took about 30 minutes to revitalize it. I can't quite understand why I did it though. I think [perhaps] because my roommates were always so skinny and fit—seeing their perfect bodies tormented me. I had learned that everyone met their sweethearts in college, and wondered why no one was interested in me. I blamed my weight.

Today, I still consider weight [control] a constant part of my routine. Now I stand at about 140 pounds but am still not satisfied with my weight. I wake up every morning and the first thing I do is look at the size of my stomach. Unfortunately, I fear that I may have an eating disorder developing—[some] mixture of starving/binging/purging. Not but 2 or 3 weeks ago, I binged on trail mix and was so disgusted with myself that I purged it out—then I did the same with a piece of cake later. Though [I know] it's impossible to be perfect, I still strive to be more beautiful than I am. Everything in my life has told me that power and happiness come from beauty, and now I feel as if I am conditioned to pursue it. Weight has become a ghost that doesn't leave me no matter what I do. It has haunted me throughout my life.

April: From Carefree Tomboy to Weight-Obsessed Fat Subject

Throughout her young life, April has heard a steady stream of pedagogical fat-talk that has taught her the essentials of femininity. Her detailed chronological exposition allows us to track how specific biopedagogical messages picked up at particular times resulted in the development of different facets of the fat-person identity. Throughout all these experiences, April has internalized the dominant biocitizenship discourse according to which a good body means a good self. Between grade school and college, this once-carefree tomboy has become a fat subject, one who sees herself as fat, believes that fat people can lose weight, anxiously exercises and diets in a never-ending quest for the "perfect" slim body, and berates herself for always failing to achieve her impossible goal. All this, even though at her heaviest April was no more than mildly overweight on the BMI scale.

By young adulthood, what began as a weight consciousness has become a weight obsession. Now a college sophomore surrounded by mostly thin co-eds, April has created a weight-centric narrative about her life in which her problems are caused by her heaviness. For April, as for many large-bodied people in the upscale, thin-worshipping areas of SoCal, the feeling of being "too big" and "out of place" amounts to a kind of daily torment. The health implications of this growing weight obsession bear noting. As a child, following the script she had learned, April put herself on a diet. Ignorant of the basics of nutrition, however, she unwittingly began a lifelong pattern of starvation dieting that not only posed severe risks to her health but worked to lower her metabolism, making it harder to lose weight in the future. Today she struggles with her weight constantly, engaging in eating practices so anorexic- and bulimic-like they pose dangers to her health. Seemingly trapped in the dominant discourse, for April, the cultural war on fat seems to have caused the very problems it is supposed to eliminate: heavy weight and poor health.

"We Don't Like Ugly Asian Girls": Tiffany's Hidden Struggle

Tiffany is a twenty-two-year-old Chinese American from a middle-class family in Fountain Valley, where the municipal motto is, ironically, "a nice place to live." Unlike April, who experienced the cultural commentary about the body as an informative biopedagogy she must adhere to in order to fit in, Tiffany is the victim of biobullying so vicious it leaves her traumatized, with no idea of how she might gain social acceptance, let alone happiness or power.

Mean Girls on the Attack

I come from a large Chinese family of six, with one older sister, one younger sister, and one younger brother. [As a young child], weight and body image were not important to me. It wasn't until I transferred to a public school that the notion of body image began to affect me.

I remember in fifth grade, I was always bullied by the other students and I was never sure why. One day, while I was waiting in line to get into class, I finally confronted two of the girls who were picking on me. When I asked them why they were being so mean to me, they responded, "Well, we don't like ugly Asian girls with your *hair* and ugly *face*. So you can't be our friend. No one likes you." I was devastated by their words. However, it got worse. I asked why they liked this other girl who had the same hair as I did and they responded, "She's cute, and you are *fat and ugly*." I still remember those words; they stuck with me, always in the back of my mind. I never told my mom about what happened; neither did I share this with my sister. I was scared they would laugh at me or even agree with what those girls said. Out of [my entire] elementary school [experience], I remember this incident best.

Going on into middle school, I remember I went on a diet. At that time I did not know what calories were. All I wanted was to not be fat like those girls accused me of in elementary school. My diet was simple. Since I am Chinese, I would eat rice every evening. So I measured [what] I ate by only having one bowl of rice. I followed that diet for a year. I remember running into [former] school teachers who would comment, "Wow, you have lost a lot of weight! You look so much better." That simple phrase just boosted my confidence. I was so happy that people were noticing that I was losing weight.

Middle school went by much better than elementary school for me. I was not picked on by people, and no one said anything negative about my body image. If I commented on my image, my friends would always coo, [saying] "Nooooo! You are so pretty and not fat at all." They would always be reassuring me that I looked fine. Things changed when I entered high school.

Betrayed by a "Best Friend"

Everything ran well in my freshman year until, midway through, my "best friend" at the time came up to me and said she had something important to say. What she had to say was that all throughout middle school, one girl whom I considered a "best friend" was just using me, and thought I was a "fat and ugly bitch." That one little comment brought back all the memories of my elementary school days. It sucked, honestly, hearing that being said about me. It really hurt. That one little statement made it really hard to not look at myself and wonder, "Am I really that ugly? Do I look that fat? What is everyone else thinking right now?" I became very paranoid from then on. I never wore anything tight, I hated clothes that showed the stomach, and I was afraid of the beach. I was so scared of being judged, I was terrified of other people's opinion.

It was hard trying to make it through high school. I really began to struggle with my image. It wasn't always about my weight; it was how people saw me. I was scared to be ostracized like I was in elementary school. I would try to wear clothes that never showed a stomach "pooch" and I would always suck in my stomach. Then at lunch I would not get anything to eat. I would only drink water so I could avoid that after-lunch stomach bulge.

Accusing Eyes All Around

I remember the doctors. I hated to go. My weight wasn't bad, much of it [was due to] the muscle mass I had acquired in my arms from all the conduct-ing [in the marching band]. However, my doctors would always look at my weight and say, "Your weight is creeping up, but you are OK still. Just keep ex-ercising." In the last three years it's gotten worse. This year when I went for my annual check-up, my doctor specifically told me, "That one to two pounds may not look like much, but it all adds up. Watch your weight, exercise every day, and watch what you eat." She never said I was fat, but she implied it, which, I felt, was worse. This is when everything got worse everywhere. After this incident, I felt my struggles really escalated. Before I would worry on oc-casion; now I felt like there were accusing eyes around me saying, "You are fat. No one likes fat."

The worst part of this was when those accusations came from home. My mother tried to boost my confidence and tell me that I was still young and anything can happen. It was my little brother and father who really made everything seem like a reality. At the dinner table, my little brother would always chant, "You are fat and ugly. No boy will want you." Before I would just take this as a jest and brush it off. My mother would always scold him and my father wouldn't say a word. Only recently, in the past few months, has it all picked up in pace. Now when my little brother points at me and screams "you're FAT!!," my father says, "He's not wrong." That is crushing. When I think about it, and as I'm typing, I'm trying my best not to cry. It re-ally hurts and it makes me wonder if that is how everyone perceives me. Am I really that fat? Am I that unappealing? Is that why I'm so lonely and have barely any friends?

I always thought that family was supposed to be there for you and to sup-port each other. All my life, I've believed in my father, looked up to him, and trusted him, and then he says something like that to me. I don't know how to react to his statements. I've tried to talk to my father about what he said, but he doesn't listen, claiming it's a joke. To me, when someone says something repeatedly, it becomes a truth for them and eventually they will believe what they are saying.

I don't think they realize there is a consequence to their words. I'm now a vegetarian and I tell people it's because I love animals. But to be completely honest, it's because of what they have said. Being a vegetarian means I eat much less, feel full much easier, and look healthy while I try to battle with my body image. I don't ever want to become anorexic, nor do I want to be stick thin, but it seems like I'm following [a well-worn path to] becoming an anorexic. It scares me, because all I want is for the name-calling and the fat comments to go away. I'm just desperate for those comments to disappear, and the only way, it seems, to become unfat is to lose all the weight no matter [the risk to my health].

Tiffany: Biobullying and a Crushed Sense of Self

In this disturbing account, Tiffany is the victim of biobullying so vicious it simply crushes her sense of herself as a good, socially worthy person, leaving her vulnerable to others' judgments. Moving chronologically, Tiffany's essay tracks a series of incidents in which significant people in her life have called her "fat and ugly" in deliberately attacking, hurtful ways. What stands out here is the cumulative nature of the abuse and social ostracism. With every additional incident, she grows more traumatized and paranoid about being judged, eventually slipping into a mind-set in which others' remarks determine her reality. From the very first assault, Tiffany is afraid to tell even close family members about it. This leaves her alone with her horrible fears, which then grow and fester. When her brother and father take up the verbal abuse, her world falls apart. In the absence of supportive body comments from anyone (except her mom), these verbal assaults have worn away Tiffany's self-esteem to the point that she now deeply believes the weight-centric narrative people have imposed on her— that it is her "ugly fat body" that explains why she has so few friends (if indeed she does). Although Tiffany's weight falls far below obese levels, in her desperation to make the comments stop, she embarks on an anorexic-level weight-loss program. Once again, societal efforts to reform the overweight have backfired. Tiffany has lost her excess weight, but only at costs to her health that one hopes will be short-lived.

All They Can See Is My Fat: Binh's Story

Binh is a twenty-two-year-old Vietnamese American from a middle-class family in the Silicon Valley city of San Jose. In his essay, Binh charts a long history of fat abuse and encounters with less-than-helpful purveyors of biopedagogical advice. Yet unlike April and Tiffany, who internalize the dominant message about weight and selfhood, Binh sloughs it off, telling a different story about his life.

Mocked in Middle School

During middle school, I was what a person would call "fat" or "chubby." A combination of my overweightness and a penguin-like wobble in my walk resulted in mockery by my peers as well as members of my family. My brother and his friends would often walk up to me and call me "fat boy," and tease me endlessly. My mother would hug me and joke, saying "oh, wow, my arms can't reach around you; I can't hug you all the way." It made me sad because I knew I wasn't bothering anyone, but at the same time [I] did not speak out against everyone's criticisms and jokes.

The only one who tried to protect my feelings was my Aunt [Hue]. On Wednesday and Thursday afternoons, when she would drive me to my tutoring lessons I would ask her, "Auntie, am I fat?" She would always reply in a matter-of-fact tone, "No, honey, not at all," like I had nothing to worry about. I was always grateful to her because she was the only one who didn't make me feel like crap, and [she] picked up on how everyone's comments made me feel. Of course a part of me knew I was overweight at the time, but she was the one who saw how bad it made me feel just being poked and prodded when all I did was sit in a room.

At thirteen years of age, during my period of puberty, I saw that I had gotten taller and my clothes fit better. Everyone was looking at me differently. I was getting more compliments, and girls were actually, *actually* attracted to me as well as talking to me. This brought me joy, but my mentality and fear of looking fat stayed with me. I would often ask my friends: "Do I look fat?" It was my worst fear, to return to that state where I wasn't like everyone else, where just by looking different I was to be ostracized and mocked. During my high school career, I spoke with my gym teacher, and asked her what I could do to lose weight. She laughed, looking at me and told me I had nothing to worry about. I assured her that if I were to take my shirt off right then and there she would think otherwise, but of course, out of fear of being looked down upon because of my large belly, I did not. After taking her suggestions to heart, I would find some increments of time during the week to do some form of physical activity, such as go on long walks or run on the treadmill, in order to stay away from looking fat. Unfortunately, I felt like I could never swim without my shirt; I had to hide what made me different.

The Freshman Fifteen: My Worst Fear Comes True

Slowly [but surely], the mentality and fear [receded] in my mind. Before coming home from my first year of college, I gained the [infamous] "Freshman Fifteen." It was not my fault I had to sit on my butt every day to study and all there was to eat was fast food. I could not find time to go to the gym either, due to my struggles to stay afloat in the competitive sea that is the School of Biological Sciences. People from home would often come up to me, poke at my stomach, and tell me how fat I had gotten. My gain in weight was all they could see, not their old friend Binh who [had] treated them so nicely before college, but just some new random fatass coming home from college. The news spread, and I even received comments on pictures on my Facebook, stating how huge I had gotten.

Often when I am depressed or stressed, I find myself eating sweet and junky food because I seek some pleasantness or satisfaction. I felt that I could eat what I wanted because I was upset and it was okay because it was all for making me feel better, but unfortunately that was not the outcome. The outcome was simply more weight gain and, in turn, more stares and criticism by those close to me. I realized that was not the way to go about bringing control back to my life.

My mother took my brother and me to see a doctor just for a check-up. I was already afraid the doctor would measure my weight, and he did so as he is required to in a normal check-up. He told my mother that according to the BMI, I was considered overweight and was just over the borderline of satisfactory and overweight. My mother had not thought so of me until she heard this from the doctor, and since then she has taken every [opportunity] to show her disappointment in me and to remind me to exercise and lose weight.

Intimidation and Deviance: Biocops in the College Dorm

Currently I am living with four other guys who all happen to be some kind of athlete. They always talk about how hard they work out or how much fun they have playing a sport. Unfortunately I don't share their passion. Naturally, I try to fit in by working out at least once in a while to appease them (and make myself feel healthier). They always encourage me to go swim, play basketball, or bike ride with them, but at the same time they criticize what I eat.

I mostly eat food my mother buys and cooks for me and, being Vietnamese, our food is less than what most health fanatics would call healthy. One of my roommates mentioned that in order to lose weight I would need to throw out a lot of the food my mother cooked for me. I refused to do that. Who are they to tell me to throw away the [only] kind of food [my mother] knows how to make? Living with these guys, I often feel like I have to eat in seclusion when they are around, or if they're coming into the kitchen I immediately need to hide the food I am about to eat because I know they like to compare my habits to theirs behind my back. They often ask me why I don't find the time to exercise. I reply because of my busy schedule, but when I do have time I like to spend it relaxing and doing nothing. They often tell me that my way of thinking is weak and all I come up with are excuses.

A Stealth Attack on Christmas Day

On the morning of Christmas Day last year, I woke up to find that my family and relatives had all gathered in the kitchen. Groggily yet happily, I walked into the room and greeted everyone. From across the room, I received a friendly smile from my uncle's father-in-law. Naturally, I smiled back, [never guessing] what he was going to say. The old man smiled at me all warmly, and then yelled out to me: "You're fat.!" My smiling ceased. I looked at him for five of what were probably the longest seconds in my entire life. My eyes turned to my uncle, who was looking at me already, and laughing wholeheartedly at what his father-in-law had said. Everyone heard it and laughed. My aunt who had tried to protect me all those years ago [now] said with a big smile, "You probably shouldn't eat so much junk, Binh, heheh." I felt that it was the most embarrassing moment of my entire life because it was Christmas morning, and I didn't even know the old man that well. I was also very upset because my damn relatives just let me take it.

After that I didn't even eat, I just stayed up in my room, except to go on a walk with my uncle and his wife. We walked for a good thirty minutes or so, and he asked me if I was tired. I replied, "[Do you say that] because I'm fat?" "Well, no," [he replied,] "not at all, but clearly you are. I think you need to lose some weight too." [My comment] was very vicious but I think he got the message. No matter what anyone in our family said, he told me, it wasn't meant to hurt me. I didn't agree. If they know that saying such things does hurt me—and they can tell it does—why do they continue? All of that just makes me feel like that is all everyone sees and that's all I am. No one in my family cared that I had worked so hard in college, or that I was a big brother figure to their kids, or that I was one of the most, if not the most, responsible and loyal kids in the family. All I was and still am in their eyes is "the fat one of the family."

Binh: Resisting the Fat-Boy Label

Binh lives in a world of virtuous biocitizens, all of whom tell the same story: that he is overweight and bad, it's his fault, and he's responsible for changing it. Unlike April and Tiffany, who internalize the fat-girl message, Binh rejects the fat-boy identity. What is fascinating is how, in the process of defending himself from this succession of attacks on his worthiness, Binh slowly stitches together the pieces of an alternative account of his life in which he does not deserve the condemnation and he has socially worthy identities outside of his weight. In childhood, he claims that he does not deserve the abuse because he can't help that he looks different and he did nothing to hurt anyone. In college, rather than accepting his roommates' account of his personal failures, Binh insists that it is not his fault—he has to study all the time, he deserves comfort food once in a while, he does not enjoy exercise—and that he doesn't deserve the abuse. Also noteworthy is how, in his constant search for support for his counternarrative, Binh seems to remember every incident in which someone protected him emotionally, affirming that he was a good person and "not fat at all." Despite the relentless message that he is a bad person for failing to lose weight, by holding fast to this counter-story Binh is able to resist the fat-person identity. In the end, Binh neither accepts personal responsibility for his heavy weight, as a good fat person would, nor sees himself as abject, either morally or physically. Nor does he take up the corporeal practices of the fat subject that everyone presses on him, constant dieting and exercise.

The differing response appears clearly related to gender. For girls like Tiffany and April, identity and self-worth are closely tied to appearance. Socialized to rely on external acceptance to inform their identity, girls are more vulnerable to others' opinions. For boys, identity and self-worth are measured more in terms of abilities. Protected from fat selfhood by the culture of masculinity, Binh holds onto the notion of himself as a good person with other, noncorporeal identities—a kind cousin, a good student. His essay relates his profound sadness and bafflement at a world in which everyone looks at him and sees not his fine qualities but only his excess weight.

A Flawed Diagnosis and a Spoiled Identity

In the narratives presented so far, young people became fat persons in response to a growing chorus of biting fat-talk telling them they are huge, ugly, and disgusting. The process was usually slow and ragged, unfolding over several years and multiple encounters with mean kids, thoughtless relatives, and concerned biocitizen parents and physicians. People can also become fat persons through diagnosis by a doctor who informs them for the first time that their BMI score places them in the category of over-weight and unhealthy. This diagnosis produces an instantaneous—and traumatic—change in their sense of self, from healthy and normal to un-healthy, abnormal, and in need of remediation. With this new under-standing of themselves as unhealthily big, these kids begin to develop the characteristics of a fat person. In this section, we meet three youngsters—Alexis, Annemarie, and Ryan—who developed fat identities through medical labeling of this sort. What is troubling about their stories is that they were all very healthy, strapping athletes. They felt healthy and fit, but the doctor said they were unhealthy and fat.

"Approaching the Red Zone"—a Spoiled Identity for Life: Alexis's Story

Alexis is a Caucasian girl raised in a well-to-do family in the upscale coastal town of Santa Barbara. Her essay brings out the confused and distressed subjectivity of a young girl who at the age of five was diagnosed as border-line overweight. Although the medical label turned out to be a poor index and even poorer predictor of Alexis's actual health and fitness, the labels "too big" and "unhealthy," attached to her at so tender an age, infected her deepest sense of self.

A Life-Altering Moment

It all began fifteen years ago at my annual check-up. I was an active and healthy five-year-old girl living what I believed was a healthy lifestyle. My family was very healthy and active: my sister danced and my mom and dad were both marathon runners. I had recently joined the Santa Barbara Swim Club and was attending daily swim practice [and competing in] swim meets every two weeks. [That day, as] I sat in the doctor's office listening to her run through a list of things to check up on, I remember her pausing at my weight. Her eyes stopped [moving down the list] and she pulled out a [multi-colored] chart, on which she measured something with her fingers, point-ing it out to my mom. [Turning to me,] she explained that I was nearing the "red zone," something that a few minutes earlier had meant nothing to me.

She [proceeded to] explain that I must go on a healthier diet, with no sweets or treats during the week, no candy, no soda, no "wasted calories" [of any sort].

I can vividly remember this moment, as it literally began to change my life. My mom, who had always cooked healthy but [kept] a few treats in the house, began to flush out anything that might [count as] "wasted calories" or sweets. My lunches started to consist of apples, carrots, and turkey sandwiches with no mayo and—most importantly—no goldfish or tiny bags of cookies. I grew envious of my friends' lunches, and developed longings for that small Twinkie wrapped in tinfoil. None of this made sense to me. I could not understand what had caused the change and why it was affecting only me, not my friends.

I'm Fat!

This is when I began to develop a concept for the word fat. Until then, I had been a free-spirited child who spent most of her time in the water and running around in the backyard. It was true that I had always been a little rounder than my friends, but it was just something I had never truly noticed. As I edged on six, I remember one of my best friends asking why my stomach was "squishy" and why my legs touched when I stood straight. This was when it hit me: I was fatter than they were. Things began to make sense as each reference or small insult piled on top of the others. I went home from school after this, sat down to go to the bathroom, and noticed a few rolls form on my stomach. I remember grabbing these rolls and telling myself over and over again that I had to go on a diet—and I'm pretty sure I had no idea what that meant at the time.

At the time, my sister, who was 12, was a dancer and very skinny. Sitting across from my sister at the dinner table was when the concept of dieting, or "restricting," came across my mind. At six years old, I had no concept of calories, or burning them for that matter. I only understood the concept that food made you fat. I would watch my sister eat and try to mimic her every bite, chew, and movement at the dinner table. I felt that if I could eat the way she did, I could look the way she did—skinny.

Diagnosis: Anxiety Disorder

Living with this distorted perception of reality contributed to many body issues as I was growing up. I always had the feeling that I was not thin enough compared to my peers. This continued way into high school, when I shot up 10 inches in one year, reaching six feet by the time I was a sophomore. Being taller than the rest of my peers gave me the sense of being larger than them, which further skewed the perception I had. I continued swimming, becoming a distance swimmer for my club and high school teams, and making it to the Junior Olympics and California Interscholastic Federation (CIF) [a championship tournament] on multiple occasions. I was a strong, healthy, and athletic girl on the outside, but on the inside I remained a very insecure and fragile creature.

Since then, I have battled my insecurities constantly. As I have grown older and into the person I am now, I feel as if I have matured and come very far. I am no longer completely concerned with my weight, but I still maintain an obsession with eating healthy and working out. I was diagnosed with anxiety problems a few years ago, when I would have anxiety attacks each time I didn't have time to get on the treadmill or complete my daily workout routine. Since then, I have developed techniques to reduce my anxiety problems and I have watched them slowly subside as I have become more comfortable in my own body.

[After all this time] I have begun to understand the effects that doctors can have on one's personal life. If it wasn't for the doctor telling me I needed to "diet," who knows where I would be now? If they had known that I was going to grow to be 6 feet tall, maybe their reaction to the chart would have been different. It was frustrating to be labeled "unhealthy" when I was actually very healthy and active. This labeling ended up contributing to a spoiled identity that I have carried with me for most of my life.

Alexis: Olympic Swimmer Diagnosed as "Overweight," "Unhealthy," and "Anxiety Disordered"

In her essay, Alexis tells a fall-from-grace story in which her active, carefree young life came to a sudden end the day the doctor announced that she was overweight and unhealthy and her mother leapt to action. In her confusion and sense of deprivation, the five-year-old Alexis begins to develop a consciousness of herself as "fat" and to narrate the events in her life around this new story of her "fatness." When she shot up 10 inches in one year, her new height only magnified her feelings of being bigger and fatter than her peers, thus intensifying her desperation to control her diet and exercise. Even as she developed into a Junior Olympics–level swimmer, Alexis became a fat subject, with all the attributes described earlier.

The ironies hardly need stating. In Alexis's case, the mistaken diagnosis had disastrous effects, transforming her happy, carefree life into the miserable life of a weight-obsessed, emotionally traumatized fat girl. The diagnosis also produced serious iatrogenic illness: an anxiety disorder that flared whenever she was unable to work out. Alexis's story highlights the potential problems with applying the BMI to growing children and shows how its use at too early an age can devastate a child's life, with effects that can last into adulthood.

BMI = Boost My Insecurity: Annemarie's Story

Annemarie is a twenty-two-year-old middle-class Mexican American raised in Granada Hills, in the heart of the San Fernando Valley. She was a strong, healthy, happy athlete with a rock-solid body whose perfect world fell to pieces the day a nurse administering a state fitness test declared sternly that her BMI was far too high and that she absolutely had to lose weight.

On the whole, the body mass index has been the source of many sleepless nights and dreadful days in my life. Weight has always been a very particular issue of mine, despite the fact that I have never been fat or obese, just "solid," as my mother likes to call it. I've been an athlete my whole life, with the exception of my college years, but even when I was in the best shape of my life, I was still "solid." However, I can easily pinpoint one specific moment in my life when the knowledge of BMI warped the image of my existence in society, and from that moment on, I believed myself to be a BMI number, a number in the upper 20s, which may as well have been 100 in my book. BMI was a concept that changed my whole existence, and until [recently] I basically believed that BMI was the word of God, unwavering and immovable. Realizing the faults with the BMI has brought me a whole new level of happiness. Like age, BMI is just a number, but to look back at the amount of time that I spent thinking about my BMI and the ways to get my BMI down, and whether or not I would ever reach my [target] BMI, is astonishing and essentially quite sad.

I would say that age 12 was a good age. I was carefree, happy, wore no makeup, didn't have mind-numbing cramps, and had a "boyfriend" who didn't pressure me to do anything except sit with him at lunch. Not only was I young, I was athletic and I was happy about it. Basketball was my sport, along with softball, track, and swimming. I played basketball every single day and had a very intense tan on three-quarters of my body. I loved school, I was very good at it, and I was happy to be me.

The Red Number

Then, in seventh grade, I was expected to pass some sort of fitness test in my PE class. I ran my mile in under 8 minutes and did well over my required number of sit-ups and push-ups. My PE teacher was very happy with my performance and constantly used me as an example for my classmates, much to their annoyance. Then came the time when we were supposed to be measured and ultimately weighed. At the age of 12, I stood 5'7" tall. My weight was not a problem that I thought about at all. So the day came when we were supposed to be weighed, and I happily stepped up onto the scale and then stepped aside as the nurse quickly calculated my BMI, something I had never heard of. She gave me my number, which was written in red, and explained to me that I was overweight and that I had to lose weight because my BMI was much too high. I had been to the doctor before and he had notified me that my weight was a little high, but because he knew I was an athlete, he didn't particularly tell me to change anything except maybe to stop eating at night after practice. Because of this, the nurse's words were news to me, and when she sternly looked at me and told me that I absolutely had to get my weight down, I was stunned. As I walked out, I realized that there were many other kids who had never heard of BMI and they had the same staggered look on their faces that I did.

After heading back out to my class, I ran into a classmate who had just recently been weighed and measured as well. Now, my classmate was quite overweight, much more than I was, and was just about the same height as me, yet she reported that her BMI was only 1 number higher than mine! I could not understand this phenomenon at all and started wondering if I had been delirious about my true body image all along.

From Athlete to Fat Girl in an Instant

I had never seen myself as fat, but from that moment on I started comparing myself to the thin, beautiful eighth-grade girls who wore short skirts and a size 0. In fact, I remember a moment when I just wanted to melt right into my seat because I felt so fat. This moment consisted of a very pretty girl walking in front of me, while boys noticeably started staring at her in her short miniskirt. I looked down at my large thighs, my big feet, and my size 6 tan skort and felt so inferior and enormous that I wished more than anything I was either invisible or just as beautiful and thin as that girl.

From that moment on, my weight was constantly on my mind. It became difficult for me to even walk in front of a class without feeling the "spotlight effect" and thinking that everyone was staring at me, discussing how big I looked, how fat I had gotten, and how high my BMI was. Things only got worse when I came to college, where the dreaded Freshman 15 (more like 25) entered my life and completely took over. Despite the fact that I grew another inch (reaching 5'8"), my BMI just continued to climb and climb, making my terror increase and my self-esteem plummet. Because of the way my body is shaped, even at my very heaviest I never looked fat, and if people knew how much I really weighed they would be astonished. However, this dissonance between my appearance and my rising BMI only made my weight a much more confusing concept for me. Being able to wear the same clothes I'd always worn, while knowing that I was overweight according to my BMI, made me doubt how "good" I really looked.

While this story does not necessarily have a happy ending, it does have a brighter future. My weight has [now] taken a backseat to my health, which I measure by how much better I feel and whether or not I fit into my favorite jeans. BMI is not only an inaccurate measure of the amount of "body fat" on an individual, it is a teenage girl's worst nightmare and an obsession that makes perfectly sane girls insane and feel guilty about anything and everything they eat. I find it incredibly disturbing that 11- and 12-year-olds are being taught that BMI is a medical fact and is irrefutable. My life was shaken by BMI and the fact that I did not know that because I was very athletic and muscular, my BMI did not accurately reflect the amount of body fat I actually had.

Annemarie: A Life Shattered by a Flawed BMI

In Annemarie, we have another case of a strong, happy girl athlete crushed by a BMI score. No longer was Annemarie a star athlete whose trained body made her feel powerful and in control of her life; the number said that she was just another overweight girl who needed nothing so much as to go on a diet. Although Annemarie received her diagnosis at a later age than did Alexis, the result was virtually the same: emotional shock followed by an instantly altered identity. From a happy, healthy, high-performance athlete, Annemarie transformed into an unhappy young woman obsessed with her weight. In no time at all, she acquired the typical characteristics of the fat self.

Annemarie's essay sheds disturbing light on the multiple layers of confusion a young girl feels when her own longtime perceptions of her body and health diverge from the conclusions of the science of weight. The news that her much heavier friend has a BMI only 1 number higher than hers leaves her baffled, wondering if she had been hallucinating about her true body image all along. The dissonance between her rising BMI and the normal-weight body she sees in the mirror leads her to doubt how good she actually looks and, more generally, to question whether she can accurately read the signals from her own body. Such experiences have long-term effects, undermining young people's trust in their ability to know, and thus manage, their own bodies. At yet another level, the essay implies, Annemarie was left deeply perplexed at how something that was supposed to make her healthy—sports and exercise—had the opposite effect, resulting in a diagnosis of unhealthy and a tortured, weight-obsessed adolescence.

The Match I Could Not Win: Ryan's Story

Finally, we meet Ryan, a twenty-year-old from Long Beach whose relatives emigrated from China via Vietnam. Ryan tells an endearing story of a family that loved him deeply, yet in its ignorance of American culture was unable to protect him from a quintessentially American trauma. Like Alexis and Annemarie, Ryan is an athlete diagnosed as "unhealthy" by a doctor rigidly applying the BMI. From there on, though, his story diverges from theirs in ways that will color the rest of their lives.

A Big Dose of Chinese Culture

I was raised by my grandmother while my parents were off looking for jobs. She had immigrated to America right before I was born, so she raised me with a lot of Chinese culture. One of these customs was to keep me fed as much as possible. She would steam rice every day with delicious vegetables with pork and beef marinated in all sorts of sauces. She made it mandatory that I finish off everything in my bowl at each sitting. I was led to believe by her that however many grains of rice were left in my bowl were how many warts my future wife would have on her face. So I was not hesitant to oblige.

This continued until, around the age of 10, I began living with my parents again. My mom would ask me to eat just about every time I passed her way, or walked into the kitchen. Now it has come to the point where it is quite annoying because she would ask me to eat in about seven different [ways]. I have grown to understand that in Chinese tradition, women show their love through their cooking, and nothing pleases them more than to see a husband or family member with a full stomach.

"Buddha" Joins the World of Sports—and BMIs

It was not until I joined the wrestling team in high school that I became so self-conscious about my body. Before joining the wrestling team I was the victim of many jokes among my peers about my roundness. They even gave me the nickname "Buddha," since I had a bald head and an equally round stomach. That was what motivated me to join the team, since it was a very rigorous sport that puts a lot of [emphasis] on the issue of weight, since wrestling is split up into weight classes. I walked on the team at about 135–140 pounds. In about three weeks I dropped over 10 pounds to make the 125-pound weight class. My doctor applauded me for my healthy life-style and for my particularly excellent BMI. This idea was reinforced as I got compliments from my coach, my fellow wrestlers, and even the girls at school about how good I looked.

Despite feeling very good about myself for changing my body, I hated my life in many respects. I hated eating salad for dinner and drinking nothing but water the entire day. I also hated not being able to eat my mom's dinner, along with the attitude she gave me every time I would reject her offerings. I would go work out constantly at the gym down the street. I felt like I had no control over my own body, let alone my life. I didn't get much support from my family. They didn't go see a single one of my wrestling matches. It was hard for my parents to understand what I was going through. At my age, they emigrated from China to Vietnam, just as the Japanese were invading. From there, they snuck their way onto ships that eventually made it to America. My father was held at gunpoint at one time and was almost killed over a bag of rice. As young adults, with no grasp of the English language, they hopped onto the bus to go search for jobs. They spent their teenage years trying to survive, while I'm complaining to them about "eating too much." On top of that, they don't know the pressures of American society simply because they aren't a part of it.

During my preteen and teenage years, it is safe to say that I felt very alone. My brother was in the Marines and was in boot camp getting ready to go to Afghanistan and Iraq. Obviously, he didn't care too much about my kiddy problems either. I did not feel comfortable talking about it with anyone, especially my friends. I didn't want them to think I was some girl obsessing about my weight. I was supposed to be a "guy," and act accordingly.

After a year of wrestling, I decided that I had had enough. I still wanted to keep up my physical shape, so I decided to join weight training class. Throughout my sophomore year I worked out vigorously. I didn't deprive myself of delicious food and gained weight steadily. A week after quitting wrestling, I went from 125 pounds to about 135–140 again. I thought I looked good and I felt even better. I worked out four days a week, resting for three days, and I ran on weekends. My family loved how I had changed, and my mom loved it as I ate her meals heartily.

Diagnosis: Overweight

So, as I walked into my doctor's office that year for my annual physical, I was quite surprised at his diagnosis: "Everything looks good, Ryan, you are quite healthy. But there is just one thing. You're a little heavy for your height. Your BMI is a little high." I looked down at myself wearing nothing but boxers. I saw my biceps, my big chest, and my six-pack. I saw my toned body and I looked up at him. In my head I was thinking: "Are you seeing the same thing I am?" He proceeded to hand my dad a pamphlet titled, "How to Deal with Your Overweight Child." My dad chuckled out loud as he saw it, but he respectfully listened to the doctor as he was instructing him how to go about [overseeing] my "treatment."

At that moment, I knew what it felt like to have a spoiled identity. I knew how healthy I was, but the doctor's words got to me. I was standing there in front of him with the body of an Olympian. I know because I was training with one. My training buddy and best friend is a short track skater who won two bronze medals at the Vancouver Olympics [in 2010]. When I told him [about the BMI score], he laughed so hard. He told me my doctor was crazy, but I hated how the doctor got to me. Just because he has a white coat, he is supposed to be the expert. He was right and I was wrong.

To this day I have a skewed image of doctors. I hate going to doctors and I hate how society puts them on a pedestal thinking they are all-knowing, omnipotent people. Every time I go in, they still tell me I have a high BMI and need to lead a "healthier lifestyle," but in my head I just think they are full of it. I still feel that I'm in the best shape of my life, and I will not change anything just because a guy in a white coat is labeling me from a chart on a piece of paper.

Ryan: Rejecting the Man in the White Coat

Like the two young women, Ryan is given an inappropriate diagnosis by a medical professional rigidly applying the BMI scale to a muscular, fit, high-performing athlete. Even when the doctor's verdict flies in face of compelling evidence from his own body, Ryan finds it inordinately hard to reject the judgment of a man in a white coat. The result is a severely spoiled identity—a feeling that he is defective in some very fundamental way. Yet unlike Alexis and Annemarie, Ryan is able eventually to reject the label, dismiss the doctor as an illegitimate teller of bodily truths, and claim the right to tell his own truth about his body and health. The residual attitude of disbelief and hostility toward medicine may well stay with him for life.

Why was Ryan able to eventually reject the identity when the girls were not (at least until many years later)? One reason could be that his parents did not jump on the diagnosis, as Alexis's mom did. As recent immigrants, Ryan's parents remain innocent of the mystique of medicine and BMI scores. Another reason is related to gendered body ideals and gendered differences in the world of sports. Being thin is such an essential part of feminine identity that the two girls, told they were overweight, immediately take up the diagnosis and begin efforts to shed pounds. Their entire social worlds uphold the idea that slenderness is more important than anything—evidently, more important even than being a strong, competitive athlete. Ryan is offended by the diagnosis, too, but he has support from his world of sports—his training buddy who is an Olympic athlete and thus a body expert in his own right—for the idea that the BMI is problematic. With the backing of his buddy, Ryan is able to resist taking on the fat-subject identity and retain his confidence in his body, despite the elevated BMI.

How Overweight People Become Fat Subjects

In this chapter we've traced the strange process by which young people who are merely chunky or chubby, by growing up in a world of virtuous biocitizens and weight-concerned docs, wind up taking on the characteristics of a fat person—everything but the excess poundage.

A Biocitizenship Society, Continued: The Key Role of the Physician

This chapter adds to our growing understanding of the workings of our biocitizenship society the critical role of the physician and other medical professionals, including nurses who conduct school fitness tests. Healthcare professionals are major agents in the transformation of children into fat subjects. Merely by delivering the news about a bad BMI, a well-meaning doctor can abruptly end a carefree childhood, turning a happy, self-loving child into a weight-obsessed, self-doubting child. When the doctor's diet-and-exercise orders are taken up and enforced by responsible biocitizen parents, which they almost always are (in this chapter, Binh's and Alexis's moms, but not Ryan's dad), the intervention in the child's life is all the deeper. And when the child receives the bad news at a very young age, he or she cannot possibly comprehend why his or her world has come undone. All the child understands is that he or she is fat, fat is bad, and so he or she is bad. Alexis's case provides a particularly poignant example. In diagnosing a weight-based "disease" and urging diet and exercise for weight loss, the physician also spreads two biomyths: first, that certain weight categories constitute diseases, and second, that weight is under individual control and people are heavy because they are irresponsible about eating and exercising. With the physician's endorsement, these biomyths become ever more firmly entrenched.

Becoming Fat Subjects: The Differing Roles of Pedagogical and Abusive Fat-Talk

In this chapter we've seen how young people who are only slightly chubby come to see themselves as fat and therefore biologically problematic and socially unacceptable. In the first pathway, the two types of fat-talk worked together to transform the three heavy-set youngsters we met into fat subjects. The pedagogical fat-talk (including that delivered by doctors) was productive of new identities and practices, setting out weight-based identities, informing people of their status, teaching that weight can and must be controlled, and educating children and their caregivers in what practices they must adopt to achieve normal weight. Whether critical or complimentary, the incessant body-size commentary, because of its ubiquity and force, also taught young people that their body weight was an essential component of their personal identity and social acceptability. The fat-abuse, by contrast, was destructive because it was experienced as an attack on the self. For the two young women (April and Tiffany), fat-abuse worked to erode their self-confidence and undermine alternative identities based on other, positive attributes (personal values, achievements, and so forth), rendering them vulnerable to the new weight-based identities being thrust on them.

As they struggled with this new socially and medically imposed identity, these three young people developed all the attributes of fat selfhood. First, they saw themselves as "bad"—biologically flawed, morally irresponsible or unworthy, socially inferior, and/or aesthetically unappealing. Second, they engaged in size-appropriate body practices (dieting and exercising) in an effort to lose that degrading weight. When those didn't work, as they usually don't for people with resistant biologies, the fat subject often takes them to the extremes—self-starvation, binging and purging, or (in cases presented in later chapters) excessive exercise—in a desperate attempt to lose the weight. Although these practices may pose serious dangers to their health (such as lowering metabolism and blood-sugar levels, as in April's case), after years of insufferable insults, developing a full-blown eating disorder is seen as the price they must pay to finally rid themselves of that intolerable identity. In some cases (such as April's and Tiffany's), by college such dangerous practices had become daily routines.

Third, they withdrew socially. Faced with incessant ridicule and social rejection, the fat subject retreats from his or her peers, skipping beach parties (Tiffany) or eating in the privacy of his room (Binh) to avoid people's rude and insensitive judgments. The anticipatory fear of fat abuse altered their personalities, leading Tiffany to be distrustful and Binh to be fearful of the traps set by weight-obsessed roommates and relatives. Finally, the self-perception of fatness invariably brought emotional suffering—including depression, low self-esteem, and pervasive insecurities—combined with vivid fantasies of radical bodily transformation. For some of the young people (especially Tiffany), memories of cruel fat abuse in grade school were long lasting, producing fear of similarly abusive comments in young adulthood. For these young people, brutal social rejection in childhood left them with enduring emotional scars reflected in deep-rooted insecurities and drastic weight-loss practices that had become a way of life.

Labeled "fat" again and again, all were forced into life-consuming identity struggles, internal battles over the extent to which they would accept the demeaning label as applying to them. The three young people resolved these in different ways, creating a continuum of identities that ranged from high to low fat identification. For April and Tiffany, fat became their dominant (although probably not only) identity. Binh was subject to withering fat-abuse, yet he stubbornly refused to follow the diet, exercise, and weight-loss script set out for him. Protected by his maleness—which made appearance only one of his many defining attributes—Binh managed to resist becoming a fat person and hold onto his definition of himself in terms of positive achievements (good relative and good student).

Young Athletes: Flawed BMI, Spoiled Identity, and Iatrogenic Injury

One of the central biomyths in the war on fat is the notion that the BMI is a good, or at least workable—or at the very minimum, safe—measure of fatness and indicator of health risk. Although physicians may recognize the limitations of this one-size-fits-all measure, because it is measured by a health professional ordinary people generally believe that it tells the scientific truth about their weight and health. This unquestioned trust comes out in the essays. For Annemarie, the BMI "was the word of God, unwavering and immovable." Alexis's mom instantly accepted the red-zone diagnosis of her child and completely changed her diet. Ryan trusted his first doctor as the "expert"; he harbored doubts about the second doctor but had a hard time shaking the diagnosis off.

In the last set of essays, we see why the shortcomings of the BMI matter. Despite their healthy weights and superlative health, all three young people were diagnosed as overweight and unhealthy by medical workers who applied standardized scores, failing to factor in the heaviness of muscle tissue. Standard BMI scores are not only poor indicators of health and disease in such cases, they have effects that are often counterproductive or even damaging for those mislabeled "unhealthy." Despite their physical prowess, all three athletes developed spoiled identities as fat subjects—perceptions of themselves as flawed, permanently damaged people who might not ever be able to live a normal, successful life. And the transformation from fit, strong, self-confident athlete into unhealthy and self-doubting overweight kid was instantaneous. For these young people, the diagnosis was nothing short of life-shattering.

The stark contrast between the doctor's "unhealthy" BMI score and the young people's lived experiences of their bodies also left the young people intensely confused about their actual health, undermining their confidence in their ability to know their own bodies. The encounters with the doctors were disempowering and deskilling at best. Far from helping to improve these athletes' weight and health, the BMI scores produced iatrogenic injury. In one case (Alexis's), the trauma was so severe that she was later diagnosed with an emotional disorder. The young people's later realization of the wrongs that had been done led in turn to anger and hostility toward their physicians. Ryan may well never get over his skewed image of doctors and his anger about what he considers the illegitimate power they possess. Others simply dread going to the doctor. Few were neutral about their physicians. This general hostility, wariness, and disbelief in medicine—worrying for patients and doctors alike—is another unfortunate yet little remarked effect of the war on fat.

In the next chapter, we leave behind the heavy groups targeted by the war on fat to meet a category of people who are labeled diseased according to their BMI scores but who are largely neglected by the medical world. These are the "underweight," and they have no end of complaints about how the world treats them.

5

"UNDERWEIGHT"

My entire obsession with weight in my opinion is caused by peer pressure and what I see in the culture. In my head a man should be muscular not skinny, tall not short. I see big, muscular men around me and I feel that in order to be a man, I need to also be muscular. So I try to gain weight and become more muscular. [Last] year I started going to the recreation center and working out. I was eating five meals a day and drinking protein shakes. I was doing all I could to gain weight.

ELWOOD, FROM HIS ESSAY "THE INFO ON THE SKINNY" [SC 86]

Given the celebration of thinness in our society, one might expect the very thin to live charmed lives. But such is not the case. As everyone of slight build knows, there is a fine line between "thin" and "*too* thin" that, in SoCal at least, falls around BMI 16 or 17 for girls and somewhat higher for boys. Those just above this line are envied as "attractive" people with "to die for" bodies, while those below it are scorned as just plain "skinny" or "scrawny." Skinny people—the term my informants use for themselves—have long been the butt of jokes, but the medicalized discourse of the war on fat makes their condition something else—the "disease" of underweight. The discourse divides the full spectrum of the lower weights at 18.5 and says that all those with a BMI below that are "underweight" and in need of medical treatment to bring them within "normal" range. (Someone 5′6″ tall weighing 114 or less is "underweight.") The medical discourse that dominates the war on fat has thus created a new weight-based identity and a new target of surveillance, intervention, discipline, and control.

With all the concern about excess weight, the plight of those deemed "underweight" has been woefully neglected—in popular culture and even in medicine. (The exception, of course, is the field of psychiatry, which treats eating disorders.) As a result, we know little about what causes underweight and how it might be "treated," and even less about the lived realities of those who get that label. Even the cultural basics remain elusive: How disparaging is the label "underweight"? Is it as degrading as "obese?" Do very thin people take on the new medical identity? More generally, how is life lived at this end of the weight spectrum? We simply do not know.

We've seen that, in our biocitizenship society, virtuous biocitizens have the right and the duty to monitor those who have weight-based "disorders" and seek to coax or coerce them into becoming "healthy," normal-weight biocitizens. In SoCal, my research reveals, the duties of the biocitizen to watch and work on the "abnormal" extend to the underweight end of the spectrum. For underweight targets, the key mechanism of persuasion is *skinny-talk*, a variant of fat-talk with assumptions, biomyths, and moralities that closely parallel those of the much more common fat-talk. Unlike overweight people, the number of underweight people is small. Of the 234 ethnographies I gathered, only 7.2 percent (17 in all) featured the travails of underweight subjects. But their experiences are important—not only because they suffer a form of weight-based discrimination that is poorly understood but also because of what they reveal about the larger consequences of the societal war on fat.

In this chapter, I present the auto-ethnographies of seven young people who suffer from the "disease" of being too skinny. Again, I ask three sets of questions. First, what kinds of skinny-talk do these young people hear and from whom? More generally, how does biocitizenship work at this end of the weight continuum? Second, do those labeled "underweight and defective" internalize that identity; if so, what are the attributes of the "underweight" or "skinny" subject? Third, what are the larger consequences of these dynamics for the health, well-being, and lives of uber-skinny young people?

Once again we find a range of responses. Some young people take on the degrading identity of the skinny subject, an identity that, because of its preoccupation with weight, can be considered a variant of the fat subject. These people accept the demeaning label and live miserable lives struggling to find ways to gain weight and be "normal." Others continue to work to achieve "normality" but find ways to deflect the demeaning discourse so it does not invade their sense of self. Still others manage to see outside the medicalized discourse that labels them ill to grasp how that discourse does its work. Goaded by a sense of injustice, they channel their anger into developing critiques of the BMI-based approach to deciding who is normal.

The problem of skinniness plagues some categories of individuals more than others. While being overweight is especially difficult for women, for whom thinness is essential to femininity, being underweight poses major challenges for men because the norms of masculinity make bigness, strength, and muscularity the signs of "real manhood." Thin men must struggle to prove not only their "normality" but also their masculinity. Ethnicity is also important here. In the United States, the idealized (or hegemonic) masculine figure is white (and tall and buff). Nonwhite males who inhabit subordinated masculinities cannot hope to change their skin color or height, but they can try to get closer to the ideal masculine form by bulking up.

Yet there's a further complication, for within nonwhite groups, some racial/ethnic groups are more biologically predisposed to being skinny than others. Asians are much more likely to be rail thin than members of any other racial/ethnic group. CDC statistics show that Asians are at least twice as likely to be underweight as Americans of other ethnic groups (in 2010, 4 percent of Asians but only 1.4 to 1.8 percent of other groups had underweight BMIs).[1] There are also big differences among Asian groups: 10.9 percent of Vietnamese and Japanese were underweight, compared to 5.7 percent of Chinese, 3.9 percent of Koreans and Asian Indians, and 1.6 percent of Filipinos (figures for 2004–2006).[2] It is no coincidence then that none of the African Americans, Middle Easterners, or Latinos I worked with were "too skinny" but goodly numbers of the East, Southeast, and South Asians were. Ethnic differences in parent-child relations play a role in the formation of skinny-person identities as well. While virtually all parents are concerned about their kids' health and well-being, in some groups fat-talk (and its skinny-talk variant) is a routine and, for the targets, mortifyingly public part of family conversations. As we've seen in previous chapters, in East and Southeast Asian families, parents routinely comment on their kids' weight, berating them if they are "too fat" or "too thin." In these groups, where parents are the major (or at least earliest) deliverers of the skinny-talk, it seems to be especially difficult for young people to reject the perception that they are indeed too skinny and that something is seriously wrong with them.

Skinny Asian Guys: What Is Wrong with Me?

Popular culture portrays thinness as highly desirable, consciously chosen, and deliberately achieved by eating little and/or exercising much. Thin people, the story goes, have achieved the cultural ideal and live happy, successful lives. The accounts of Jason and Huy show us just how wrong this story is. Subject to relentless biobullying yet unable to gain weight, these two young men come to see themselves as "skinny and defective." They endure intense emotional suffering because the world they live in tells them they are bad sons and bad Americans, yet there is nothing they can do to improve their lot.

Yellow Swan: Jason's Life as a Skinny Male

In this essay, Jason, a naturally rail-thin twenty-one-year-old of Chinese descent, writes of the sadness, frustration, and anger he has felt being the butt of humiliating skinny jokes his whole young life. Internalizing the skinny-talk, he now believes that something is biologically wrong with him. Jason comes from a financially struggling family in the Glendora section of Los Angeles.

I am currently 5′8″ and 117 pounds [BMI of 17.8]. I'm completely aware that I'm really skinny. Unfortunately I've been told that I was skinny all my life, and it's really started to piss me off. I've struggled with attaining a normal weight ever since I can remember. I really don't know what's wrong with me. I eat normally—about as much as my friends who are normal weight—so why can't I gain weight? I'm going to share my feelings in this essay, something I've never done even with my family. I've never even talked about it with my closest friends because, frankly, I'm a "man" and something like this, and the frustrations I would like to share, could make me come off as—pardon my language—a "pussy."

The Handball Champion Gives
Up His Game

Back in elementary school, I was the school's best handball player. I loved playing that game and I really was known school-wide as the "handball champion." I was the third grader who could beat the fifth graders. It really helped my self-esteem because that was probably the first time I got recognition for being good at something. I had one of the deadliest serves around. Some people couldn't believe how far I could hit the ball, to the point where it was almost impossible for my opponent to return it. My secret was to start off gently throwing the ball at the wall and then run as fast as I could, timing my strike so that I would be using my entire body's momentum to bash the ball as hard as I could into the ground after the first bounce to send it soaring into the sky.

I made many friends playing that game. Quite frankly, I also made some enemies. I was, as you could guess, very skinny. The reason I was able to hit the ball the way I did, according to the bullies—whose names and faces I still remember very clearly—was not because I knew the basic concepts of physics but because I was skinny. I didn't have any "cushion" in my forearms so, according to them, I had a distinct "advantage" because I didn't have any of the fat that normal kids had that could prevent the ball from going as far as it did. These bullies made fun of me for it. I'm not trying to come off as a giant crybaby, but it sucked, it really did. My outlet for success and recognition on the school playground was becoming a venue for bullies to make fun of me. I quit handball when I started the fifth grade. I didn't want to be made fun of anymore.

Every time I socialize with other people, I'm always wondering what they think of me. Do they think I'm too skinny? Will they not want to be my friend because I'm too skinny? Especially now in college, I'm just worried that the fact that I'm not the most visually appealing male will impede my objective of getting to know as many good people as I could, in order to build up my network of people I can turn to for help when I become a real adult.

Thankfully, it hasn't been that much trouble. I know I'm skinny and I know people think I'm skinny. Some people even give suggestions on how to gain more weight. Now, I completely understand that people just want to help me when they give tips and diets for me to try to gain weight, but it pisses me off when people do that. I'm not pissed at the other person, I'm pissed at myself, because, frankly, when people tell me to eat more, do they seriously think that I haven't been trying that for the past few years of my life?? I always think to myself, what else could I do [to gain weight]? I've stayed awake in bed at night thinking about this. I've even dreamt about being normal weight. I still don't have the answer. The media sure as hell hasn't helped me feel any better; my family definitely has not made me feel any better. Every time I go home—about every three weeks—it's almost guaranteed that at one point in the weekend, my mom will tell me that I'm too skinny and that I need to eat more. In fact, I've kind of made it into a little game in my head where I'll try to guess when she's going to tell me that, and I've nailed it quite a handful of times, ha ha.

Responsible for Parental Loss of Face

Now I'm going to share something that really made me angry. My parents—my mom, specifically—is always telling me that I'm too skinny and that she wants me to get bigger so that I can "save face." Well, my aunt from my father's side recently came to visit from Taiwan. I've never seen her before; I didn't even know who she was. I had to ask my father how I should address her. Guess what the first thing this aunt said to me after I gave her a hug and introduced myself. YEP! She said in Mandarin, "Wow! John (my father), why is your son so skinny?" Great first impression, Jason, good going! Right when I heard that, my heart sank, I was so close to just yelling a big F*** YOU! right then and there. But I didn't. I wanted to "save" whatever "face" my father had left by not verbally destroying my aunt so that she couldn't bundle up my being skinny and completely rude and use it against my father. My father understands me. He was really skinny when he was young, too, and he immediately knew how I felt after my aunt said that. He pulled me off to the side and said, "thanks," because he saw my subtle facial expressions and my fists clenching. I teared up a little when my dad thanked me; in fact, I'm a little teary writing this now.

I really am trying to gain weight, though mostly not for myself but for my mom and dad, because I'm tired of having them hear "your son is too skinny" from church friends and family members. One of my most distinct memories is of when my father introduced me to his church friend who is also our insurance agent. I really remember this occasion clearly because it sucked. I'm not sure how much lower of a low-blow you could possibly execute to someone. This male church friend, after my father exchanged introductions, stated, in Mandarin: "John, you have to stop focusing on your business and start feeding your son." This comment doesn't seem too bad, right? Until I tell you that my father is the owner of a restaurant. So this church friend told my father that he had paid too much attention to feeding his customers and neglected feeding me. You can only imagine how much rage [I was feeling]. I'm a pretty sensitive guy. I try my hardest to not hurt anyone's feelings. Unfortunately, the majority of the rest of the world doesn't [seem to care about others' feelings].

I'd say that one of the most amusing incidents I've encountered that had to do with my skinniness [occurred] at a party. One of the girls, who actually was fairly attractive, told me that she was jealous of how thin I was. In my head, I was, like, "Wait, what did you just say?" I wasn't pissed at all because she told me so in a different way than I've been told my entire life. I told her that she didn't want to be at my level of skinniness, but I think she genuinely did, which is a little messed up, ha ha.

Humph, I just remembered something that someone said in class that I'd like to share. In one of the class discussions, a female stated that she doesn't like Asian guys because we're too short and skinny. I wasn't really hurt by what she said, as it's not that big a deal, but I will probably remember for a very long time that someone said that, because it kind of describes me, ha ha. I haven't seen the [2010] movie *Black Swan*, but from what I've heard, it [features a ballet dancer with a] significantly low BMI. I hope my experiences of being a skinny Asian male—a yellow swan, as it were—provide some insight into how brutal society can be toward people who aren't of normal weight.

Jason Becomes a Skinny Subject

In this account, we see how the bioabuse meted out to skinny people can exacerbate the social and bodily problems of a very thin child. Unable to take the mockery of the grade school bullies any longer, Jason gave up handball, the one thing in his life that had given him self-confidence and, one must imagine, improved his physical stamina, coordination, and general health. On top of the biobullying, Jason was the recipient of unsolicited biopedagogical advice on weight-gaining diets, none of which he appreciated because he had tried them all with no success. Through it all, what angered him the most was the assumption of the bullies and pedagogizers alike that his weight was under his control. His experience said otherwise.

Jason's essay documents the process by which pole-thin youngsters, subject to relentless skinny-talk, come to adopt the identity thrust on them. In Jason's case, being a skinny person involves the feeling that he is physically defective and unappealing for reasons he does not understand. Buying into the biomyths underlying the war on fat, Jason assumes that he should be able to gain weight; because he cannot, he figures, his body must be defective. The social and emotional world of this skinny self is fragile indeed. Despite the essay's self-effacing "ha-ha"s, it is clear that Jason is deeply insecure about his appearance, always wondering about what others think of him, fearing social rejection because of his weight, and worrying about his future in a society in which good looks are essential to career success. Although as a "man" he has never been allowed to publicly express his feelings about his weight, this essay reveals an emotional world full of rage, sadness, humiliation, and hurt.

This essay provides fascinating insight into the dynamics of biocitizenship in the Chinese American community, where the individual is decentered in favor of the group. Whether the result of poor parenting or poor biology, Jason's stubborn skinniness causes his parents serious loss of face in front of their relatives and friends. Jason is only too aware of this. His shame is their collective shame, and he would do anything in his power to make it end. Jason thus suffers a double dose of shame, the first for bringing dishonor to his parents and the second for bringing disgrace on himself.

"Skinny," a Label as Hurtful as "Fat": Huy's Story

In this auto-ethnography, we meet Huy, a twenty-year-old Vietnamese American who was born in Vietnam but raised in San Diego, where his parents struggled to make ends meet. Like Jason, Huy is naturally small and skinny. Subject to overwhelming social and media pressure telling him that he is biologically defective and eating-disordered, Huy comes to see himself in those terms, despite the absence of any relevant symptoms.

Many people think being skinny is an easy thing, but that is not true. It is as hurtful for a skinny person to be criticized as it is for a fat person. Being skinny my whole life, I assure you it is not easy, especially when you are a boy.

[In my home country of] Vietnam, where access to food and healthcare is often limited, it is normal for children to be skinny. In that context I thought of myself as normal. However, after moving to the United States, it was apparent that I was not normal, for I was much thinner than the boys of my age group. In school, [no one said it out loud] but there was a faint social implication that I was an outcast. Back then, though, the [discrimination against other-bodied people was not so blatant]. I remember thinking that maybe when I grew up, I would just grow out of it and be normal like everyone else. But that would not happen.

Fast forward to today, when I am still as thin as ever. Whenever my friends complain about how they are dissatisfied with their weight, I find it funny because losing weight is so easy [for me]. I can lose three pounds a week if necessary. Gaining weight, on the other hand, is much harder. My friends have no idea how much I want to be fat, and I mean it. I think that, for a boy, being fat is much better than being skinny, for at least when you're fat you know that you can just always work out and turn [the fat into] muscle weight. But if you're skinny, where will you get that excess weight from? For me, gaining weight is seemingly impossible and I hate it. I have tried eating dinner before bed, eating ice cream before bed, and eating junk food, but [the result is] nothing—no changes, still the same weight.

Becoming "Anorexic"

On top of that, facing the criticism alone is hard. To be honest, I do not think of myself as an anorexic, but the people around me keep saying it over and over again, so that sometimes it is like, "Hey, if everyone thinks you are, then it must be true." At some point, my self-perception completely worsened. Suddenly, I grew conscious of myself, which was funny because I had never cared about looks before. It was especially hard in high school because everyone falls into different social categories, and it is better to fit into a certain category than to be in no category at all. Now, looking back, I think that during that period I took up this identity of being skinny to fit into the perception that others had of me. I do not have an eating disorder, but the attention that people showered on me was all that mattered. It is silly and totally shallow, but for once people paid attention to me and I was not completely invisible. [To tell the truth], the idea [that I have] an eating disorder is completely absurd because I like to eat and I do not purge or anything. Still, the criticism went on and it hurt [because] being called skinny is tantamount to the shame of being called fat.

For me, the only really bad experience with losing weight occurred during my first quarter in college. My family economic background was not the best, so to go to college I had to take out a lot of loans. I was doing badly in school, so I felt like my life was spinning out of control and I had no power over anything anymore. It sucked. I do not know why, but I took it out on my eating habits. I do not know what I was thinking, but I just figured that food is the only thing that I have under my control. Instead of gaining the Freshman Fifteen, [though,] I lost ten pounds. When I came home to visit, my family became worried and I told them what happened. They told me that I should not worry about it and I should take care of my health. I did and was able to gain back the weight I lost, but I just could not gain more than that. I think losing weight was like a cry for help.

A Disappointment to Everyone

The worst thing about being skinny is that people think it is easy to gain weight, but it is not. People just do not understand when I say I cannot gain weight. They think I am just not eating, but I am, it is just that I cannot gain weight no matter what. This feeling of being unable to gain weight becomes so overwhelming that sometimes I just want to give up. Sometimes it feels like you are a big disappointment because you cannot gain weight like normal people. It makes me feel like I am defective or something, and that certainly does not help boost up my esteem.

In the end, skinny or fat, it is the same thing: [both bodies are flawed]. The thing skinny and fat people have in common is that we do not fit into the standard that society glorifies. [In America] people say that being different is good, but being skinny is definitely not good in a place where everywhere you turn, you see abs rippling, [buff] movie stars rescuing their love interests, [and] college guys wearing their V-necks so deep it looks like their pecs are trying to escape from their shirts. It is those blatant images that make [me look at myself and ask]: "Why am I not like them? Am I abnormal?"

Huy: Acquiring a Defective Sense of Self

In Huy we have an immigrant boy who wanted nothing more than to fit in and be accepted by his new peers. But that was not to be. He was different simply because he was skinny, and nothing he tried—not eating all the junk food in the world—helped him pack on pounds. The result was a radical rupture in his identity; from feeling normal in his home country, Huy went to feeling abnormal in his adopted one—"all alone" as a skinny guy in a world of larger, muscled males.

In illuminating how the pervasive skinny-talk and muscle-imagery work to alter a young man's sense of self, Huy's essay reveals the extraordinary power of social discourse to remake subjective reality. Subject to constant criticism, in high school he became acutely self-conscious of his skinniness. Repeatedly taunted about his putative "anorexia," Huy began to fit into the social category others applied to him simply to be accepted and to gain social visibility. Sadly, being eating disordered became a positive identity for Huy because it brought him attention and recognition. Huy makes clear that his identity as a skinny anorexic is a detestable one. Declaring skinniness to be worse than fatness, he views himself as defective, a bad biocitizen who cannot gain weight "like normal people." In the end, he sees no way out: he cannot gain weight, and he cannot escape the comments and media images that establish the norms and define him as outside of them. Trapped by the biomyth of individual weight control, yet unable to see its mythic nature, all he can do is ask himself over and over why he ended up so weird.

Skinny Asian and White Girls: Weaklings and Weirdos

It might be better to be a skinny girl than a skinny guy, but the assumptions about twig-like girls are demeaning nonetheless. Here we meet three uber-skinny girls, a Vietnamese girl, Linh, and two white girls: Sabrina, who is rather short, and Ariel, who is rather tall. All three endure constant biobullying and, in response, become self-conscious about their weight and obsessed with putting on pounds. In the end, Linh comes to believe that she is abnormally and unhealthily small, while the white girls seem more able to deflect the comments and eventually accept themselves as they are.

Although we can't be sure why Asian girls like Linh are more likely to internalize the shame, it could be because Asians already suffer discrimination as minorities, and the maltreatment they get on account of their bodies comes as more of the same. Asians might also suffer more because their demanding families and high-pressure communities are obsessed with their thinness and constantly badger them about it, whereas the families and communities of white girls like Sabrina and Ariel express less concern about their thinness. This relative freedom from skinny-abuse by intimates may have allowed the white girls to step outside their own lives and develop a wider perspective on how the larger cultural world of skinniness works.

More Than Just Some Numbers: Linh's Declaration of Personhood

Linh is an ultra-thin twenty-two-year-old Vietnamese American who grew up in a financially struggling family in Westminister, the center of Orange County's large Vietnamese community. Although Linh hates her thinness and is trying frantically to gain weight, the social world she inhabits interprets her life through the dominant discourse, which holds that thin people actively choose to be thin. In her essay, Linh describes the frustrations she endures living in a world in which the reality of her struggles makes no cultural sense.

> I have a BMI of 17.9 and yes, I do know I am underweight. However, that does not seem to stop people from perpetually drawing that fact to my attention. I am not anorexic and have never been drawn to the "cult of thinness." Contrary to popular belief, I do eat, at least three meals a day to be exact. I do not frequent the gym religiously and do not partake in the diets

endorsed so powerfully by celebrities. No matter how many times I tell people that I am healthy (I have the doctor visits to prove that), and that I do not harbor some obsession about my weight, they still assume I live my life around a set of numbers: BMI, weight, and caloric intake. Yes, being thin is a positive thing in the supermodel world, but in real life—in my life—being thin presents more challenges than advantages. Many times people tend to focus on my weight more than who I am as a person.

"A Weakling"

Despite my accomplishments, people still think of me as mentally and physically weak, a quality that my family members assume comes with being thin. Whenever I go to family [functions] there will always be comments made by my relatives about my weight. They always assume that I am on a diet and tell me to eat more. They also advise me to take easier courses [in school so] as to not increase my stress and my chances of being sick. In addition, they also assume I am not physically and mentally strong enough to [handle] the stresses of graduate school and thus should settle for a more passive path, a path more [suited] to my physique and my female status. It is also very bothersome that my mother constantly worries about my health whenever the weather changes slightly. It is as if she thinks I would faint at the weakest of breezes or that I would catch a cold when the temperature is slightly below normal solely because my thin body cannot withstand the weather.

Even though size discrimination is getting more media attention, people tend to neglect the fact that thin people as well as fat people suffer discrimination. When I applied for a job at a local pharmacy where my sister once worked, I was rejected. It was not until I talked to my sister, whose friend knew the hiring manager, that I discovered that my size was the reason that I was not accepted for the job. According to the manager, I was passed over in favor of a young, normal-weight man, not because of my qualifications but because she felt I was too thin to lift boxes, type and stand at the computer, and talk to customers for a whole work period. My weight has always led people to underestimate my abilities when it has come to finding and performing in jobs.

"It's Your Choice"

The belief that being underweight is [something I have chosen] due to vanity or some sick obsession with anorexia is quite common but utterly untrue. My mom has put me on high-protein, high-calorie diets along with medicine that supposedly increased my appetite. All this was to no avail, not because I chose to be thin but because there is just some part of me that cannot gain and maintain healthy weight for a long period of time. I do not like being so thin and I despise all the disadvantages that come with it. If I had a choice, I would choose normal weight because I know I would be much happier being normal. Still, to this very day, I am on a diet plan to increase my weight. I despise the fact that I still look like a child or a waif from the "heroin chic" days of Kate Moss. I despise the fact that all the clothes that I would like to wear do not fit me. I despise the fact that people still mistake me for a lost child whenever I walk alone by myself. For me, being thin is a curse, not a choice. I am pursuing every option available to me to not be as thin.

The media are obsessed with fad diets and slimming techniques linked to the "cult of thinness," but there is little help for people who are thin and want to gain some weight. When I receive my magazine subscriptions to *Women's Health*, I always see some sort of diet or exercise tip on the cover, but I have yet to see an article with advice on how to gain weight in a healthy manner. I also do not like the fact that most depictions of thinness in the media appear in the modeling industry with models who are anorexic and harbor an obsession with thinness because of vanity. I want to be able to read articles that suggest a healthy method of gaining weight instead of the unhealthy way most people suggest, which is mainly gorging oneself with fatty foods. I want to be able to gain weight without having my risk of having a stroke or heart attack increase later on in life. I know the subset of thin people who want to gain weight is small, but it does exist and it should receive more [and more sympathetic] attention.

Linh: The Curse of Thinness

Linh's essay brings out the costs imposed on thin people by the treatment of underweight in the dominant obesity discourse—both its diseasification and its neglect relative to the problem of obesity. Linh's world is full of virtuous biocitizens, from her relatives, who urge her to eat more and pursue a modest career, to her mother, who puts her "diseased" daughter on special diets and medicines in hopes of inducing weight gain. Not only do the treatments not work but all this attention to body size has damaging effects. This obsessive attention to Linh's weight imposes a skinny-person identity on her, reducing her to her weight and ignoring the accomplishments that might form the basis for more positive, non-weight-based identities. The dominant discourse also makes assumptions that are woefully wrong—what we might call the biomyths of skinniness. It assumes that Linh's skinniness is associated with disease (anorexia) and that her thinness is a voluntary condition that she could reverse if she just tried. (These very same assumptions were applied to Jason and Huy.) Employers (and relatives) presume that Linh's thinness makes her weak, inviting discrimination based on size.

Facing all this pressure, Linh responds by adopting most of the identity imposed on her. She sees herself as abnormal but, lacking the notion that thin can be healthy and have biological or genetic roots, she has difficulty explaining what is wrong with her. Deeply affected by all the skinny-talk, and by her lifelong experiences of cultural denigration and economic discrimination, her goal is to gain weight and become "normal." To that end she adopts a host of healthist practices associated with biocitizenship. Although Linh is in many ways a believer in the dominant weight discourse, her essay is also a plea for a broadening of that discourse to recognize the problems faced by thin people and provide them with healthful ways to become "normal." Most of all, Linh is trying to reclaim her personhood, to define herself as an able and worthy person despite her thin body.

Too Tiny a Dancer: Sabrina's Quest for Normality

Sabrina is a twenty-year-old dancer from a well-off Caucasian family in Santa Barbara County. At 90 pounds, she is definitely "underweight," a fact she hears from everyone in her world—as though she did not already know. She eventually figures out how to navigate around the comment, but not before taking on the identity of a "skinny person" possessed by the desire to pack on pounds.

> [I am a dancer and dance is known to encourage slender bodies.] I went into high school at 5'2" and 90 pounds. I was extremely tiny, and although my calves were muscular from ballet, I had tiny chicken legs. Most people I know are afraid of becoming overweight, but I am always worrying that I am too skinny. I have always said that I just want to be normal. I know that people think they are being nice when they say, "Oh, my gosh, you weigh like nothing." But to me that is actually an insult. I have constantly had to deal with the astonishment of people remarking on how skinny I was.

Snacking Up to Normality?

When I was a sophomore in high school, I wasn't having much luck dating guys. I had gained close to ten pounds since freshman year, but my self-confidence was at an all-time low. At the beginning of the school year I found out that my long-time crush didn't share the feelings I had for him. I became very depressed and told my best friend that I knew it was because he thought I was too skinny. I went straight to the cupboard and grabbed a bag of bread rolls. I ate six of them in a row. I just shoved them in, one after the other. I didn't become crazy or anything, [but] I would always try to eat more at meals. I always insisted on having three meals a day. If I didn't get three meals, I would feel like a failure. I never ever tried to eat healthy because I felt like I didn't need to.

Over Christmas break of my sophomore year I stayed home the entire time and literally stayed in bed every day watching "Fat Camp" reruns on MTV. I kept a few bags of chips and other snacks by my side and ate the entire time. I gained 4 pounds in two weeks. That was quite a lot for me. I was now 5'3" and 103 pounds. Every pound counted for me, and I was constantly obsessed with weighing myself.

When I was a senior, I had my first official boyfriend. I started to feel a lot more comfortable in my own skin. [I was still trying to gain weight, though. Just like anorexics constantly check Pro-Ana sites for advice on becoming skinnier,] I would often look up which foods had the highest calories or were really fatty, and try to eat those. I never counted calories, but I would purposely try to eat hearty (that is, fatty) foods. And I would try to wear more flowing tops to cover my stomach, which I always thought was too skinny.

Who's the Alien? Dealing with the Skinny Abuse

During my senior year in high school I [finally discovered] how to handle people's comments on how thin I was. Some of those people would make me seem like an alien for being skinny in order to make their own heaviness seem normal. Why do I have to be the weird one, I wondered? Why is it so odd to be thin? I [learned to] just smile, laugh, and say thank you. I realized that most of the people who made these remarks were self-conscious about being overweight and would kill to be me.

When I went to college I was disappointed that the Freshman Fifteen did not exist for me. Since I was on the college dance team and a dance major, I was always exercising, so gaining weight was basically impossible. I remained at 103 pounds. This year, though, [her sophomore year] I quit dance team because I wasn't happy with the coach. I have been skipping more meals because I'm caring less about having three meals a day. I've also been snacking a lot on fast food. I weighed myself and discovered that, out of nowhere, I have gained three more pounds. I am now 5'3" and weigh 106 pounds [BMI of 18.8, at the very bottom end of the normal range].

I honestly believe that this is a very healthy weight for my height. An ideal weight would be between 110 and 115 pounds, but I am very happy now. I think the difference between me and anorexic girls is that I am much more muscular and have some small curves. It really bothers me how they make tons and tons of bigger clothing sizes, but it is so hard to find really small sizes. And they make diets for overweight people but there are no diets for people who are trying to gain, other than body builders. [The world needs to stop discriminating against tiny people and start finding ways to help them.]

Sabrina: Becoming a Bad Biocitizen in the Quest to Become a Good One

Subject to skinny-talk her whole young life, Sabrina early on took on the identity of the abnormally skinny person. Her whole life since then has been spent wanting to be normal, obsessing about her weight, and strategizing about how to gain pounds. Internalizing the negativity around skinniness, Sabrina seems to measure her self-worth by the number of pounds she gains. Although she eventually figures out a way to deflect the hostile comments, her weight remains the single most important part of her identity.

Focusing on overweight Americans, the war on fat conveys the message that they became fat by overindulging in high-calorie and high-fat junk foods and that they must now eat healthfully and exercise to get down to normal weight. Sabrina has heard these messages and believes that, because she is underweight, she doesn't need to watch what she eats. She believes that eating fatty, high-calorie junk food can help skinny people put on pounds and become more "normal." In college she is thrilled to discover she has gained weight—by quitting dancing and living on fast food. Ironically, in her single-minded focus on gaining weight and becoming "normal," Sabrina has become a bad biocitizen whose poor diet is surely bad for her health.

Stick-ing Out—Growing Up Skinny in High School: Ariel's Story

Ariel is a twenty-one-year-old Caucasian from a middle-class family in Pomona, an upscale community in northeast Los Angeles County. As an exceedingly tall and skinny girl, in high school Ariel was the target of relentless biobullying that made her feel like a "freak."

An Outcast and a Freak

I am 5'10" and 110 pounds, and people are [constantly] staring at my height and criticizing my weight [BMI of 15.8]. I lost count of how many times people have said, "Wow! You're tall! How tall are you?" It gets annoying. I mean, I cannot go around and say to people, "Wow! You're fat! How fat are you?" or "Wow! You're short! How short are you?" Those are seen as rude, while the tall comment is seen as perfectly acceptable.

My growth spurt [occurred] in ninth grade, the awkward grade for most of us. I went from a "normal" 5'6" to 5'10" in about one summer. While my height went up, my weight stayed the same. Great. I was a stick. Most of the time, a stick is seen as unhealthy. Nevertheless, I was healthy. I ate right and attempted to exercise. However, my classmates thought otherwise; they assumed I had an eating disorder. In high school, appearance is important, and my classmates would constantly comment on my weight and height. One incident really stood out.

During gym class—one of the worst hours of the day—one of my classmates would not stop bugging me. In gym class, the popular jocks rule over the scrawny book nerds like myself. I could not throw or catch a ball to save my life. That cruel classmate [was named] Mack. He was ugly and fat, so of course picking on the skinny, defenseless girl was the easy thing to do. Whenever I would pass him, he would go, "EWWWW!!! How disgusting! It's all stick and bones." Or he would shout out: "Go eat something!" Whenever I would hang out with my guy friend, Mack would shout out, "He doesn't like you! No boys do." Yeah, these things were not so creative, but at 14, it hurt [to be criticized]. I did let Mack, along with others, get to me. People in gym class would stare at me; the shorts and shirt that were too big did not help. I felt like such an outcast. Nobody wanted me on his team.

The stares and whispers also ruled the hallways. I towered over the majority of my classmates. Girls would look at me as I ate lunch to make sure I was eating. I remember I sat with some girls and one screeched, "Oh, god, you're so skinny!" I did not know if she was complimenting or insulting me because after that comment she stared me down and left. The stares and whispers made me feel more insecure until I began to think of myself as a "freak."

Since my growth spurt occurred so rapidly, people were shocked to see "the new Ariel." Well, "the new Ariel" also shocked Ariel. My height and weight did not match up. Whenever I would look at myself in the mirror, I would just see bones. I could actually see my bones popping out. My freshman year [in high school] was horrible. I knew I was lanky and there was not much that I could do about it. It also did not help that my older sister was 5'2". With our height difference, people thought it was hilarious that the little sister was taller by far than the older sister.

Learning to Accept Imperfection

I knew I could not shrink my height and my metabolism did not allow me to gain a lot of weight, so I learned to accept my height and weight. I mean, it does not help to obsess over our height and weight. If we do that, then we do not have time to do other things. I feel like whether you are too fat or too skinny, people are going to judge. If you are fat, then you are lazy, and if you are skinny, then you have an eating disorder. It is hard to determine what is the perfect height and weight. It varies from person to person and no matter what your height/weight combination, somebody is bound to criticize it. So, no one is perfect, and that is ok.

Since my freshman year of high school, I have become more comfortable with my body. I still get the occasional stares and comments, but I have learned to not let them get to me. In fact, the other day I was walking to class and a girl loudly whispered to her friend, "OMG! Look at that girl, she is so skinny!" And you know what? I laughed to myself. That girl probably said it out of jealousy. I feel like girls constantly have to criticize others' bodies in order to feel more secure about their own. Society makes it hard to accept different body types. Each body type comes with its own stigmas. But the only thing we can do about those stigmas is ignore them. If I had ignored my classmates' comments earlier, I would have had more self-confidence earlier and not felt so insecure about my body. [We should] accept our bodies because they are the only ones we've got!

Ariel: Ignoring the Skinny-Talk

Ariel's essay offers fascinating insight into the culture of skinniness in high school. She documents the kinds of viciousness that biobullies routinely mete out in gym class, in the hallways, and in the lunchroom. Earlier chapters revealed how overweight kids are routinely called "abnormal," "ugly," and "lazy." Ariel shows how underweight kids like herself (and Sabrina) are placed even further beyond the pale—they are called freaks, weird, and alien. Those words and the social exclusion that goes with them wormed their way into Ariel's consciousness, altering her sense of self, lowering her self-confidence, and making her feel like a reject from society.

What is unusual about Ariel is that she is able to shed the identity of skinny outcast. She comes to understand that judgment about bodies is ubiquitous, that perfection does not exist, that her body size cannot be changed, and that it is smarter to simply ignore the biobullies. Although Ariel gives no hint about what enabled her to rise above the insults, the fact that her bodily "flaws" were not fatness and shortness but, rather, skinniness and tallness—both of which are valued in our culture and so subject to less derogatory weight-talk—undoubtedly helped her eventually escape the weight-based identity.

Mislabeled and Mad: Blasting the BMI

Very thin youngsters face not only cultural pressures telling them they are "too skinny" but also the medical label of "underweight." For those with BMIs under 18.5, such as Seth, the young man we meet here, the label "abnormally skinny," backed by medical authority, tends to cement the feeling that there is indeed something biologically wrong with them. Unlike the others we have met, however, Seth knew from the signals from his own body that he was in fact thin and healthy. Angered by the constant comments and weight-gain practices imposed on him, he not only rejected the label, he developed a larger critique of the BMI itself.

Diagnosis, Underweight . . . and under Suspicion: Seth's Story

Typically, doctors use the BMI scale to diagnose a youngster as overweight or obese. In some cases, however, they use it to diagnose a child as "underweight," a label that invariably brings on suspicions that the youngster is concealing anorexia, a much more serious disease. In this essay we meet Seth, a twenty-two-year-old part-Caucasian, part–(East) Indian, with roots in northern California. Seth's auto-ethnography relates what happens when, at the age of twelve, this rebellious young boy became the target of overzealous medical labeling—by his very own physician-mother.

I have chosen never to acknowledge that I was pushed into feeling as though my weight were an issue while I was growing up. My mom is a physician. In fact, she's a pediatrician who is currently an active spokesperson for the childhood obesity "epidemic." In my opinion, doctors genuinely try to help their patients as best they can. However, certain scales hardly paint the entire picture of somebody, and doctors all too often rely on scientific, quantifiable methods to diagnose a patient. Around my puberty years—age 12 or so—I remember going to the doctor thinking I was healthy inside, only to receive a ho-hum, you-could-do-better reaction to my weight. My mom made it painstakingly clear that my weight was an issue, and her concern grew exponentially over the next five years. Yet my issue was not that I was obese; it was that I was too skinny.

Losing the Game of Life—by Middle School

I can't recall what number I was on the BMI scale—it was somewhere on the borderline between "normal" and "underweight." All I can remember from that period was that this newfound attention to my body was unwelcome and the birthplace of a few insecurities that I've had to battle to this day. Before being labeled underweight by a medical authority, I never thought twice about my body or that it was slender. I ate three times a day, got lots of exercise, and usually had well-rounded meals. The label "underweight" [stemmed from] an irrational concern of my mom and my doctor that I wasn't eating enough. From there it went downhill, [and everything I ate was] monitored and micro-managed by my mom.

At first I began to believe that I was too skinny and there was indeed something wrong with or unhealthy about me. My developing mind didn't know any better and it is natural to believe what your mom tells you about yourself. I started feeling insecure and self-conscious about my skinniness. The breaking point came when my mom began to suspect I was anorexic. My mom would interpret any little food-related issue as a sign that I was indeed anorexic. For example, if I was not hungry for dinner she would see it as my forcing myself not to eat. If I was picking at my food, she would see proof of my anorexic tendencies. Being suspected of having anorexia, I felt like already, by middle school, I had lost at the game of life. That label truly spoiled my identity, and I had lost control over my life to medical authority.

From Distress to Anger at the Society-Wide Attachment to a Faulty Scale

The anorexia suspicion crossed the line, however, since anorexia is indeed a serious disease. After years of forced protein shakes, huge bowls of pasta, and ample amounts of 39-cent McDonald's cheeseburgers, [I grew irritated at the constant reminders about being too skinny] and grew tired of being nagged about something I could not change. I changed my attitude and accepted that I was slender and healthy, and shifted my focus from internalizing the medical diagnosis to rejecting it in its entirety. I am also stubborn, and being stubborn about my perception of my body is what helped me ultimately reject the medical [view] that I'm unhealthy because I'm underweight. I became infuriated and disappointed by the fact that my mom seriously believed I had a medical problem. That, in retrospect, was the most [deeply] affecting and heart-breaking realization that I came to. I knew that there was nothing wrong with me, I knew that I'm naturally on the slender side, and I knew that I had a healthy, active lifestyle. Interestingly, my dad, who is also a physician, never once thought that there was something wrong with my weight, [probably because] he was also incredibly slender when he was a teenager. Yet my mom, who is supposed to be there and support me, jumped onto the medical bandwagon and declared me to be somehow unhealthy. This was all a direct result of that physical exam that revealed my BMI number. I've spent years overcoming the irrational insecurities that developed from the label "too skinny."

The point of this brief glimpse into my life is not to bash my mom or the medical world. It's to bash the importance of the BMI scale in modern medicine. If less emphasis were put on a person's BMI reading, there would be a more balanced and accurate approach to labeling somebody as healthy or unhealthy [and eating disordered]. I know my mom was looking out for my best interests and she simply wanted me to be healthy and happy. Her medical training, however, failed to let her see the effects such diagnoses have on a patient. My mom did not intentionally harm me, and I forgive her and still love her for who she is. In fact, had this experience never happened, I probably wouldn't be half the person I am today.

From "Anorexic" to Critic of the BMI: Seth's Transformation

Seth's story provides a compelling example of the profound transformations in identity that can be wrought by a medical diagnosis of the diseases of underweight and possibly anorexia. From a healthy, happy, active boy who thought nothing about his weight, Seth became a worried, insecure youngster who thought his low weight meant there was something wrong with him requiring medical monitoring and correction. Seth's narrative illuminates how much damage well-meaning physicians can do by rigidly applying the BMI scale and treating thinness as a disease. Young

Seth suffers iatrogenic injury—not just his identity as damaged goods but also long-term insecurities (not named) and a feeling of being betrayed by his own mother. Unlike most youngsters, who internalize their diagnosis and endure in shame, Seth is able eventually to see the medical label as flawed. This realization fuels his outrage and anger at medicine, leading him to reject the diagnoses and become an ardent critic of the BMI and its tendency to create disease where it does not exist.

Becoming a Skinny Person

These essays open up an entire world of skinniness—identities, bodies, and lives—that few Americans even know exists.

Skinny-Talk and Practices: The World of the Uber-Thin

Regardless of gender or ethnicity, everyone we've just met reported similar experiences of being skinny in a fat-obsessed world. All were subjected to a constant barrage of unwelcome skinny-talk. Acting as responsible biocitizens who seek to coax—or ridicule—the abnormally thin to become normal, the people in their social worlds felt compelled to remark on their skinniness, as though that were the most important thing about them. Some of the comments were pedagogical (compliments, diet tips, and encouragements to eat more), but many more were abusive. Meantime, the wider culture of media images, clothing offerings, and so on provided constant reminders that those with skinny bodies did not belong to mainstream society.

Underlying the comments and cultural images is a set of assumptions about ultra-skinny people that appears to be remarkably widespread. These assumptions parallel, almost point by point, the assumptions and biomyths we uncovered about obese people. Skinny people are presumed to be abnormal, unhealthy, and closet anorexics. Skinniness is deliberately chosen, the result of a willful decision to undereat or remain on a diet, not an uncooperative biology. Not only can they gain weight, it is easy for them to do so. Because they are not gaining, evidently they are bad Americans who, through inattention or vanity or sickness, do not take proper care of their bodies. Thinness is deemed a moral defect through and through.

Just as obese people are assumed to have character and other flaws, some of our thin informants are subject to a further set of assumptions about their character defects. Linh, in particular, was believed to be physically and mentally weak, incapable, childlike, and unable to take care of herself. Whereas obese people are said to be irresponsible, abnormal, and lacking in self-control, at least they remain part of the human community; others can relate to their putative weaknesses. Skinny people, by contrast, are placed beyond the pale into a category of the not-quite-human. From the stares and whispers Ariel endures to the "constant astonishment" Sabrina experiences to the blanket rejection of people like Jason simply because they are small and skinny, these young people are made to feel like outcasts (Huy), aliens (Sabrina), or freaks (Sabrina). Whatever the term, what they all signal is that no one in their social worlds can fathom why skinny people would "choose" to remain so unappealingly thin; their experiences are so far outside the norm that no one can empathize with or relate to them.

Just as fat-talk is associated with a set of practices aimed at eliminating the disease of obesity, skinny-talk is attached to a set of practices designed to name, address, and fix the opposite "problem." Doctors diagnosed my young informants as underweight and anorexic and began surveilling and managing their eating to correct their "disease." Several of the moms put their kids on special diets and medicines intended to increase their body weight. Schoolmates placed them on "anorexia watch" in the lunchroom, eyeing them closely to make sure they ate (Ariel). One (Linh) was subjected to outright discrimination in the workforce because a potential employer thought she was too "weak" to do the job. And worst of all, from their perspective, the anti-obesity campaign has been so focused on helping heavy people lose weight that it has created no diets, medicines, or other techniques to help the underweight add pounds and become "normal." No wonder these young people feel ignored, "left behind" by society and the medical world alike.

Skinny Selves: The Inner World of Skinny Personhood

Living in a world that is constantly telling them they are flawed and unacceptable, it is not surprising that most of these young people take on the identity of the skinny subject, at least for several years. In a now-familiar pattern of identity formation, as children most never cared about or noticed their low weight. When people started making fun of them, they became self-conscious about it for the first time. Then, as the skinny-abuse and pressure to gain weight persisted year after year, they came to see themselves as abnormal, skinny people who needed nothing so much as to gain weight and become "normal." One (Huy) even took on the identity of "anorexic" to fit peers' perception of him and to gain attention. Just as, for many girls, fat is a dominant identity, for these guys and girls, skinny is a dominant identity, one that seems to crowd out other important aspects of who they are. The essays reveal a continuum of skinny identification, however, from those who identify totally as skinny and unhealthy (the Asian boys and Linh) to those who are able to grow out of it and see beyond it (the Caucasian girls and Seth).

The characteristics of the "skinny person" were remarkably similar to those of the "fat subject." First, like being overweight or fat, being skinny was considered a despicable condition that was bad in almost every way. Every one of these young people hated being skinny and felt that their skinniness made them deviant, flawed, and sickly. Some admitted that they felt unattractive and even disgusting. One felt like a big disappointment. Clearly, the BMI discourse that defines underweight as a disease has done its work. Although two of the young people (Jason and Seth) knew that their dads had also been skinny as young men, they were so trapped in the discourse of personal responsibility for weight that they did not put two and two together to realize that being skinny was most likely in their genetic cards. This insight could have saved them a lot of heartache.

Being skinny also brought a host of negative emotions that ranged from hurt to anger, humiliation, shame, low self-confidence, and poor self-esteem. None reported any positive feelings about being uber-thin. If these six cases are any indication, skinny people are also subject to some social exclusion, although less than that suffered by the very fat. Although none reported a lack of friends, several said they felt isolated and alone, misunderstood by everyone around them. Finally, all were obsessed with their low weight and preoccupied with body practices to increase it. Just as fat personhood involved obsessive dieting and exercising to lose weight, skinny personhood involved constant struggles to eat more to gain weight. Exercise was not part of the program because it was seen as dangerously weight-shedding.

Larger Consequences of Pathologizing and
Stigmatizing Skinniness

What, then, are the effects on their bodies and lives? Evidently, all the
skinny-talk of the concerned biocitizens in their worlds did not work to
turn these young people into good biocitizens. Not only did no one gain
weight and keep it on, in the face of so much pressure some turned to
patently unhealthy eating practices in an effort to add pounds. Believing
that high-calorie and high-fat foods make people fat—a widely publicized
warning meant to get heavy people to avoid them—several of these young
people sought to stuff themselves with such foods to gain weight. In a per-
verse logic, Sabrina was thrilled when she gained weight, even though the
added pounds were the result of dropping her exercise routine and snacking on junk food. So obsessed were they with their skinniness that, ironically, some of these youngsters became bad biocitizens—that is, people
who used *un*healthy practices to change their weight—in effort to achieve
normality. Put another way, they prioritized their weight over their health.
At least one, however, sought to gain weight in healthful ways—by eating
regularly and well and remaining fit (that was Linh). Yet, despite mighty
efforts over many years, no one was able to become a normal-weight person. And with no advice available, no one saw any way out. Clearly, their
weight, far from being wilfully chosen, was biologically based.

The essays make clear that, for these young people, skinniness is not a
disease but just another way of being in the world; as they insist, and the
evidence they present suggests, they are skinny *and* healthy. Yet in a world
where all bodies are understood through the medicalized language of the
obesity epidemic, they are treated not just as diseased but also as freaks
simply because they are "too thin" rather than the much more common
"too fat." The larger effects on their lives are worrying. Skinny youngsters suffer not only emotional distress from all the stigma and biobullying; their lives are diminished in many ways. Linh's life prospects seem
especially dimmed. Facing a family that pushes her onto less difficult life
pathways and workplaces that actively discriminate against her because
she is "weak," she will have to fight hard to realize her true promise.

Others suffer damage to their mental and physical health. Seth's experience of being labeled unhealthy and anorexic by authoritative figures left

him with insecurities that he is still fighting years later. Facing constant bullying, Jason was forced to give up his favorite sport, handball, the one thing that brought him recognition and built up his physical prowess and coordination. Those who undertook diets of high-calorie, high-fat junk food jeopardized the good health they already had in a futile effort to add pounds. The field of medicine suffers too. Seth's account suggests that physicians lose credibility and authority when patients misdiagnosed as unhealthy and anorexic discover the mistake and become hostile toward a field that uses a limited measure to deliver an inappropriate and damaging diagnosis.

If overweight and underweight young people all suffer so much on account of their body sizes, surely those at medically normal weights feel good about their bodies. Or do they?

6

"NORMAL"

People I know seem to use the word "fat"—or "fatass"—very often to describe themselves. Yet the majority of my friends are a size 4 or 6. Is that what fat is? I believe that it is the average body size for a female; average body size is normal. Yet normalcy does not seem to be acceptable. Females want to stand out, to be complimented, and to be different. Being skinny and thin can [bring them] one step closer to perfection.

MELINDA, FROM HER ESSAY "THINK THIN" [SC 59]

The overriding emphasis of the war on fat is getting people in "abnormal" weight classes to shrink down to "normal" weight. What about those whose weight is already "normal," that is, whose BMI falls between 18.5 and 25? (For a 5'6" person, a weight of 115–154 is "normal.") Are they happy with their weight and bodies and selves? Are they socially rewarded for achieving a medically normal weight? Do they even see themselves as "normal"? We really don't know. Given their achievement of "ideal" bodies, one would expect their experiences to be celebrated in the media. In fact, they are ignored. Not only is there no reality show called "How I Became Normal," "normals" don't have a public presence at all—they don't talk about themselves and their lives in public spaces. The odd result is that we seem to know an enormous amount about obesity but almost nothing about normality.

In this chapter, we turn finally to the question of "normality," aiming again to learn three things. What social and cultural pressures, if any, are "normal" weight people subject to? Do people self-identify as "normal," and if so, what are the characteristics of normality? What are the broader consequences of being "normal" for young adults' health and lives?

The public discourse on the obesity problem leaves normality as an unmarked category, a blank with little content. The implication is that once people achieve normality, as long as they continue to be reasonably virtuous biocitizens, they will be content with their bodies. The California essays tell a different story. They suggest that few people who fall into the medically normal weight category are satisfied. Why? Because, in addition to the medical norm of normality, there are cultural norms of the ideal body and the cultural norms have much more force than the medical ones. In the "flawed" weight categories we have examined, the two norms largely coincide: being too fat or overweight is considered both medically dangerous and culturally unacceptable. The same is true for underweight. In the "normal" range, however, the two sets of norms diverge. In popular culture, the medically ideal body is deemed too chunky for girls and too scrawny for guys.

In southern California, where the motion picture, television, and recorded music industries play outsized roles in defining the cultural norms surrounding the body, no one wants to be merely normal. In the popular mind, normal goes with ordinary, plain, uninteresting, and lacking in distinction of any kind. Instead, as Melinda notes in the epigraph, everyone wants to stand out. Girls and guys want to stand out in different ways, though. Girls want to be ultra-slim ("size 0" or "perfect"), while guys want to be hyper-buff ("strong" or "manly"). As we saw earlier, all the good things in life are believed to go with these body types—and to a certain extent they do.

In the first two sections of this chapter, we meet some of these medically normal but deeply dissatisfied young people. Although they are the targets of much less weight-talk than those we've already met, in their self-perceptions and bodily practices these normal-weight young people who see themselves as "too fat" or "too scrawny" are almost indistinguishable from the overweight and underweight people we encountered earlier. The reason is that the women see themselves as *virtual fat persons*, who are little different from real fat persons, or as *at-risk fat persons*, who are consumed by fears of getting fat. For their part, the men see themselves as *virtual skinny subjects* or *at-risk skinny subjects*.

In the first section, we encounter two normal-weight women who, viewing themselves as virtually fat or on the verge of becoming fat, are miserable about their extra pounds and devote huge amounts of energy to excising them. We also meet a normal-weight man who is so distressed about his "small, skinny" body that he becomes an obsessive body-builder. The war on fat may not have fostered the identity "normal," but it has certainly encouraged the emergence of a new (or newly heightened) identity among some normal-weight people: that of the *health freak*. For those who claim it, health freak is a positive identity that denotes a person who dedicates his or her life to the pursuit of "optimal" health. A health freak is someone who is hooked on the science of diet, exercise, and other bodily disciplines and devotes much of his or her life to becoming a kind of hyper-healthist super-biocitizen. If we look more closely, however, we see that what drives the obsessive healthism is a deep fear of bodily failure, in particular, of gaining (or losing, for men) significant weight. Underneath the proud health freak, then, is an at-risk fat (or skinny) person who fears nothing more than becoming fat (or skinny). In the second section, we meet two striking examples of the health freak. Although both are able to lower their weights and maintain them within normal levels, their auto-ethnographies highlight the inordinate amount of work that is required to keep bodies that are prone to gain weight within the bounds of "normality" and the price young people who see themselves as potentially fat pay to stay on the right side of the BMI line.

In the last section we meet two of the rarest young Californians of normal weight, those who are comfortable with their own normality. Rejecting the public health notion that there is an ideal weight, they celebrate the beauty in all bodies. Readers may not be surprised to learn that both are what we might call *post-fat subjects*, people who once viewed themselves as fat but then, in a transformative moment, came to see beyond the culture of ideal weight to embrace a more accepting view of their own body and more positive, non-weight-based identities for themselves. We read their auto-ethnographies to see what allows some fortunate young women to escape what Kristen, one of my informants, calls the "beauty monster" that eats up so many girls.

Normal: Still Not Thin (or Man) Enough

In southern California, where beautiful bodies are de rigueur, most young women at the middle or higher end of the "normal" BMI range feel too large. They feel, in other words, like virtually fat subjects. Marissa, our first subject, is an Asian American, whose community defines thinness as the sine qua non of feminine beauty. Lindsey, our second, is a Caucasian who is comfortable enough with her normal weight but, after a recent weight gain, is consumed by fears of losing her healthy, fit body. Our third subject, Brandon, thinks his stubbornly short, skinny body makes him unmanly, marking him as a virtually skinny person. Despite their medically desirable weights, all deeply believe they are flawed (or at risk of becoming flawed) and commit huge amounts of energy to getting the body society says they should have.

SoCal, Where Size 0 Is the New Normal: Marissa's Story

Marissa is a twenty-one-year-old Chinese American raised in the largely Chinese community of Monterrey Park. Although struggling financially, her parents have the highest expectations for their children. This essay, by a close friend, brings out the extraordinary power of the media as a biopedagogical force. Through stories like the one of a star's fashion gaffe, the media teach us what counts as a desirable body and what we must do—or not do—to achieve it.

Media Messages

[For the body-conscious, it is hard to forget the Jessica Simpson mom-jeans incident. In early 2009,] the tabloids and gossip blogs had a field day when an unflattering picture circulated of Simpson dressed in high-waist "mom jeans." Simpson has always been known to be a little on the curvaceous side, but when this picture appeared, people began to speculate that she [had] gained a little weight. The media puts a spotlight on her noticeably fuller figure, further supporting our society's perception that being thinner is more attractive. When women and young girls see this image bombarded all over the media [with captions such as, "Jessica Simpson Shocks Fans with Noticeably Fuller Figure"], they are led to believe that a curvy, full-figured body is unattractive. In order to be accepted as beautiful by society, they have to look like the rail-thin celebrities and super-models.

My friend Marissa was extremely horrified at this disastrous fashion ensemble. She deemed the high-waist mom jeans a major fashion no-no. She went on to proclaim that mom jeans can only look "right" if you have a "long torso and long legs;" otherwise, you'll end up looking like you gained several pounds. Marissa fully believes that the extra baggage on people's body [keeps] them from being considered beautiful.

Parental Pressures: Mediocrity Not Allowed

"My mom has always told me since I was little that if I was skinnier, I would have been pretty, and I think that's true." Growing up in an Asian American household, Marissa has always felt that the standards are different from those of normal American households. "You can never be mediocre," she explained; "if you are, that means you're not trying hard enough." Marissa's parents immigrated to the U.S. when they were in their late twenties and they have always worked hard to try to move their family up the social ladder. They have always been extremely hard on Marissa and her siblings. Her parents have always tried to push her academically by enrolling her in after-school tutor programs, piano lessons, violin lessons, and art lessons. And in return, she has always been obedient, trying to please her parents by getting the best grades, becoming the captain of the tennis team, and joining several clubs and organizations on campus. But one area in which she fails at pleasing her parents is weight.

Since she was younger Marissa's relatives would always comment on her weight. They would compare her to her female cousins, commenting that her arms are a little thicker and pinching the extra fat that hangs off her body. Marissa remembers distinctly one of her aunts telling her mother, right in front of her: "It's such a shame that she is fat; she could have been pretty." These [constant] attacks on her weight and body have lowered her self-esteem. Whenever her mother took her shopping Marissa would always stick to oversized sweaters and t-shirts. Even when the weather was hot, she refused to take off the sweater or jacket she was wearing because she felt self-conscious about her "overweight body."

A Life That Revolves around Weight

As a young adult living on her own these days, Marissa has learned to stay away from junk food, not only because it is unhealthy but most importantly because she doesn't want to gain any more pounds. After entering college, Marissa gained the Freshman Fifteen. When she had added an extra 13 pounds to her 125-pound frame, Marissa decided to try the "Special K diet" that she had heard about from one of her dormmates. According to the Kellogg website, a person can lose up to 6 pounds by substituting a bowl of

Special K cereal for their daily meals for two weeks. On the eighth day, Marissa caved. She couldn't stand to eat cereal for another day and went out to buy an In-and-Out hamburger.

After discovering a street-fashion blog one summer, Marissa tossed her oversized, plain t-shirts and jeans aside and began to consciously dress more fashionably. These fashion blogs [only made her more self-conscious] about her weight. One of the major things she notices on these fashion communities, such as LOOKBOOK.nu, is that only super-skinny girls can look good in certain [fashion] trends. She believes that she [can't wear them] because she is "too fat" and "they wouldn't look right on me."

"According to the BMI charts, if I gained another five pounds I would be considered overweight," said Marissa. Standing 5'3" and [weighing] 135 pounds, Marissa is tremendously unhappy with her body [BMI of 23.9]. She tries to live a healthy lifestyle by exercising three times a week and avoiding eating out whenever she can. But she is disappointed that she hasn't [achieved] any significant weight loss in the past year. Sure, she has more curves than those stick-thin models and her stomach may stick out now and then over her jeans, but she is certainly not overweight. To be sure, there are those whose weight borders on the morbidly obese, but what about those Americans who aren't a size zero and who aren't obese? There is still negativity shed on those who don't have a toned and slim body. Marissa's story exemplifies how her life pretty much revolves around the issue of her weight. Weight is a burden on her life and holds her back.

Marissa: A Failure Twice Over

In this essay, a concerned friend describes how the media and the ubiquitous weight-loss advertisements work to deepen people's self-consciousness and anxieties about their weight by defining curves as unacceptable, trumpeting the benefits of weight-loss products, and featuring fashions that look good only on ultra-skinny bodies. As media frenzies develop over the bodily faux pas of the stars, producing a cascade of biting commentary, the effect is to reinforce the dominant thin-is-in norm and create a whole new class of virtually fat persons unhappy with their not-quite-perfect bodies.

As a Chinese American, Marissa suffers a double dose of pressure: from the wider culture and from her family. In Chinese American culture, ordinary is never good enough. The constant criticisms Marissa heard as a young girl still weigh on her mind, leaving her with a damaged identity, a sense of herself as "too fat" and a disappointment to everyone. Although her BMI puts her in the high-normal range, as a southern Californian and a Chinese American, she experiences her life as a virtually fat person because she lives in an environment where any woman who is not size 0 is by definition "overweight." In college, Marissa becomes a virtuous biocitizen who reorganizes her life around weight control. But her quest to achieve a pencil-thin body founders, leaving her feeling like a failure in life. In our weight-obsessed society, where cultural standards for the acceptable body are much harsher than medical ones, almost everyone who has some "imperfection"—and who doesn't?—is at risk of becoming a virtual fat subject.

At Risk of Losing My Normality: Lindsey's Fear

In this essay, we meet Lindsey, a twenty-year-old Caucasian from a middle-income family in Alameda County, in the Bay Area. A multisport athlete during her early years, Lindsey finds in college that she has no time to work out and is vulnerable to gaining weight. Unlike Marissa, she is not obsessed with being skinnier than "normal." But she has another body-based fear—a dread of becoming fat—that keeps her equally preoccupied with her weight.

Weight is something that I have thought about a lot more than I needed to. Ever since I can remember, I have been involved in multiple sports. In elementary and middle school I played softball and basketball. Then in late middle school and throughout high school I focused on volleyball and played both school and club again. It got to the point where I would have some kind of practice or tournament almost every single day. When I was playing sports, weight was something I consistently thought about but never had to worry about. I could eat anything and everything I wanted, knowing that I could burn it off almost instantly.

Coming to college showed me a whole new side of things. This was the first time I did not have planned-out practices where I would get my daily and weekly exercising in. Now, going to the gym is an extreme struggle for me. I am now so unmotivated and lazy that getting ready to go work out is a chore on its own. That mind-set of being able to eat anything is now coming back to haunt me. I am in the "normal" range according to the BMI. The problem is that I now put on weight based on what I eat. I try to be careful about eating sweets and junk food. I also try to have a healthy diet. However, I see and feel the effects of eating unhealthy much quicker than I used to. I will sometimes slip back into not thinking about [what I eat] and then realize I am gaining weight.

Now, because of the media, women are expected to be perfectly fit and extremely skinny. We are put under such a harsh scrutiny to fit this almost impossible-to-reach goal. People judge you based on your weight. If you do not meet society's standards, you are almost looked down upon. Now that I am gaining weight [for the first time in my life], weight seems like a big issue. [Although] I am a "normal" weight I am always concerned about not passing this point. Weight now has become almost a fear for me. I am always worried about losing that healthy weight. I do not want to be the girl that people look down on or make fun of based on something as superficial as weight. My goal now is to lose this fear. Yes, I want to still eat healthy and exercise, but I do not want to let it take over my life. I do not want to define myself by what I look like.

Lindsey: Twice Guilty

Lindsey is a classic, and acutely self-conscious, at-risk fat subject whose goal is to keep from gaining weight and losing the healthy body she has enjoyed her whole life. She faces a problem familiar to many American adults: work or study keeps them so busy they have little time for exercise. Given the obesogenic environment in which we live and a willing body, unless she constantly works at weight control, she will put on pounds. Although she watches her diet carefully, she cannot bring herself to exercise, and so the fear of weight gain preys on her mind.

Lindsey reflects on the oddity of someone of normal weight not relishing the achievement of a culturally valued status but, instead, being consumed by the fear of descending into abnormality (fatness) and being subjected to the stigma and ridicule that status brings. She is keenly aware of the contradictions society imposes on young people—and especially young women—of being defined and, in turn, defining herself by her appearance and weight, while at the same time resisting being defined by something so shallow. Her hope now is to escape, to rid herself of the fear of weight gain. So far, though, she has found no way out. As a result, she suffers a double dose of guilt—the first for gaining weight and the second for letting her weight define who she is.

Addicted to Bodybuilding: Brandon's Struggle to Escape Normality

Brandon is a twenty-two-year-old Filipino American from a middle-class family in San Diego County. Although his weight is normal by the standards of medicine, by the standards of manhood in American society his body falls badly short. Just as the women viewed themselves as virtually fat, Brandon sees himself as virtually skinny, an identity so intolerable that he throws himself into a body-modification regime that quickly takes over his life.

Feeling Skinny and Inferior

Hello, my name is Brandon. I am a male of Filipino descent who was always considered skinny. My earliest memory of thinking about my height and weight was around the fourth grade. Among the boys, those who were wider and taller were [considered] tougher and stronger. I remember thinking, "What if I don't get to be that tall?" I also realized that I was skinny. In my middle school years, I felt inferior to the other boys who were able to get girlfriends and be popular. [I wasn't sure] what it was based on—handsomeness, height, weight, or some mystery [ingredient]. My inferior body was one of the main things I suspected. I [was so concerned I avoided getting into fights or arm-punching matches with boys who were bigger than I was].

I had my final growth spurt—to a height of 5'7.5"—at the end of sophomore year [in high school]. I was proud of my height for a while, but my closest friends kept growing and eventually got taller than me. In high school a lot of our identities were defined by what naturally happened to our bodies. For most of my friends and me, we tried being as lazy as possible in PE and we ate what we felt like eating. I weighed about 130 pounds throughout high school, so my BMI was about 20, which is in the normal range, but I always felt too skinny.

The first difference between the guys I wanted to be more like and me was that they had abs. Another difference was that my arms were thinner than those I compared myself to. My surroundings told me that I was too skinny and that shaped me to think less of myself. The second semester of sophomore year, I took weight training as a PE substitute. During this year, I was most proud of myself being "the bicep guy" among friends also taking the course, but the older guys were still much stronger and bigger. I was able to reach a weight of 140 pounds while taking this class. In junior and senior year, I thought less about my weight because I was busy with more social activities.

Becoming a Bodybuilder

In college beginning the spring quarter of junior year, I started working out consistently. During my first 12-week plan, I gained a great amount of mass. I started off around 130 pounds and now weigh 165 pounds, which makes me overweight on the BMI chart. I looked toward the online community for advice. I came upon Bodybuilding.com, which gave advice and a simple workout regimen to follow. I only took a few key points away from the site: eat more, eat often, work out consistently, and sleep well. Diet has always been hard for me. It's hard to eat often when you have classes that are back to back. Buying the "good" food is difficult; it must be cheap, and if it's cheap it'll need to be prepared. Working out is easier, but it takes time—at least an hour and thirty minutes each time. I stay consistent for the most part, going out of my way to make sure I get my workout. The guys I see [at the gym] all the time look like amateur bodybuilders. I get inspired to work hard by knowing that I might be able to get there.

I've taken a plethora of supplements in my efforts to gain mass and strength. I would guess that I've spent over $400 on supplements since last year. I consistently buy a whey protein which costs $30 per month. I'm not entirely sure if any of the supplements actually work, but I continue to invest a lot of money in them. I am probably just another victim of the advertising for supplements.

I've thought of myself as skinny all my life, so now that I have the time, I work to not be my former self. I'm 165 pounds and still not satisfied. It's a kind of addiction for me to keep working out and getting bigger. I probably have a warped idea of how my body is. It takes a lot of time to prepare all the meals in the day and it takes time out of my day to work out. I like the times that I work out because I feel like I'm doing something more productive than just sitting at home [playing video games]. I am still a beginner bodybuilder in my eyes [with much farther to go].

Brandon: The Skinny Story of my Life

In this essay, Brandon documents how his identity as a virtually skinny person emerged: in grade school he developed a consciousness of himself as being too short and skinny and, then, in middle school he began to see himself as inferior because of his twig-like arms, small stature, and overall weakness relative to other boys. Brandon crafts a skinny narrative about his life, in which his major identity is his extreme thinness and his problems in life—his inability to get a girl, his lack of popularity, and so on—are all due to his pole-like shape. By college, this appears to be the dominant story of his life—all this despite the fact that his weight has always been medically normal!

Believing the biomyths that everyone can achieve the ideal body and that a perfect body will bring a perfect life, Brandon adopts a host of healthist practices in an effort to gain weight. He develops a passion for bodybuilding, which, once it shows results, develops into a time-consuming and expensive addiction. Despite a substantial weight gain—to a medically overweight level—he keeps obsessing because he cannot shake his childhood view of himself as skinny and inadequate. Brandon sees himself as a virtuous biocitizen who is willing to spend the time necessary to prepare all those meals and to work out all those hours because it is so much more "productive" to be building one's body than engaging in other "wasteful" activities, such as gaming. Brandon is somewhat aware of how the culture has trapped him—he notes his distorted body image and his victimization by the supplement advertisers. Yet in his obsessive focus on fitting in and becoming a "real man," he is unaware of the costs this life project has imposed on him. The biggest cost may be the loss of other identities and pursuits that he might find more satisfying in the long run.

Health Freaks: Extreme Biocitizenship and Its Costs

Many American are concerned about diet and exercise, but some take these concerns to an entirely new level. Often guided by the popular science of nutrition and sport they find on the Internet, they micromanage their food intake and exercise in an effort to optimize their health and bodily appearance. Although the motivations are complex, the desire for a slender body is central, marking these people as at-risk fat subjects whose body projects are driven in good part by a desire to avoid becoming fat. In this section, we meet two self-identified health freaks, Jade and Sarah, who are able to maintain trim, fit bodies only by becoming extreme biocitizens who devote much of their life to the pursuit of that agenda and build their core identity around this project. We will see how young people can become so entranced by the promise of science to remake their bodies and lives that they reorganize their entire life around the quest. We see, too, some of the hidden dangers of their pursuit of "health" at any cost.

Health Freak and Proud of It: Jade's Story

The protagonist of this unusual story, Jade, is a twenty-year-old Chinese American brought up in a middle-class family in San Diego. After a childhood as a chubby, junk food–addicted tomboy, Jade's life is completely transformed by a high school health class, whose scientific discourse on health and weight becomes the guide for her life.

I have never had an eating disorder and I have never been morbidly obese, but I have been obsessive about my weight. If you ask any one of my friends to describe my current dieting behaviors, they will immediately say "health freak," and yes, I have to admit that it is true. It is a blessing and a curse, but in the end I am glad that I'm a meticulous eater because I know that in the long run, my body will be functioning at a healthier level. Eating healthy at a time like this where we are constantly surrounded by fast food chains and sweet temptations has not been easy. Achieving the balance that I have today with diet and exercise was incredibly difficult because I spent most of my life struggling with weight.

A Round-Cheeked Tomboy

As a fourth grader, my round cheeks and protruding tummy didn't exactly scream healthy. I was pretty much a tomboy who never wore any super-tight clothing or cared about how I looked at school. I never read nutrition facts, and my parents never told me what [foods were] healthy or unhealthy. I never figured that burgers, pizza, soda, or cheetos would do me any harm. Around sixth grade, I grew a few inches taller and the weight began to distribute more evenly. My massive cheeks and round tummy shrank and I was in better shape as I became a playground monkey. [Neither my] weight nor my diet was ever on my mind.

In middle school, things started to change. I was entering the teenage world where girls began wearing make-up and getting boyfriends, and the "popular crowd" began to form. I started becoming more feminine and realized that I had an appearance to maintain. In addition, my older brother was taking a health class in high school. He started telling me about how soda and processed meats were unhealthy and he himself began to be health conscious and avoid those foods. [With friends] I started watching MTV, VH1, and TV sitcoms. [For the first time,] I [began to notice] women and how they were portrayed.

Becoming a New Person

[During] freshman year [in high school], I took the same health class as my brother. By the end of the year I had become a new person. I began the sport of tennis and ended up making the team sophomore year. I put hours into vigorous practicing on the court with my coach, who put me through the most physically challenging [regimen] of my life. That year my body also took a drastic turn. My legs were no long unshapely sticks; they became toned and muscular. I gave up fast food and soft drinks and most of the time I ate health food at home. I read nutrition facts often and went from reading not only the numbers on the label but also the ingredients in the foods. Despite my change in diet, I was still dissatisfied with my weight. During my junior year, the most stressful time in high school, my weight rose to almost 140 lbs. And I am only 5'4". I spent that year wearing a large sweatshirt because I couldn't stand my thunder thighs and lower gut. I graduated high school dissatisfied with my weight and figure, despite my change in lifestyle.

Today, as a [twenty-year-old], my weight fluctuates constantly, with the main contributors being stress, school work, and lack of time. However, [my weight] is more controlled than it has ever been. I have to say that I am proud that I became a health freak. It was something that I achieved on my own and it has benefitted me in ways that I could never imagine. My diet has helped me do better in school and kept me on my feet. In addition, my workouts have helped my asthma, which was very severe [when I was] a child.

A World Full of Challenges

My aim in writing this essay is to express [how] difficult it is growing up in this world. I know that eating healthy is good for my body, but I think in the back of my mind, one of my main motivations was to be skinnier. I have always put so much pressure on myself to be in great shape and I have always wanted to do it the right way—meaning eating healthy and exercising. Sometimes I ask myself, "Why am I like this and who am I doing it for?" Surely, I don't see any of my roommates eating these high-fiber cereals, brown rice, or soy protein. I have to say that this is a personal issue of mine. For many years now, I've suffered from a visible genetic skin condition for which there is no cure. I want to be healthy and fit so that I can look at my figure and see that I am beautiful despite my skin. Moreover, as a chubby teenager, I always feared that I was perceived as someone who was lazy and lacked control. I have always wanted people to perceive me as someone who is in control of her life.

At this point, I believe that I will forever be a health freak who constantly weighs herself and reads nutrition facts. Re-reading this essay makes me feel ashamed at how much I have valued appearance. I think there are many aspects of who I am that greatly outshine my physical appearance. However, it is a difficult journey to discover happiness and contentment with one's body.

I have to admit that today I am not completely satisfied with my body, but I am learning to love it more and more.

Jade: An American Success Story

In this fascinating essay, Jade relates how she acquired her identity as a totally disciplined biocitizen who takes heroic biocitizenship as her core identity. In framing her story, Jade draws heavily on the dominant obesity epidemic discourse on Americans' personal responsibility and civic duty to manage and optimize our own health. She frames her narrative around the tropes of the American success story: personal courage, self-control, individual struggle, and eventual if always tentative triumph. In her account, she has undergone a long struggle to become thin and fit into an environment full of challenges—ignorant parents, a naturally heavy body, a deforming genetic disease, and a world full of fast food and sweets. Through years of courageous personal struggle, she has overcome the obstacles and prevailed to achieve a level of body management that allows her to proudly claim the identity of health freak.

Jade represents the epitome of what the anti-obesity campaign is trying to produce: biocitizen subjects who take the pursuit of health and normal weight as their central task and follow the latest science in that endeavor. More than any other young person we will meet, Jade takes it all in, earnestly making biocitizenship her core identity and major life project. This wholesale adoption of the dominant paradigm is evident throughout Jade's essay. For example, she assumes she is responsible for her weight, she employs a machine model of her body (which "functions at a higher level"), and she views bodily control as a cardinal virtue. And reflecting the assumption that all Americans should scientifically manage their diet, she is critical of her parents for not being nutrition-savvy.

Jade notes that being a health freak is "a blessing and a curse," but her essay lists only the blessings. Yet one can find hints of the curse. Her extreme obsession eats up her life, precluding the development of other identities or activities that might bring her more intrinsic happiness and better prepare her for adult life. Moreover, the biocitizenship model might not in the end produce thinness or health. Will Jade wake up some day and realize that she gave up her youth to the pursuit of an impossible goal?

Heeding the Experts: Sarah Becomes a Health Fanatic

Next we meet Sarah, a nineteen-year-old middle-class Chinese American from Temple City, a largely Chinese town in LA's San Gabriel Valley. A self-aware, smart young woman with a rebellious streak, at a tender age Sarah discovers the seductive online world of nutrition, exercise, and weight gurus. Ignoring her parents' cautions, she makes herself over in the experts' image, with decidedly mixed results.

Secrets of the Body Only One Click Away

My parents had *Yahoo!* as their [Internet] homepage, and one day [when I was in grade school] I stumbled upon an article about health. It intrigued me. I wanted to know more about what is "healthy" and what is not. What foods, looks, body types, and lifestyles were considered "healthy?" I searched and found *Yahoo!'s* health page, [where I] read about BMI, superfoods, exercising tips, and so on. At the time, I had no idea what the BMI was or what it was for. For [the next] few years I read more and more, [absorbing] personal stories, tips from doctors, and explanations of nutrition labels. My thoughts and opinions on health, fitness, and the perfect body were being shaped by the articles I was reading. I felt knowledgeable, and I was determined to shed some pounds because the articles told me to.

When I turned 11, my body began to change drastically. I began gaining a lot of weight and [watched as] my face got rounder and my stomach bigger. My parents would say in Chinese that I was getting fatter, but in a positive tone that meant I was healthy. But at one point those comments [took on] a negative tone. I was getting *too fat*. Because I was already reading health articles diligently at that point, I knew the steps [I needed to take] to reduce my weight. I vividly remember making monthly and weekly charts for exercise, diet, and weight: 93, 95, 96, 98, and the deadly 99. I felt saddened when my weight increased, not knowing it was all a part of physical growth. I could not possibly pass the 100 mark at age 12—I had to diet and exercise.

As I continued through middle and high school, I [remained] very physically active while watching what I ate. I counted calories from age 13 but never religiously. I learned what anorexia and bulimia were, but I knew I [could not develop] those diseases because I loved food too much to not eat or to throw it back up. Instead, I used my interest in food to cook healthier meals. [Meantime], I had very low self-esteem for those six years, wearing baggy clothes to hide my fat. As I matured, the fat started to balance in womanly areas. My friends would tell me I was not fat, but I knew I was. I was determined to lose weight, even after I learned more about the BMI and found I fit into the "normal" range.

Misplaced Faith in the Popular Science?

At the end of my high school career, I had more time on my hands. I got a [gym] membership and started to vigorously work out. I felt like I was becoming more toned and was burning more calories. My self-esteem shot up when people started to notice my new figure and my family members praised me for my good work. However, my weight did not drop; rather, it rose due to the added muscle mass. Even though I [understood the connection], I continued to work toward losing weight. I suspect this is because I had grown up believing I had to lose weight. The articles, doctors, and television shows all told me so. [At the time] I was [totally] fine with my obsession with health and fitness. I enjoyed learning scientific information like what chemicals went into processed foods. When I read an article, I looked at it as an opportunity to learn and expand my knowledge, not as "laws" I had to abide by.

Today I realize that biological factors do play a part in how much fat I carry. [Although] I have adjusted my eating and exercise habits to have a healthful lifestyle, I still count calories and get upset when I see the fat around my abdominals. In my own eyes, I still need to lose those extra 5 pounds because I want to run faster and be less at risk of some sort of medical disease in the future. I know [now], though, that there is much more to health and beauty than weight. When I was growing up, I disregarded most of [my family's] comments because I was rebellious. But because I had faith in doctors and people who dominated their professions and were well educated, I fell into their traps instead. In the end, after all the restrictions and long hours of exercise, I am very glad that I am open-minded enough to realize that not everything doctors and nutritionists say is true. [So now] I will eat that red velvet cupcake if I want to, but then go running afterwards, of course!

The Seductions—and Dangers—of Popular Science:
The Lessons of Sarah's Life So Far

In Sarah's tale, we can see the incredible allure of the scientific story about diet, exercise, and weight, which is a ubiquitous part of our culture and, of course, a centerpiece of the war on fat. As a young girl not yet ten years old, a curious Sarah was seduced by the scientific fairytale that holds that there exists a "perfect" and "healthy" body, and that everyone can achieve that ideal body by following the expert advice (a core biomyth in the war on fat). Trusting the well-educated experts, like Jade she remakes herself into a health fanatic who obsessively tracks her diet, exercise, and weight in a relentless effort to optimize her body.

While noting the subtle pleasures of being a virtuous biocitizen—the intriguing information; the belief that one is leading a better, more productive life; and the comfort of knowing that one's actions are helping prevent future disease—Sarah's story also reveals the dangers of exposing impressionable young children to scientific stories such as these. Such dangers are legion. As an eleven- and twelve-year-old, Sarah begins exercising even more vigorously, not realizing that her weight gain is a normal part of adolescent development. In middle and high school, although her BMI is normal, she diets obsessively to achieve an imagined optimal body. After high school, she works even harder to lose the extra 5 pounds, even though that additional weight was the result of growing muscle mass from excessive exercise. Sarah's reading of the expert advice made her think she was on her way to success, when in fact her project was bound to fail because the ideal body, if such a thing exists, is unattainable and because there are limits to our ability to control our bodies. Sarah used up a large part of her young life learning these hard lessons.

Post-Fat Subjects: When Normality *Is* Good Enough

Among the essays, there were a handful written by young people who had transcended the culture's—and their own—weight obsession and learned to be comfortable with their bodies, "flaws" and all. In some cases, there came a point in a young person's life when the accumulated pressures to achieve a rigorous body ideal became so onerous that the person was finally able to see how they had trapped him or her for so long. Our first writer, Megan, fits this profile. In other cases, an intimate partner's abusive comments spurred a moment of rare insight, in which a girl was able to see through the shallowness of the cultural obsession with skinniness and give up the ideal of perfection. Our second autoethnographer, Kristen, exemplifies this pattern. In both cases, the journey was one from fat subject to a post-fat subject who has transcended body hatred and fat personhood and arrived at a place from which she can see the problems with our culture's fat obsession with special clarity. Coming to terms with their own bodies allowed the young women to stop basing their identities on their bodies and to embrace other, more rewarding identities instead.

My Journey as a Female: Megan's Story

Megan is a twenty-one-year-old Caucasian who grew up in two of the epicenters of the cult of the toned, thin body in SoCal: San Diego and the wealthy OC coastal enclave of Newport Beach. An unusually self-aware young woman, Megan documents how parental and other pressures turned her into a perfect biocitizen and, then, how she came to reject that obsession with bodily perfection in favor of other identities that felt more authentic to her.

I'm a 21-year-old white female and I grew up in San Diego [with my mom] and Newport Beach [with my dad]. I've always been pretty thin, and for the past few years weight hasn't really been at the forefront of my mind. Nonetheless looking back, [I see that] weight *has* had an effect on who I am, who I will become, and what I've thought of myself through my journey as a female.

Parents Pushing Biocitizenship

My first issues with weight began when the Atkins Diet became very popular. My mom has always been a bit obsessive about her weight, and as soon as she heard that there was a diet which would help you start losing pounds in just a week, she was all over it. The Atkins Diet emphasizes that you radically cut back on consumption of carbohydrates. At this point, I was in middle school, around seventh or eighth grade. I thought her dieting woes were silly at first, but when she told me she was actually losing weight, I remembered my friends talking about their own weight and wondered if I was skinny enough. My mom encouraged me to go on the diet, too, even though I was already pretty skinny. I decided to join her. One day, when I visited my dad, my step-mom saw the list of foods I'd eaten that day with the carbohydrate and fat content [written] next to them. The list was [so] short, she [expressed] concern about how little I was eating. I told her the diet was largely popular, so I knew it was safe. But [that diet] didn't last long.

I remember when I was first introduced to the Body Mass Index. I was still in middle school and stood at a lofty 5'9″ and weighed about 125 pounds. When I calculated my BMI, it barely met the cutoff for "healthy weight." Most people would have been happy with this, or perhaps a little concerned that they should add a few pounds to their body. But me? I was upset. Pissed. Depressed. Healthy weight? That puts me in the same category as people I considered "chunky." I didn't want to be healthy, I wanted to be underweight. I had the height, but I was sad that, according to the scale, I didn't have the weight that the models and celebrities I saw in ads and on TV had. I needed to be skinnier, but I was unwilling to starve myself to get there. At the time, I also lived in a "bad" neighborhood in San Diego, so going outside [for exercise] wasn't an option.

Fast forward to high school. I decided to move to my dad's house in Newport Beach and attend high school there. This gave me a new sense of freedom. I could go for walks, stroll to school, and explore the outdoors that I'd always loved so much without feeling unsafe. As I continued living at my dad's house, he forced me to get involved in a sport and go to the gym. I've always been more of the creative type, finding more joy in photography and reading than running and trying to get a ball in a hoop. But my dad is very stern, and I ended up joining my high school's basketball team. I was only on the team for a year because the athleticism it took exceeded what I was willing to give. But that didn't mean that I would be allowed to give up the gym. My dad was always pushing me to do something athletic—basketball, tennis, dance, running, or becoming a gym rat. I couldn't escape it.

As I look back on my life, I realize just how much both of my parents pushed thinness on me. My family is full of tall, lanky people, and I am no exception. I've never reached a point in my life where anyone could have called me "fat" or anything close to it—except my parents and grandparents. I remember visiting my grandma one afternoon and having her tell me that I looked "fatter than before." Her comment sent me to the living room crying. My mom came up to me later to try and comfort me. I told her that I felt my nana was out of line with her comment. My mom agreed and consoled me, saying, "I think she just meant that your legs look a little fatter, but your stomach looks good!" That was my mom's kind of comfort.

Free to Be Me

Finally, the day came when I started college. Finally, I would escape this madness. I could do what I wanted and be happy with who I was, without a parent or family member reminding me of my imperfections. As soon as I started at UCI, however, I joined a sorority, which emphasized physical looks over anything else. The cycle continued. During my time in the chapter (I'm no longer in the sorority, in part for this reason) I tried to uphold all the standards it set. You know how women's inner thighs can get a little fatter near the crotch area? I had that and wouldn't wear shorts because of it. I was 5'9" and skinny as can be but couldn't wear clothes that showed my "fat."

I was a slave to the institutions that continued this cycle: the family members who ridiculed me, [the sorority that valued looks above all,] and the media that made me want to be someone else for a majority of my life.

Last year, I made the decision to free myself. Now, I'm about 135 pounds, but I feel beautiful when I look in the mirror [BMI of 19.9, still very skinny!]. I don't have the ripped abs I had once done 500 crunches a day to achieve, but I've finally ripped off the chains that kept me from reaching this liberation. Sometimes, I still see models or friends with that "perfect" body and wish I had it, too, but I know there are much more important things than looking like them. Whenever I go home, my mom comments on her own weight: she's too fat, she can't drink orange juice because it has too many calories and so on. And now I feel bad for her. I hope she can escape this trap, too.

Chains That Chafe: Megan's Journey to Self-Awareness

In her essay, Megan deftly charts the forces that turn young women like herself—white, naturally tall and thin, relatively well-to-do—into, as she puts it, "slaves" to the institutions of contemporary feminine biocitizenship. She describes how a young girl who loves creative endeavors and is subjected to her parents' and grandparents' continual criticism of her "imperfections" develops a raw self-consciousness about the softer parts of her body. As early as middle school, young Megan scorns the idea of being in the same "normal, healthy" weight class as girls she views as "chunky," aspiring instead to be underweight like the super-models and celebrities. Unlike the vast majority of girls in SoCal (and elsewhere), Megan's 5′9″ height and her white skin allow her to dream the impossible dream—of actually achieving our culture's anorexic-like ideal of pale feminine beauty.

Like quite a few SoCal parents—especially economically privileged ones—Megan's are harsh biocops, with each parent pushing one plank of the biocitizen program on her. Going to college, Megan finally escapes her parents' pressures, only to become trapped in a similar set of pressures from her sorority. Feeling imprisoned yet again, she made up her mind to free herself from the harsh, now largely internalized demands of bodily perfection and accept a low-normal weight body as just fine for her. Whether she could have cast off the body obsession if she was heavier is unclear; it seems doubtful. Megan experiences this change-of-direction as a giant liberation that will allow her to claim other, more creative identities that were buried in the avalanche of biopolitical demands during her childhood and adolescence.

More Than Just Looks: Kristen Finds Her Own Path

In this inspiring essay, we hear the sweet voice of Kristen, a twenty-year-old Japanese American raised by middle-class parents in the LA South Bay city of Gardena. Kristen is the rarest of young women—one who managed to escape the beauty trap and define herself as much more than a body image. Here is her tale of entrapment and escape.

Ever since I was little, I watched shows like "Power Rangers" and "Sailor Moon" and wanted to be the beautiful character. The character with the longest legs, the prettiest face, the nicest hair, the skinniest waist, and the best body shape—that was what my friends and I aimed to look like and to be in life. Our thought was: "If I look like that, I am bound to be successful." Now that I'm older, I realize that looks are not necessarily everything, and although I still find myself buying make-up, contemplating diets, and so on, I try my best not to give into the judgments of society. As I look back on my past, I am glad I did not give into the beauty monster that society turns so many young girls into.

I come from an all-Japanese family, but my grandparents and parents were born and raised in Lima, Peru. From there my parents immigrated to LA. When I was growing up, my mom and dad never really chided me for my weight. They just wanted me to finish my food so I didn't waste any of it. I remember comments like: "She sure finishes everything on her plate," or "Your daughter is very good at eating." I did not think much of it, and I still do not. Luckily, my parents did not make me see such comments in a negative light. It was not even until middle school that I had any [thoughts of] weight loss, dieting, or exercising.

The BMI Score: "Too Average"

I guess I never really knew the ideas [that were prevalent] in our society. In seventh-grade PE class, though, I [was] weighed and measured for my BMI. I remember this because at first I had no clue what BMI even meant. When all my friends were gathered in the line to take the measurements, they were whispering and chattering on and on about how this girl *had* to be a certain BMI because she was so big or so skinny. It was then that I encountered my first feelings of fear about my image. Since I did not exercise regularly and I ate whatever I wanted, I was very afraid that I would be classified as having too much body fat, that my ratios would be all off. When I got measured, I was relieved to find that I was perfectly average. However, that feeling did not last long. Some girls around me looked at my paper and said, "Yeah, you would get average; I mean, you're not fat, but you're not skinny [either,] you know?" It was then that I began feeling the need to diet and exercise because I was too average. In order to be perfect, I needed to have almost no body fat. The girls in my class all exclaimed at the girls that had dangerously low body-fat ratios. They were the pretty ones whom everyone envied.

Although this event shook me quite a bit, it did not affect me as badly as it did others. I remember trying to exercise, but my laziness got the best of me and I ultimately decided that I might as well [forget it and] just live my life and be happy. [But] my other friends, especially the boys, got hit hard. I remember that my friend Johnny [simply] stopped eating. I tried to talk him out of not eating, but he wouldn't listen. He told me that he was a man and could take care of himself. He got really skinny, and no one else ever said anything about his eating habits.

The Boyfriend: "Saggy and Ugly"

The next instance of [extreme] image-consciousness came during senior year of high school. I had just been asked out by this cute guy. He did not eat much and was quite skinny. I was the opposite! I always ate something every few hours! I felt so awkward and ashamed that I stopped eating in front of him. On dates, I asked him to not look at me while I ate. I said it jokingly, but something inside of me really meant it.

I remember going to the mall with one of my guy friends and hearing him say that I did not have as curvy of a figure as before; [in particular,] my butt was no longer existent. Although he meant to make fun of me, it backfired [and I started drastically dieting]. That boyfriend would always [comment on] how saggy my arm fat was or how ugly I looked a certain day. He would even point out any blemishes or acne marks on my face, when he himself had imperfections! [Eventually] I broke up with him because I wanted to rid myself of anyone who would put me down because of the way I looked.

Although I still get ashamed and embarrassed about how I look, I try my best to reflect the person I am inside. It is hard to not fall into the "normalities" of society. But I feel that I can try to provide a good example for my younger cousins and show them that being a girl is not about being an image. We are all so much more than looks. I am glad I found the right path to approach beauty and weight, and I hope I have the courage to help anyone who [struggles with these issues] as [much as] Johnny and I did.

On a Mission: Kristen Commits to Making the
World a Less Weight-centric Place

Kristen may be the most fortunate young person featured in this book. Whether they were simply relaxed about their daughter's weight or, as recent immigrants, oblivious to the cultural anxiety about obesity, diet, and exercise in children, Kristen's parents treated her weight and its management as nonissues, giving her the space to figure out her relationship to her body on her own. Because her parents never made her weight part of her identity or made her feel that her body was problematic, Kristen seems to have emerged from childhood with a genuine confidence in herself, a sense that she was good just as she was. She was certainly subject to her fair share of cultural and peer pressures to be thin; her essay highlights the role of school fitness tests in inducing a weight obsession among young girls and boys, and the damaging effect of peer culture, which taught her that she was "too average" to ever be popular. Yet, through her own life experiences and observations, Kristen was able eventually to step outside that culture of thinness and see its limits. What she concluded is that she— indeed, everyone—is more than her weight or body, and that people who judge others harshly because of their appearance are not worth having as friends. What is heartening is not just that Kristen has the wisdom to transcend the body-obsessed culture of her peers and the courage to break up with a bullying beau but also that she has taken it as her mission to help others see that we are so much more than our bodies and our weights.

No (Self-Identified) Normals Here!

Normality, a medically idealized but culturally invisible category, turns out to be highly complex and productive body status. Because their bodies are not especially remarkable, normal-weight kids are largely free from biobullying, but they receive biopedagogical advice from many sources. Three stand out in these essays: the media, popular science, and school fitness tests. In our media-saturated world, the media are arguably the most important source of biopedagogical advice on the good body, teaching us what kinds of bodies are desirable and whose bodies we should emulate. This is especially true for today's young people, who grew up with the media as major forces in their daily lives. Kristin documents the power of children's TV to turn tiny viewers into Cinderella and Prince Charming wannabes. Others describe the impact of pop stars. With their seductive images of the beautiful bodies and exciting lives of the stars, celebrities, and super-models, the media teach that medical normality and cultural acceptability belong to two separate universes. For women, they instruct, the culturally desirable body is twig thin and large breasted; for men, it is tight and buff with ample musculature. Unless one has these attributes, a medically normal BMI score will bring praise from no one except, perhaps, the doctor. The media also teach that normality—whether medical or cultural—is nothing to be aspired to. To gain social approval, we need to look superlative, distinctive, special. That may be why, compared to fat-talk and skinny-talk, there seems to be little that might be identified as normal-talk. There was only one example—when Kristin's classmates berated her for being "too average"—and it reinforced the negativity around normality.

Advertisements for foods and health and beauty products (from "lite butter" to "low-cal breakfast cereal") have long taught us how to identify and fix our bodily "flaws." Today, however, a major source of the critical information needed to be a virtuous biocitizen is the popular science of diet, nutrition, and exercise that is almost inescapable on the Internet and in print media. As the stories of Jade and Sarah suggest, the popular science of the body, with its aura of objective scientific truth, is hugely tantalizing to children and teens looking for ways to fit in and gain the holy grail of "health." The ability of youngsters to find and absorb all these scientific facts in the privacy of their bedrooms is one of the many attractions. Impressionable young children are easily seduced by the fairytale that, simply by following the advice of the experts, they can create the perfect bodies that the world so admires. Little do they know, such articles are often infotainment, sponsored by food corporations and ghost written by paid writers with a profit-making mission. For the unwary, dangers abound. Many experts are self-proclaimed only. Far from being cut and dried, the science is often contested. What appears to be hard fact may be fuzzy fiction. Not only may the promised solutions not work but, as we will see next, they may also pose bodily hazards. And when the scientifically recommended practices take over young lives, the result may be anything but the promised health and perfect body.

We have seen the importance of health-care professionals in inducing weight consciousness in children. This chapter has elaborated on this by illuminating the role of school fitness tests in creating weight worries among grade and middle school youngsters. Kristen documents the troubling impact of these tests on children as young as ten. Surrounded by an aura of scientific authority, the tests teach children that some bodies are good, while others are bad and must be fixed. As they receive their BMI results, then, youngsters also receive the message that their weight is a moral matter. More generally, the tests induce body-consciousness in children who rarely thought about their bodies before. Administered in public, they also give scientific weight to the everyday practice of comparing bodies while creating a new hierarchy of good and bad BMIs, deservingness and lack of it. For young children, who want nothing more than to fit in, the tests establish a new pathway to inclusion or exclusion. The tests teach children that not just schoolwork but also their weight, over which they have little control, is a critical measure of their performance and suitability for inclusion in the categories "proper pupil" and, by implication, "proper American." These tests may help the schools promote fitness (by providing data needed to measure and monitor health status), but in the process they produce body anxieties and weight obsessions that, as the essays suggest, can last for many years.

The outsized pedagogical role of the media helps us understand why, despite the war on fat's goal of normality for all, in southern California normality scarcely exists as a culturally meaningful social category or personal identity. Not one of the young people we met here saw him or herself as normal or put his or her energies into becoming a normal person. Instead, responding to the wider culture of biocitizenship, they all became fat subjects of varying kinds. This happened in three ways.

In the first, young women with high-normal BMIs, who saw themselves as "too large," began to craft fat narratives about their lives and eventually became virtual fat subjects who dieted and exercised obsessively to lose weight. In a parallel process, the normal-weight young man we met, who deemed himself "too skinny," created a skinny narrative about his life, gulping down supplements and exercising obsessively to gain muscle mass. In the second pattern, kids of high-normal weight became health fanatics who devoted their lives to the pursuit of "health." Far from identifying as normal, the two health addicts created an alternative, morally superior identity—that of health freak who, through intense commitment and hard work, is able to pursue and achieve higher, more worthy goals than most mortals can imagine. Yet beneath the preoccupation with health was a deep concern about weight. At heart, they were at-risk fat subjects whose obsession with healthist practices and heroic moral subjectivity were driven in good part by a deep-seated fear of fat. In the third pattern, some young people, who had been subjected to pointed fat-talk and identified as fat, were able eventually to transcend that experience and learn to accept normal weight for themselves. They didn't identify as normal, but they gave up the obsessive body practices and were able to make weight a secondary issue in their lives. They became post-fat subjects who were fashioning identities based on attributes other than weight.

Of the manifold effects of these new identities for the young people's bodies and lives, two are especially important. First, despite their corporeal normality—which should bring *relief* from the culture-wide obsession with weight—these young people are just as obsessed with their bodies as their peers who are over- or underweight. In the most extreme cases, the health freaks, the quest for bodily perfection leads to extreme practices that endangered their health. With their narratives of achieving moral superiority through super-biocitizenship, they were unable to see the costs the impossible quest for "perfect health" or the "optimally managed body" was imposing on them.

There was one encouraging effect, however. The handful of young people in my study who were able to overcome a history of biobullying and accept their merely normal bodies as fine were able to see beyond the cultural obsession with bodily perfection to the damage that obsession does. One sought to draw on her own life experiences to make the world a better place, a place where all bodies are seen as beautiful and where the measure of human value is broadened to include much more than looks. Her transformation contains hopeful possibilities for a post-war-on-fat future.

Part 3

Uncharted Costs and Unreachable Goals

7

Physical and Mental Health at Risk

My closest friend [is beautiful] but she always thinks she needs to lose more weight. A few weeks ago, she went on this diet called the "lemonade diet." For ten days she had nothing but this lemonade that she had to prepare with organic lemons, cayenne pepper, and organic syrup. She would also take a laxative tea every night to flush out everything in her stomach. Struggling to fight her hunger, she was torturing herself in order to lose a few pounds. After only a few days, she looked so weak. The liquid diet was taking a toll on her mood as well. And still she pushed herself to go to the gym. After ten days she had lost ten pounds, and was so excited to find that the diet worked. Now her habits and practices have rubbed off on her friends, who are trying the diet too.

GABRIELLE, FROM HER ESSAY "10 DAYS, 10 POUNDS" [SC 178]

The essays we've read reveal how the societal war on fat is producing a generation of young Americans with spoiled identities whose members no longer see themselves as good, socially worthy persons. The dominant narrative on obesity expresses worry about the harm obesity does to the nation's health, health-care costs, and productivity. This narrative about what counts has become an unquestioned truth that has hardened into a kind of dogma, crowding out other ways of understanding the obesity problem and keeping us from seeing things like the shrunken selves of young people as issues worth attending to. In this chapter, we explore a possibility that has been almost inconceivable in terms of the dominant discourse: that the fight against fat has not only diminished selves but has also damaged the bodies and health of some of the most vulnerable members of our society.

Hints of such adverse, iatrogenic effects can be found in the public health and medical literatures. For example, the research on fat stigma reviewed earlier provides powerful evidence that weight stigma, which has increased in recent years, is deeply damaging to its victims. A second area of concern has been eating disorders, described by S. Bryn Austin as a "blind spot" in the push for childhood obesity prevention.[1] Until very recently, obesity researchers have essentially ignored the possible connections to eating disorders. In the eating-disorder community, however, there has been growing concern about the possible iatrogenic effect of childhood obesity-prevention programs on the development of risk factors for eating disorders.[2] The research of Dianne Neumark-Sztainer and her colleagues reveals a striking prevalence of dieting, self-weighing, and disordered eating among middle and high school students.[3] These researchers have traced such behaviors in part to weight teasing and diet encouragement in the family.[4] Another study suggests that school-based obesity-prevention programs could be worsening disordered-eating patterns.[5] The possibility that the national campaign to fight fat might be inadvertently diminishing the well-being of fat people and exacerbating disordered eating is worrying enough. But might the damage go even further?

In this chapter, I draw on the California essays to show that the battle against extra pounds is also inadvertently yet systematically harming the physical health of American youth—the very thing it was devised to improve. Such risks to young Americans' health are not only pervasive, I believe, but endemic, built into our approach to the national epidemic of obesity. Although very few are able to achieve long-term weight loss, overweight young people are badgered to lose weight and stigmatized and marginalized for failing to do so. Public health messages and medical advice urge weight loss above all. Believing they are improving their health, and subject to unremitting cultural pressures, heavy youngsters are pushed to go to extreme—and often physically risky—lengths to shed pounds. Bodily damage often follows.

In this chapter, I first cull evidence from the full set of essays on the use of extreme weight-loss practices and the resulting bodily harm. Because they present historically ordered narratives about individual lives and describe the (conscious) motivations for the use of weight-loss practices, the essays allow us to see connections between specific pressures to lose weight, particular weight-loss practices, and various forms of bodily harm in individual lives. Unlike statistical data, these essays allow us to connect the dots between the war on fat and the development of bodily harm.

I then turn to some individual cases to examine those connections up close and personal. I share cases of young people who suffered short- or long-term harm as a result of extreme dieting, exercise, and/or drug use. I ask three questions of these cases. First, what kinds of pressures were the subjects under; are their cases unusual in some way? Second, what practices did they undertake; did they know of the dangers? Third, what are the likely long-term effects of these experiences? Are those who risked their health likely to do it again, or did they learn a difficult life lesson they won't repeat? Because the connections between the risky practices and physical effects are quite straightforward, rather than including separate discussions of each essay I analyze all the essays together in the chapter's conclusion.

We then turn to the links between the fight against fat and the development of eating disorders. Although the essay assignment asked students to write about diet and weight, more than a fifth chose to write about full-blown eating disorders. Clearly, anorexia and bulimia were on their minds and were closely connected to diet and weight. Eating disorders are quite prevalent in southern California. The surveys I conducted reveal that during the years I taught "The Woman and the Body" (1995–2011), fully 63 percent of women students (1,582 students in all) knew at least one person with an eating disorder. Roughly 10 percent knew five or more.[6] Some replied that "every girl I know" or "more than 70 percent of my friends" were eating-disordered, suggesting the prevalence of these problems in some social circles.

The essays I gathered do not allow me to systematically address the many ways in which obesity, starvation, binging, and purging are entangled. They do, however, enable me to illustrate some of the ways in which the extreme cultural and medical emphasis on getting rid of extra fat at any cost seems to be pushing some people down a slippery slope into full-fledged eating disorders. In the chapter's penultimate section, I provide an overview of the almost fifty essays dealing with eating disorders and then present three for closer reading. These essays make clear that the line between the everyday dieting and exercising expected by the culture and eating-disordered behavior can be quite fine, and that efforts to achieve an ideal weight and be a good biocitizen can easily tip over into an eating disorder, especially, but not always, when an emotional trigger is present.

Risky Practices and Their Bodily Effects

Facing both external and internalized pressures to lose weight, but with few effective means to achieve that goal, the young Californians featured in the essays tried harder and harder to "drop pounds," as they put it. With no understanding of sensible limits on these practices, they reasoned that the less food and the more exercise the better, intensifying their routines when the pounds did not fall off and turning to risky practices when safer ones did not work. The result was a veritable epidemic of extreme and potentially dangerous weight-loss practices. Extreme dieting is so common as to be unremarkable. Young children incessantly pressured to lose weight or bullied for being fat put themselves on virtual starvation diets, depriving their bodies of needed nutrients. Some reportedly did not eat for several days to a week [SC 12, 16, and 28]. Others lived on extreme diets such as crackers and water [SC 223], vegetables and ice [SC 173], water and salad [SC 1], or brown rice [SC 23]. Exercise addicts reported working out three hours a day for seven days a week [SC 30] or going to the gym twice a day, five days a week [SC 39]. Teenagers desperate to shed pounds often treat dieting as a competitive sport, inventing contests in which groups of young people egg each other on to eat less each day [SC 3 and 177]. The winner is the one who consumes the fewest calories—without succumbing to health problems.

Often, extreme diets are coupled with excessive exercise in which young people, usually men in high school or college, take on ever more difficult workout routines on the assumption that the combination of relentless exercising with eating next to nothing will relieve their bodies of unwanted pounds. Typical cases include the boy who lived on fruit and water then ran 3 miles every day [SC 25] and the girl who starved herself while attending dance practice four hours a day [SC 242]. The regular use of extreme diet and exercise practices was not only normal or common, it was normalized—considered nothing unusual. Indeed, for anyone with a little extra body fat, the use of such practices was expected, even demanded, by almost everyone in their lives. When groups of friends follow rigorous diets or exercise programs together, the attitude toward the routines is quite cavalier—because everyone's doing it, there couldn't possibly be a safety problem.

When diet and exercise don't work, or work too slowly, young people often turn to diet drugs and other quick-fix solutions. People learn about them from friends or family members—including their own moms—or from searches on the Internet, which is full of ads announcing dramatic weight-loss successes for little effort and even less cost. (A Google search for "weight-loss drugs" in July 2014 yielded 79.6 million hits.) The most frequently mentioned of these methods is laxative (or detox) teas, which are drunk after meals in order to, as one young woman delicately explained, "clear [or flush] out the systems" [SC 175]. One of the most popular is the lemonade detox, described by Gabrielle in the epigraph. Its association with celebrity Beyoncé Knowles made it a "hot" weight-loss method. For some, the "cleansing" performed by these potions is routine practice. For others, it is a less than pleasant experience not to be repeated: "Detox tea is like a tea bag that you place in hot water and then after drinking it, it creates [an] instant bowel movement. The next morning I woke up in major stomach pain and couldn't go to my classes. Instead, I spent most of the day either curled up in my bed or in the bathroom. The tea made me literally empty [everything] out [of] my stomach, from the food to the water. I reassured myself that I would not try it again, but I still longed to lose weight" [SC 48].

The use of diet pills—prescription and, more usually, over the counter—is widespread. For many if not most, the prospect of losing weight, generally through stool and water loss, silences any nagging thoughts that they may not be totally safe. One pill-taker writes, "Those extra few pounds were gone in two weeks and I felt good. Being able to walk around freely with just a bikini was refreshing and a proud time for me. Even though I hadn't done the healthiest thing to get there, I didn't care. If it meant looking good and fitting in with girls much smaller than I was, then I was willing to do it" [SC 13]. Although these pills often help eliminate pounds, they carry significant risks, such as fatigue, weakness, shortness of breath, dehydration and, in some cases, serious allergic reaction. The same pill-taker who had so proudly paraded around in her bikini decided to press her luck and try again. Choosing a different brand of pills, she ended up in the hospital with a major outbreak of hives—a frightening experience that, however, did not convince her to toss the pills [SC 13].

Still others use the stimulant Aderall to suppress their appetites. In some groups, cocaine seems to be normalized as a weight-loss strategy because, one writer explains, "Coke has been constant and consistent. It works every time" [SC 22]. Despite its addictive character, cocaine use is encouraged by media stories and the accompanying before-and-after photos of celebrities who gain the desired rail-thin body on the drug, apparently with few ill effects. The often casual attitude expressed toward cocaine use comes through in this excerpt from an essay describing a group of buddies in Long Beach: "One of my friends once tried coke for a few weeks to see how much weight she could lose in a month. My other friend who was recently arrested for possession of cocaine is going through NA [Narcotics Anonymous]. Her biggest fear is that she's going to gain weight" [SC 22].

The extent of unhealthy and potentially or actually damaging weight-loss practices in the essays I gathered was quite astonishing. A close analysis of the essays shows that in the vast majority of cases the featured subject engaged in potentially dangerous weight-loss practices. A breakdown by type of practice can be found in table 7.1.

Those undertaking these practices were oblivious to the potential for bodily harm. Nor did they understand the nutritional implications of their dieting practices. As a six-year-old, one young woman wrote, she "had no concept of calories or burning them," she "only understood the concept that food makes you fat" and so started drastically restricting her intake [SC 87]. Her case is typical. In the essays, people described in extraordinary detail their diets and exercise regimens, but not one mentioned ever thinking about the dangers or consulting an adult or the Internet to learn about them. Far from imagining harm, most believed that dieting, exercising, and weight loss, no matter how achieved, were good for their health. Some of those resorting to weight-loss pills were vaguely aware of possible safety concerns, but in their desperation to shed pounds, they accepted an unknown risk to their health in exchange for the promise of thinness.

Excessive dieting and exercising pose serious health hazards.[7] Extremely low-calorie diets can lead to a weakening of the heart and fall in blood pressure due to loss of muscle mass, interruption of sex hormone production, a slowing or even loss of bone growth and density that is irreversible, slowed metabolism, drying of the skin, and sleep disturbance. Probable psychological effects include feelings of depression, panic attacks, and heightened obsessiveness. Excessive exercise can cause severe wear and tear on the body, increasing the risk of stress fractures of the bone, injury from a poor workout schedule or accident, muscle damage, adverse cardiovascular events, and, in women, amenorrhea (cessation of menstrual periods).

Widely available on the Internet and in health-food stores, over-the-counter dietary supplements, often marketed as "natural products," are actually diuretics (or water pills), appetite suppressants, caffeine pills, or herbal supplements of little value for weight loss.[8] Nonprescription diet pills often contain undeclared (and unsafe) ingredients or have deceptive labels. They tend to cause unpleasant to dangerous side effects.

Not surprisingly, the essays were full of instances of bodily harm. Some were what we might call the everyday side effects of excessive weight-loss practices: fatigue, weakness, shortness of breath, and mood disorders such as depression and anxiety. These did not receive much comment; instead, they were treated like the ordinary and predictable, if bothersome, costs of being thin and attractive. A close analysis of the essays shows that fully three-quarters of the subjects suffered harm from trying to lose weight. Although the data in table 7.1 are but rough counts, they suggest the pervasiveness of these problems.

TABLE 7.1 Weight-Loss Practices and Their Harmful Effects

	Percentage of total
Practices	
Potentially dangerous[a]	74.2
Disordered[b]	17.0
N.A.	8.8
Total	100.0
Effects	
Full-fledged eating disorder	30.2
Rapid, extreme weight loss	5.7
Other serious harm (injuries, loss of consciousness, etc.)	20.8
Everyday harm only	8.2
Yo-yo weight gain and loss	9.4
N.A.	25.8
Total	100.1

Notes: Sample of 160 ethnographic essays with detailed information on weight-loss practices and their effects, based on the reported behavior of main subject. Table includes only the most serious type of harm mentioned in each essay. N.A., no information available.
[a]Potentially dangerous weight-loss practices include behaviors often associated with eating disorders: binging and purging; use of extremely low-calorie diets; use of weight-loss pills, laxatives, and/or diuretics; use of cocaine or other strong drugs; and severe dieting coupled with excessive exercising. Many subjects used two or more of these.
[b]Disordered practices include extreme dieting and excessive exercising.

Short-Term Harm

We turn now to the essays, beginning with forms of (apparently) short-term harm caused by unwise weight-loss practices: loss of consciousness, elevated blood sugar, and abnormal heart rate. Although such afflictions are often dismissed as passing problems that frivolous, appearance-obsessed people bring on themselves, they deserve close attention, for they could signal (or even cause) more serious and enduring conditions. Aside from the everyday side effects, blacking out is the most common form of bodily harm documented in the essays. Remember April (in chapter 4), who fainted in Starbucks after eating next to nothing for four straight days? That response occurs when the brain of someone on an extremely restricted diet is starved of blood sugar. The person becomes lightheaded and short of breath before losing consciousness. Here we meet Cheyenne, who lost consciousness as a result of starving herself of nutrients.

Americans are constantly told that obesity is a major risk factor for diabetes—and it is—but they hear little about how certain diets to prevent obesity can also predispose people to diabetes. With its reputation as a healthy food, fresh fruit is a core component of the self-made diets of a great many young southern Californians. Souri, introduced later, built an entire diet around fruit, until something happened to make her stop. Heart problems are the most life-threatening of the dangers from nutrient deprivation. Cardiac (and other) damage from starvation starts early, before the person starts to look "too thin." Finally, we meet Kym, whose experience of heart strain shook her world.

Pulling Too Much Weight: Cheyenne
Struggles to be Competitive

Sports help produce healthy bodies, but some have weight requirements that work to reinforce the societal obsession with thinness. In Cheyenne, we have an ambitious rower whose desire to be competitive in her sport led her to take dieting to a dangerous extreme. A twenty-year-old Caucasian from a financially struggling family, Cheyenne grew up in the Bay Area community of Danville; her story of extreme weight loss, however, unfolds in her college home of Irvine.

Growing up, I have always been a little bigger than most people my age. Although most of it is muscle and my body type and shape, I do have extra "baby fat," as my mother always calls it. All the women in my family have weight and image issues, so they're nothing new to me.

The Perfect Sport . . . Except for One Thing

When I got to college it was no surprise that I joined the rowing team because it's a very intense sport that is perfect for my body type. My huge soccer quads and calves were perfect for extending my legs in the boat and my softball arms and back were ideal for ripping my oar through the water. After a month I was competing with varsity girls who had rowed for three and four years. I was so happy to find my niche right away and to connect with a group of girls with whom I would be lifelong friends.

It wasn't until we were competing for a spot in the top boat for season opener that I realized the only downside to this sport: my weight. A typical female rower who's 5'9" to 6'3" weighs between 155 and 185 pounds; a female rower who's 5'5" to 5'8" weighs 121 to 130 pounds and is considered a lightweight. When I arrived on campus, I was barely 5'5" and 178 pounds. This really hurt me when my coach would adjust all our scores in the boat by our weight [which she did] because each rower has to pull her weight. I would be in the top four of the girls on my team based purely on power and how well I could row, but when weight was factored in, I dropped to the middle of the team. Ever since then I've been battling my weight and trying to drop to 150 pounds.

The lightest I remember being in high school was 160 pounds. So last season I [set] small goals for myself. In the span of the season I dropped to 169 pounds, which was almost a 10-pound drop in two months. I dropped the weight in a very healthy way: I cut a few calories out of my diet each day and worked out an extra two to three days a week on top of the six-day-a-week rowing practices. I loved getting comments from people about how great I looked. The last month of school, though, the weight stopped coming off. But I wanted more for myself the next season. That's when I set my goal at 150 pounds, to be reached by the end of the summer.

All last summer I became obsessed with my weight. I weighed myself every morning and after every workout and took my fat percentages. I was forever looking up new exercises and diets. I worked out two times a day for five days and once a day for the other two days of the week. I ate barely anything during the day. I wouldn't eat until I absolutely had to—which was usually around lunch—and then have [only] a small lunch and dinner. By mid-July I was around 163 and hit a wall. So I started becoming more extreme about what I would eat. That's when two very scary things happened to me.

Some Frightening Experiences

One morning I woke up before class to do my regular 8-mile run. I woke up super hungry but I was happy because I had dropped almost a pound from skipping dinner. I was 156 pounds, the lightest I'd been. After I came back from my run I felt kind of weak. I figured I should eat something, but only after I showered, so I could wait longer to eat. I was in my apartment alone in the shower and all of a sudden I felt like I was going to pass out. Then I was out. I woke up lying in the bathtub, alone in my apartment with no one to help me but myself. I somehow focused enough to grab my towel and crawl into my room and lie on the floor. I knew I was extremely dehydrated so I found water and a Gatorade-type drink and chugged all of it. After about 10 minutes of passing out and waking up again and again, I started to feel a little better. This was one of the scariest moments in my life. I felt so vulnerable and helpless. I never wanted to feel like that again just for another pound lost. But just a couple weeks later I did another stupid thing to my body.

I had this idea to do a seven-day detox diet. I won't go into detail, but it basically cut calories a lot, to about 1,000 per day. The third day I was super tired. I was working out about the same, burning at least 2,000 calories, and it had caught up to me from the days before. The fourth day I woke up with a terrible headache and [feeling] super dizzy. I ate the prescribed breakfast shake and proceeded to class. In class I couldn't focus. I was so tired and in such pain I couldn't stand it. I realized I couldn't do this for three and a half more days, so I had a reality check and realized this detox was not for me.

These two occurrences made me think of my mother and her battle with [anorexia] at my age. It took her years of being in and out of hospitals before she realized what she was doing to herself. Whenever I would see pictures of her at 80 pounds I would cringe and promise never to do that to myself, especially since that experience still affects her 30 years later. She gets tears in her eyes when I bring it up. This past summer made me realize I needed to stop obsessing over my weight. My eating problems may not be the same as my mother's anorexia, but they did similar damage to my mind and body. I now rest at a [steady] 168 pounds, but I do have a desire to drop to 160 pounds.

All-Fruit Diet: Souri's Solution

As an Iranian American of upper-class origin living in LA, Souri faces overwhelming pressures to be thin. At the age of thirteen, she devises her own solution to her weight problem, one that seems both super-effective and super-healthy.

> Growing up as a teenage girl in Los Angeles is not easy. As a minority child, I felt pressure to control my weight to fit American and Persian standards. I was raised around the pop culture of the 1990s [when] Britney Spears, Christina Aguilera, and Jessica Simpson were the epitome of female beauty. I wanted to look just like them. Considering I have dark hair, dark eyes, and carry most of my weight in my hips and legs, this image was impossible to achieve.
>
> I began to hate my weight. It did not help that my younger sister was so thin and her breasts were developing faster than mine. My Persian mother would constantly say to me, "Souri, if you want to find a nice Persian boy to date, you need to stay in shape and not eat so much." My middle name means "sweet" in Farsi and I was constantly ridiculed for having a big sweet tooth and gaining a bit of weight [as a result]. Around the age of 13 I started having major jealousy and weight issues. I would exercise and try to eat healthy but could never reach my sister's body size. So, I started dieting and limiting calories. I invented my own diet where I would only eat fruit. For breakfast, lunch, and dinner I only consumed fruit. I began to see results. I thought my diet was healthy [because] we are all brought up to believe fruit is good for us. Every night before I started the diet, my mom had brought me a bowl of fruit and encouraged me to eat that instead of sweets.
>
> I started losing a lot of weight [and was thrilled]. At my annual physical, though, my doctor noticed my weight loss and a spike in my blood sugar level. He advised my mom to make sure I was getting the right nutrients. When we got home I started crying and told her of my all-fruit diet. Instantly worried, Mom reassured me that I was beautiful and began cooking meals that were healthier. She also let up on the taunting. Why the instant change of heart? Because diabetes runs in my family [and] Mom was afraid I might get it.

Starving, Purging, Restricting, Binging . . . but It's
Never Enough: Kym's Life Story

Kym is a second-generation Vietnamese American whose financially struggling El Monte family seemed bent on making sure that every member—including young Kym, who had a larger body frame—achieve the family's ultra-thin ideal. Kym, now twenty-one, ended up paying the emotional and bodily price of their obsession.

I was never overweight as a child, but when I hit puberty I began to put on some pounds. Still, I had not yet reached the threshold of overweight. My mother, [who was raised in Vietnam,] would often emphasize that a woman's worth is not only her achievements but her looks as well. I remember her telling me that it horrified her when she saw people who were obese, and even those who were [only] overweight. She would ask how they lived with themselves and tell me that I should never reach that level of obesity. My family would often joke that I would end up like [those people] and die early. [Their comments] made me feel extremely guilty and angry. They would often compare me to my friends who were what you could call "stick skinny." Perhaps what happened next was a [product] of that comparison.

In middle school [there was] a time when I did not eat for one whole week. I was actually really proud of myself. I do not quite recall what made me stop, but after eating an apple one day, I got extreme diarrhea. My whole body was trembling and I felt like I was going to pass out. I could not walk straight. I felt very afraid and figured it was due to the "hunger strike."

The next thing I tried was binging and purging. This went on for about a month until one day, as I was in the middle of purging, I felt this tremendous strain on my heart. I heard a deep pounding in my ear and everything was wrong. A cold realization came over me and I felt sweaty with chills. I knew this was not supposed to happen. I had heard of models that died years later from heart attacks because they had binged and purged. An incredible wave of fear washed over me. I was not ready to die yet, and I was not going to let myself succumb just to lose weight. I promised myself I would never do that again. [Yet my struggles with food did not end there.]

When I was older my mom put me on a restricted diet. I was allowed to eat little to no carbohydrate, [only] vegetables and some meat. Sweets and junk food were out of the question. I was only allowed half a bag of noodles and she would tell me to put a lot of water in the soup so I would feel fuller. Only that did not work too well because a little while later I would be hungry again, but I knew I was not allowed to eat the other half until it was the "right" time.

When my mom started working, I was elated because I could eat whatever I wanted. I started binge eating and felt happy at first, but then this awful guilt would kick in and I would just feel so awful. I would stuff myself silly, eating so fast and so hard that I barely enjoyed [the food]. I would sometimes sneak food into my room and stash it where she could not see it. I started gaining weight and she threw a fit, accusing me of eating while she was at work and of hiding food in my room. I was so unhappy. I felt so desperate for any [way] to lose weight, but I could not bring myself to purge again. The fear was too great.

I would not say that I had or have an eating disorder. However, I do constantly monitor my weight and often feel guilty if I eat more than I should. I have lost about 15 pounds since my high school years. I am a bit happier, but there is always that thought: "if only I could lose a few more pounds I would be happier."

Musculoskeletal System and Vital Organs at Risk

Excessive exercise, especially when the body is not given enough nutrients, is a surefire way to injure the muscles, tendons, or joints of the musculoskeletal system. In the essays, boys and young men were more apt than girls to undertake extreme exercise programs. Among the essays I gathered, Farid's presented the most arresting case of physiological damage of this sort. Some of the most serious problems reported involved risk to vital internal organs (such as the heart, kidneys, and stomach) from weight-loss drugs. Travis's story is the most frightening.

Born with an Illness—Overweight: Farid's Story

Although boys are socialized to bury their feelings, deep down the harsh judgments associated with "bad BMIs" can affect them as profoundly as they affect girls. In this story, Farid, a sensitive twenty-one-year-old Iranian American from a middle-class family in Yorba Linda (Orange County), recalls a childhood so filled with traumatizing weight abuse that it spurred a drastic regimen of bodywork that left another body problem in its wake.

"He's a Big One!"

From my birth in 1989 to age 16, I was always known as the "fat kid." Even at my birth, a nurse yelling out "He's a big one!" was recorded on my father's hand-held camera. Being born at 12 pounds was not a usual occurrence, and [it] drew extra attention to me as the doctors did their routine check-up. They came to the conclusion that I was unhealthy and might be prone to certain problems if I was to continue to be overweight throughout my childhood. Just like babies who are born with illnesses such as Down's Syndrome, cystic fibrosis, or congenital heart disease, I was born with an illness: I was overweight.

As I grew older, I remained heavier than other children my age. Throughout childhood, I had a BMI ranging from 26 to 28, well into the overweight category. Not only did doctors continue to warn me about the negativities of being overweight, so too did friends, family members, and even strangers. As a child, not having too much control over my weight resulted in others trying to mold me into this highly acclaimed thin, healthy person. In some instances, people directly placed the blame on me and said it was my job to become healthy. When I was 12, people began urging me to watch after my weight. I attempted to eat healthier, but all the food I was surrounded by was high in sugar and fat. How was I to lose weight in such surroundings?

My parents, worried about my appearance, jumped aboard this public health campaign. Soon my mother went from picking up McDonalds to getting me a 6-inch from Subway for dinner. Foods began to transform from such things as whole milk to organic skim milk. Although these efforts seem to be positive the influences of others were quite detrimental. It seemed as though I was not fulfilling my obligation to lose weight, causing society to look down on me. Some people had no remorse for the fact that I was merely an adolescent. For example, at the age of 14, I wanted to try out for the basketball team at my high school. Every day at practice, a certain group of children were to run extra laps around the court for various reasons, such as not listening to the coach or goofing off. [One day] my coach came up to me and said: "Well you're running because you're out of shape." The entire gym started laughing hysterically. I ran the laps, left the gym, and never returned to basketball practice again.

Another [incident] of emotional harm also occurred in high school. It was a week before the prom dance, and I had finally screwed up the courage to ask a specific girl to the event. I took flowers to her during lunch, but she didn't even let me finish my sentence before rejecting me. Later in the day her friend came up to me and said: "Maybe she would have said yes if you weren't as chubby."

Taking Charge at Last: A New Full-Time Job

At the age of 15, I had heard enough remarks on the topic of overweight from the news, my peers, and society as a whole that I made it my absolute [objective] to become this [thin, fit person] everyone was so fond of. Starting off my sophomore year in high school with a BMI of 28, my full-time job became excessive exercising and dieting. I began eating fewer meals a day, with much smaller portions of food, and cut down on my carbs tremendously. Many days I would only eat breakfast or lunch and skip all the other meals. Overall, I had very unhealthy eating patterns. In the span of 6 to 8 months, I had gone down to a BMI of 23.7, which was well into the normal weight category. Everyone complimented my weight loss and treated me as though I were a new person with self-determination and restraint. I even ran into the basketball coach one day. He said I was in great shape and should try out for the team again.

High school passed and college began, as I continued on this goal of having the perfect male body. The perfect male body is a combination of having muscular build and being thin. [Yet] this male ideal is unattainable. Building muscle requires consuming large amounts of food, while being thin requires the opposite. In striving to [acquire that body] I would [lift weights] for hours and diet day after day, not allowing my body the rest or nutrition needed for such a lifestyle.

My excessive exercise and dieting finally caught up with me when I was 18. I developed sharp pains in both shoulders when lifting weights. [I eventually found a shoulder specialist [who] claimed that I have rotator cuff tendinosis.[9] After having been through a family doctor, shoulder physician, physical therapy, x-ray, MRI, and corticol steroid shots, still today I am in severe shoulder pain and unable to engage in any physical activity involving shoulder movement.

Through all my struggles in life and the many goals I have set, the one with the largest impact on me was the effort to [acquire an acceptable male body]. I can tell you I have the appearance of a healthy individual, but am I truly healthier now? Am I healthier now with a BMI of 23 and two injured shoulders than I was earlier with a BMI of 28 and no injuries? I guess I will have to wait and see.

A Deadly Desire: Travis Takes the "Miracle Pill"

In an era when "real women" have big breasts and "real men" big muscles, few body issues are more shameful to men than having large breasts. In this essay, we meet nineteen-year-old Travis, who is so depressed by his heavy body and fleshy chest that he falls prey to an ad for a product that promises to "free his stubborn fat." Travis's experiences unfold in his hometowns of Pomona and Riverside and his college town, Irvine.

I am of mostly Middle Eastern heritage, but with a strong presence of Caucasian ancestry. My body type is such that I have large build, a naturally muscular and large-boned frame. That is why, naturally, I tend to be heavy and have lots of mass, even if my body fat percentage is low. [As a child and teenager] I had always been embarrassed by my weight, not because of my size but because of the extra fat, the "man-boobs," if you will. I refused to go swimming with friends or go to beach parties. Or if I went, I would refuse to take off my shirt, always embarrassed by my fat.

Getting Rid of the Extra Flesh

I learned from advertisements and my parents that watching what I ate and exercising could help me lose the weight, and soon I desperately took to dieting and exercising. Once, as a sophomore in high school, I went as far as to join the cross-country team where "practice" consisted of running a daily average of about 7 miles. Sure enough, my weight went down from 180 to 160 pounds, or from a BMI of about 27 to about 23, a change big enough to take me out of the overweight and into the normal category.

Early in the [fall] during one of the biggest meets of the season, I was warming up for the race doing sprints when I tripped in a deep hole in the grass and severely sprained my right ankle. The injury was so bad I was out for the rest of the season. By then, [however], my metabolism was so accustomed to my running 7 to 10 miles a day that within one month I put on 30 pounds. I now weighed even more than I had before I started running [when I was] 190 pounds and had a BMI of about 28.

The discomfort from my newfound weight caused me to start training even harder than before, only this time it was for track. I was lifting weights, sprinting, and practicing 4 hours a day, desperately trying to get down to 160, but I only made it to 180. In the middle of all this track training, my family moved from Pasadena to Riverside. At my new high school I no longer had a competitive edge on the track team, so I was forced to quit. During the next two sedentary months of my sophomore year, I put on an astonishing 40 pounds. I was now 220 pounds and my BMI was 29.5, which is borderline overweight/obese. Since then, my weight has not changed significantly.

Recreating the Body

During the next two years in Riverside and Irvine, my discomfort with my weight really became dangerous. I had been and still was trying to completely control my eating habits. One night, when I was feeling unusually depressed about my body image, I was reading through my e-mail and came across an e-mail from the CEO of the company USP Labs, which produces supplements for weight loss and body building. In it, he offered me first dibs on a new supplement they were working on called "Recreate," which is supposed to help you "recreate" your body image in a totally new way. Normally

I am not one to fall for scams, but I felt so low that night that I went ahead and bought a bottle of that stuff. Within a couple of weeks, I had my bottle of the "miracle pill" that was supposed to "unlock the secrets of genetics" and help me "free my stubborn fat." At this point, I was a week from moving into the college dorms.

Move-in day came, and I began a new chapter in my life with new people and in a new environment. There was no longer such a thing as free time. For a while, I forgot about my body and weight. Then came winter break, and during the three weeks off my embarrassment and self-image problem came back. I wanted to bring an end to it then and there, and the first thing that came to mind were the pills, which I had bought but never used. During the winter quarter, I began a regime of [taking] those pills and [engaging in] rigorous exercise, about 3 hours a day, five days a week. By the end of the quarter, not only had my grades suffered from all the time and effort I put into exercising, but also my personal health took a [dive]. I was only 10 pounds lighter at 210 and had developed a cluster of health problems. I couldn't focus or concentrate, either in class or while studying. I became an insomniac and couldn't get good sleep. If I skipped the pills for a day, I'd vomit, become jittery, moody, and get really bad headaches. Despite all that exercising, I neither lost much fat or weight nor built any muscle.

One morning, while having breakfast with some friends, I was so jittery from having skipped the morning pill that I dropped my glass of milk. At this point I decided to go to my doctor. It turned out the reason I had all those problem was the pills had a monstrous amount of caffeine in them: about 300 milligrams per pill, when a typical cup of coffee has 90 milligrams, and I was following the instructions on the label of taking 3 to 4 pills per day! At 1,200 milligrams of caffeine a day, my doctor told me, I could actually gain weight by stressing my body with such a high dose of caffeine. My kidneys and adrenal glands could fail in months, and I could even develop heart problems. That moment was a slap in the face for me; I had been trading my health for a lower weight and false confidence. I wanted that body in all those ads—that Hollister or Abercrombie & Fitch body—so badly that I literally could have killed myself trying to get it. My only sense of self was through my body.

A New Focus for Life

Of course, I immediately stopped taking the pills and started taking better care of my health. My spring quarter was my rehab quarter. I gave up obsessing over my weight and returned to my studies. I realized that having a nice body does nothing for me. As I go [about my life] and see those ads with six-pack abs and defined chests and built arms, I think to myself that it's better to have died successful, confident in who you really were, and loved by those who mattered to you, than to have given yourself false confidence and died with no one to love anything but your washboard abs. Giving up my obsession with weight has really helped me discover who I really am and what I'm truly passionate about, and that has brought me closer to my family and friends.

From Disordered Eating to Eating Disorder

The essays also illuminate ways in which the war on fat might be encouraging the development of eating disorders. I received nearly fifty essays depicting unambiguously eating-disordered individuals. Although the situations described were complex and diverse, some patterns emerged. A number of the cases followed familiar storylines about the origins of eating disorders and did not implicate the war on fat.[10] In other cases, possible connections emerged. I detected four patterns, revolving around sports, immigration, familial weight abuse, and what I call our collective obesity watch.

Today, huge numbers of young Californians participate in school and club sports. In the 2011 survey I conducted, fully 70 percent of women and 74 percent of men said they had participated in organized school sports in middle and/or high school, while roughly 40 percent took part in club sports (based on a sample of 273 females and 61 males). Playing sports should and often does foster healthy bodies, but, as Cheyenne's story intimates, sports with rigid weight requirements heighten young people's risk of developing eating disorders. Among the most dangerous are wrestling (for boys), and gymnastics, dancing, ice skating, and synchronized swimming (for girls). From young dancers encouraged by anorexic instructors to eat cotton balls soaked in orange juice to teenage wrestlers told by "hard-ass coaches" to "cut weight" by purging or not eating, the essays of young athletes on their way to becoming eating disordered are disturbing in the extreme [SC 127, 234, 245].

In a second pattern, young immigrants to the United States who faced bullying for appearing different and bigger than their peers developed eating disorders in an effort to lose weight, stop the abuse, and "become a real American." With their citizenship already under question, having an "American body"—one with no excess fat—was essential to social acceptance. Following a pattern we've encountered before, these young people renarrated their life stories to produce accounts in which all their problems were due to their "excess weight." These stories then legitimized drastic efforts to lose it. Among the essays I gathered, there were four cases of this sort, including that of Gali, an Armenian girl, whose relatives were so busy trying to fit into American society themselves that they had no time to notice Gali's anorexia, even when she wound up in the hospital with an IV in her arm [SC 249].

A third pattern involved young people with larger bodies who were subject to unremitting weight abuse from their families and developed eating disorders in an effort to shrink down and end the abuse. There were six of these cases. Familial harassment of heavy members is not new, of course. What is new in today's biocitizenship society is that everyone has a moral obligation to be thin and heaviness is legitimate grounds for condemnation. This troubling situation is familiar from many essays we've already read, so I do not illustrate it here.

A final dynamic involves our collective obesity watch. Today people in all walks of life are so concerned about obesity and so pleased when people lose weight that they sometimes fail to notice when a pattern of what they thought was "healthy" weight loss evolves into an unhealthy eating disorder. For their part, those on a weight-loss trajectory are so encouraged by all the complimentary fat-talk that they often set more ambitious goals and amp up their diet into something more drastic. In one powerful case, a twelve-year-old's apparently healthy new diet and exercise habits so closely mimicked those promoted by the war on fat that her mom and sister enthusiastically encouraged them. By the time they finally caught on that the girl was seriously ill, the condition had developed into full-blown anorexia requiring hospitalization to save her life [SC 245].

This section presents three cases that illuminate such linkages in especially graphic ways. They feature categories of people whom one rarely thinks of in connection with eating disorders but should: men and the elderly. We meet Kasey, a former high school wrestler unable to shake his identity as a "heavy lard"; Brad, a talented graduate student from Iran struggling to become a "successful American"; and the elderly Nellie, who developed an eating disorder and died while under the care of her weight-obsessed doctor. All three essays were written by someone close to the subject.

Weighty Words: Kasey's Story

Kasey is a heavy-set twenty-two-year-old African American who grew up in a middle-class family in Paso Robles, San Luis Obispo County. In this essay, a caring friend describes how, as a young trophy wrestler, Kasey was able to brush off the biobullying about his weight with a self-deprecating laugh but then, after a huge weight gain in college, started on a drastic thinning regimen that frightened everyone except him.

"Trophy Boy" and "Heavy Lard"

During high school, one of my best friends, Kasey, [struggled with] his weight and sexuality. I remember one day walking into his room as he was standing in [front of] the mirror crying [as he looked at himself in] his wrestler outfit, which barely fit over his oversized stomach. In high school he was the class clown and, more importantly, the town "trophy boy" in wrestling. We grew up in a very small town [where] accomplishments small and wide were recognized by [everyone]. What the town didn't know was that its golden-boy wrestler champion was struggling with something deep inside that not even I quite understood.

Wrestling was a huge part of Kasey's family, [not surprisingly,] considering that his dad was the head coach of the team at our high school. Kasey was always struggling to maintain a certain weight but somehow invariably found himself either under or over his [target] weight right before a match. This usually led to his binge eating or not eating at all. He would always tell me that he thought of himself as a "heavy lard." He was bullied during high school because of this by some of his teammates. Kasey hid how much this hurt him very well. He would often join in the bullying and make fun of himself, [a move that seemed to] ease the bullying for him.

I remember after we graduated from high school and started college, Kasey wrote a blog on his tumblr that stated:

> Once I left school and went to Morehouse, I passed my driving test, which made me lazier and gave me more access to fast food restaurants. [I began] going out drinking all weekend, every weekend. Soon my weight went through the roof. I knew I was overweight, but I had a close group of friends, both male and female, and was always having a laugh. [In this way] I programmed myself to believe that it didn't bother me. [One night], while out drinking with some mates, I had a picture taken of my best mate and me. When I had it developed,

I couldn't believe how big I was. I was over 40 pounds overweight according to the BMI and looked terrible.

After reading this post, I started to check on Kasey's page on a daily basis, just to make sure he was okay and wasn't thinking about doing anything extreme. Kasey started eating more sensibly and lost two pounds within the first week after looking at that picture:

I started going [to the gym] a couple times a week, and about one month later I had lost over 20 pounds. If I could lose this much, so quickly, how hard could it be to lose even more? I started going to the gym [four days a week] and on the other days would go bicycling or running around the track. The weight was falling off me and I felt great, but I still wasn't happy. Every time I looked in the mirror I still saw the heavyset young man that I had been in high school.

After reading this post, I became worried and called Kasey, but of course he called me a "worry wart." I heard rumors from other close friends from high school that supposedly Kasey was eating less and less, and that it was showing. While most people assumed he was taking cocaine, no one took into consideration that maybe Kasey had an eating problem.

I tried to meet up with Kasey over break, but every time I called or texted him, my questions went unanswered or I got a simple response of "I'm busy, I'll get at you later." When I checked his blog the last day I was in town, his last post said: "Some days I would be starving, so I would chew gum to stop these cravings." Even though Kasey had family and friends telling him that he had lost too much weight and looked ill, he still chose to ignore them. Kasey [wrote]: "Other people were coming up to me and saying how much weight I had lost, which made me feel great, so this spurred me on. I was now eating barely anything. I was exercising every day, which consisted of a five-mile run and weight training. I was obsessed." I remember seeing this post, and thinking Kasey had completely lost it. Soon after this, rumors started to spread back home that Kasey's mom had told one of our close friends that his liver and kidneys weren't functioning right, and that he had started to develop gout in some of his fingers.

A Boyfriend Is Able to Intervene at Last

I was talking to Kasey on the phone, when I [discovered that] he was in a relationship. Patrick put up with [Kasey's eating problems] for a couple months until they got into it one night. I guess Patrick had offered Kasey some pork ribs smothered in gravy, but he had refused. They ended up getting into an explosive verbal fight and Patrick told Kasey that he couldn't handle what he (Kasey) was doing to himself. Scared that Patrick would leave, the very next week Kasey started to implement changes in his dieting behaviors. On tumblr he wrote: "I would describe it as the hardest thing I have ever done. To try and change my mindset from basically thinking that food is even [evil]. I had to get into the frame of mind that food isn't that bad as long as you're sensible with it."

Kasey started having a proper breakfast, lunch, and dinner, while still maintaining a healthy lifestyle. It took him nearly two years to realize that he had gone from being clinically obese to what he was told later was anorexic. He wrote on tumblr: "It took a long time to adjust back to what most people know as normal. With the support of my friends and family, and especially Patrick, I got through it all."

From Iran to America: Brad's Journey from Fat to Thin

Brad is a twenty-five-year-old graduate student and recent immigrant from Iran. In the interview captured in this essay, he faces a relentlessly inquisitive yet caring friend (my student) who pulls out of him the shameful reason he is starving himself nearly to death.

For this ethnographic project, I decided to interview a close friend. [Brad] was born and raised in Tehran, Iran, and moved to Irvine with his family after he graduated from high school. He is now a first-year graduate student in engineering Last month I went over to his house for the first time and was surprised that I couldn't recognize any of his pictures from Iran. The young man in the picture[s] had a very healthy body weight—a stark contrast to the still smiling, yet incredibly thin, graduate student I befriended in my classes.

We decided to meet at Panera. He ordered a cup of coffee and a cheese Danish, the size equivalent to a palm of the hand. I asked him if this was his first meal of the day. Brad hesitated before answering, "I had research all day today and it was a very busy day." Over the course of the next hour, I had to cajole him to eat three thinly cut slices of bread.

I began my ethnography by asking him [about his] BMI index:

Me: I'm asking because it is obvious you have shed a significant amount of weight since you moved to the U.S. (Brad starts interrupting to object.) I saw the pictures, Brad-y. Why do you think you lost so much weight?

Brad: Well, I started to eat healthy. After arriving here [to Orange County], I became a vegetarian. Not necessarily because of the animals, though. It's just when you don't eat meat, you feel—at least I feel, fresher.

Me: Did you worry about your weight or dieting when you were in Iran?

Brad: No, not really. In Iran, I used to only weigh myself every time I went to a yearly check-up at the doctor's office. Now I weigh myself once a week.

Me: Why?

Brad: It is good to know how much you weigh. It is a measure of your health.

Me: And do you think you are healthy?

Brad: I don't have time to really think about it. I don't have time to be hungry.

At this point in our conversation, Brad went to grab another cup of coffee while I continued writing notes.

Me: Am I the only person who calls you anorexic?

Brad: No. When we go out as a lab, my other lab members notice as well. I usually don't eat. I order coffee. My mom nags at me to eat, too.

Me: How do you feel when they call you anorexic?

Brad   It makes me uncomfortable. I don't like it. You have to understand that because I am a guy, it is worse to be thin than fat, especially here. It makes me come across as weak and incapable.

I was surprised to hear these comments from Brad, even more so because of his Uncle Alex [who] is fully assimilated within American culture.

Me: Okay, what about Alex? He is a doctor and you always talk about how close you are to him. Did he say anything when you started losing weight?

Brad: Well, in the beginning he was actually very proud. His ideology is that being fit should always be the goal. But recently, he started mentioning that I have gotten too skinny.

Me: Do you mind my asking how much you weigh now?

Brad: I was 75 kilograms (165 pounds) when I came from Iran. Now I am at 51 kilograms (115 pounds).

Me: Okay. When you first came here, you are telling me Alex said nothing about your physique at all?

Brad: Well, during my first few months living in the United States, he told me that I had gotten a bit fat and that it was bad for my health. Although I don't really agree with his philosophy concerning body health.

Me: Which is?

Brad: No, it's not something I am proud of.

Me: Come on, Brad, please tell me. What is it?

Brad: When I first came here, he told me this: "There are three things in this society necessary to be considered successful when you walk down the street. You have to be tall, white, and fit. You can't be the first two, but you can definitely be the last."

The Life and Death of an Elderly Anorexic

Finally, we meet Nellie Norwood, a white Angelena from a lower-income family who died from anorexia at the age of eighty-three. In this tragic story, we see how a physician's orders to lose weight can have unintendedly dire effects, effects never anticipated—yet also never noticed—by the doctor.

Nellie Norwood is someone dear to my heart that I truly miss. She was an amazingly strong person whom I was lucky to call my great-grandmother. Although our time together was cut short, she touched my life in ways I will never forget.

Nellie was born in 1920. She grew up in Pennsylvania, where she married and had two daughters. She soon traveled out to California with her husband and daughters to start a new life in Los Angeles. Her husband and she were from Russia and [they] raised their children to believe in the Jewish faith. Her daughters soon grew up, got married, and had children of their own.

The Norwood family was expanding quickly, but things took a turn [for the worse] in Nellie's life. Nana Nellie lost her husband in 1975 to a disease that affected his whole body. The sickness was fast-moving and killed him [before] Nana Nellie could wrap her mind around the idea of being a widow. Nellie's whole life had been her family, so when her husband passed she didn't know what to do. Luckily, she had her daughters and grandchildren by her side to help her through this devastating time.

A Fateful Appointment: Diagnosis, High Cholesterol; Treatment, Weight Loss

Everything seemed to be going fine in her life until she reached the age of 65 and went to the doctor's for a check-up. She was told that her cholesterol was really high and that she needed to try to get it down to a lower number. The doctor told her that in order to get her cholesterol down, she needed to watch what she ate and lose some weight. Nana Nellie was never a super-skinny person, but she was never super-heavy either. For her height of 5'5", she weighed an average weight of around 160 pounds [BMI of 26.6].

She started immediately counting calories. When watching what she ate didn't work, she started to take laxatives to flush everything out of her body that she was digesting. The weight was slowly [coming] off, but it was never enough for Nana Nellie. She got herself so stuck on being skinny and losing weight that she kept doing anything she could to keep her weight down. The [goal] was no longer low cholesterol, [it was] being skinny.

My nana got so picky about her food that no one could take her out to eat anymore. When her daughters would take her out to eat she would move the food around on her plate or cut it into small pieces to make it look like she ate more than she really did.

Nana Nellie would go in routinely to the doctor's for check-ups on her cholesterol level. [At none of those appointments would he notice—or worry about—] how skinny she was getting. Instead, he would support her and tell her that she was getting a lot better and that her levels were going down since she lost the weight. The doctor was feeding false information into her mind, and she believed anything and everything that he was saying. When her family would tell her that she needed to see a different doctor, she refused, [saying that] she had been with the same doctor for years now and he knew what was best for her body.

By the time she was 67 she had lost around 50 pounds. She was now down to about 110 pounds and was extremely skinny [BMI of 18.3]. Seeing herself in the mirror, she was happy with the new her. Although she liked how skinny she was she did not start eating again. She was scared of gaining any weight back and returning to the old-looking her.

Losing Nellie

Although Nellie was happy with the way she looked, her personality changed completely. My mom would enjoy seeing her grandmother, but when she started being so wrapped up in her weight, she was no longer someone fun to be around. She was moody and would not want to talk to anyone for long periods of time. When she did talk to people, she would be very short and have an attitude. Being her great granddaughter, I used to get excited to hang out with her. Sadly, she never wanted to get close to my brother or me. By the time we were born, she was a full-blown anorexic, so that all she cared about was her weight, not her great grandchildren. Although she was hard to get close to, her strength as a woman always inspired me. She was strong-willed and knew what she wanted in life.

Unfortunately, my great grandmother passed away in 2003. She was only 83 when she died. When she passed away, she weighed under 100 pounds [BMI under 16.6]. Her body was extremely bloated because it was retaining so much water. All her organs had been shutting down and were no longer functioning properly. This disease took over the [person] that so many people had loved. I know my great grandmother would want us to be happy and learn from her mistakes. Without my Nana Nellie, my life would not be the same as it is today.

Costs That Don't—But Surely Should—Count

This chapter has suggested that the pressures associated with the war on fat are actually harming the physical and mental health of many of the young people that it is intended to most help. These accounts suggest that, far from being extraordinary circumstances, it was the ordinary, everyday pressures of the war on fat that led these people to undertake extreme weight-loss practices. Featuring pressures from parents, coaches, doctors, and other authorities, the ethnographies here are little different from those in the other chapters, except that the subjects took things a little further and got unlucky.

The pervasive fat-talk in their environments—both negative and positive—played a fundamental role in what happened. Several of the cases illustrate the now-familiar role of fat abuse in motivating people to lose weight. But the essays also illuminate the importance of positive fat-talk. After losing a few pounds and receiving effusive praise from former tormenters ("you look great now!"), some (Farid and Kasey) went on a compliment-high that encouraged them to keep going, to kick their goals up a notch in the belief that, if a little weight loss could bring so much approval, then greater weight loss might yield a near-perfect life. In this pattern, which we've encountered before but not yet commented on, it is the compliments—a form of positive fat-talk—that motivate aspiring dieters to set the more unrealistic goals that require extreme measures to achieve.

The young people whose stories we've just read evinced no awareness of the dangers of the extreme methods they used. The sole exception is Kym, who thought (erroneously) that "some models had heart problems and died from purging" (those models died from self-starvation). In almost every case, they thought that what they were doing was actually healthy and beneficial, that by pursuing those practices they were being virtuous biocitizens. Souri fully believed that eating only fruit was good for her. Travis and Farid had no doubt that intense workouts were good for their bodies and for weight loss. Travis knew at some level that the makers of diet pills often make false claims, but he was so desperate that he traded the small risk of side effects for the bigger promise of weight loss.

My research suggests that the silences in the public health messages about weight bear significant responsibility for the ignorance of these young people and their parents about the dangers of extreme weight-loss practices. Americans are constantly bombarded with warnings about the health risks of overweight and obesity. Yet aside from the occasional admonitions about weight-loss drugs from the FDA,[11] little information is made public on the health risks associated with the common treatments for heaviness: dieting, exercising, and drugs (I discuss surgery in chapter 9). A search of the websites of the major U.S. government agencies devoted to protecting our health turned up no systematic information on problems associated with weight-loss practices.[12] The sole focus of those sites was on encouraging Americans to lose weight. More information is available on the worldwide web. A Google search for "dangers of weight loss practices" turned up 16 million hits in July 2014. Few of the items recovered actually dealt with these issues, but some sites, especially health-oriented websites such as LiveStrong.org, WebMD.com, FitDay.com, and LifeScript.com, carried the occasional article with a title like "Six Things Never to Do to Lose Weight."[13] Websites dealing with eating disorders also describe the risks of excessive dieting and exercise routines. But I could find little discussion of the potential dangers of the sorts of "routine" dieting and exercising that do not lead to full-fledged eating disorders.

Although some information is available to those who want to find it, in a climate where the stress of the public health field and wider culture is on the urgency of weight loss, few would think to look up the *dangers* of weight-loss practices. Children are the least likely to imagine they could be harmed by the sorts of practices that their parents, teachers, coaches, and doctors are urging them to undertake. Nor are they likely to understand the nutritional implications of their self-made dieting practices. Remember Alexis, who as a six-year-old had no concept of calories but knew that food makes you fat and fat is bad? Or April, who in middle school put herself on starvation diets to eliminate her excess flesh? These cases are far from atypical.

Warnings about anorexia, on the other hand, have come through loud and clear. After all the celebrity deaths, the images of wasting female bodies are seared into people's—or at least young women's—minds. But the message that teenage girls and their parents have gotten seems to be that anorexia is something qualitatively different from ordinary dieting, that anorexia is a "disease" while dieting is just everyday behavior. A theme that came through repeatedly is that anorexia is something only "other people" get; "we" know about it and so are protected. There is little consideration that one might lead to the other. And so the abuse of young bodies continues. Another problem is that the message that people pick up is that anorexia and bulimia are problems primarily—or only—of girls. No one suspected that Kasey or Brad might have an eating disorder until they were well developed. Nor did Nellie's doctor imagine that his elderly patient might have a full-blown case of anorexia—until it was too late.

The warnings about anorexia aside, the essays suggest that the dominant public health message young people receive today emphasizes weight loss above all, without establishing limits or pointing to the dangers of extreme practices. Children are taught not just that everyone must and can achieve a narrowly defined "normal" weight; they are also taught that excess weight marks them as unhealthy. They are also told that dieting, exercising, and losing weight are virtually always good and that, if they do these things, their health will improve. As in most public health campaigns, in the anti-obesity campaign the effort to convey the big story—that excess weight is unhealthy—has led to the neglect of important nuances and hard-to-pin-down lines, such as the line between healthy and unhealthy dieting and exercising. Although warnings are issued when tragedy strikes—for instance, when a celebrity falls ill—the evidence suggests that children are not routinely advised that there are limits to the sensible use of these practices or that there are risks associated with extreme dieting and exercising.

This ignorance of health risks is concerning because, aside from the cases of Farid and Travis, the frightening experiences of bodily harm did little to deter young people's weight-reducing efforts. For Farid and Travis, who sustained serious injury, the experience was so shocking to their sense of how the world should work that it jolted them out of their life-long assumptions about the necessity of losing weight at any cost. These young men learned a hard lesson and swore off extreme weight-loss methods, probably for life. As long as the months of high-caffeine pills caused no permanent damage, Travis will be one of the fortunate few who is able to turn a near-tragedy into an opportunity to ask himself what really mattered in life. But Travis's case is unusual because the bodily damage he suffered was life threatening. For young people whose injuries were less serious, the response was more ambivalent. Two—Cheyenne and Kym—remain extremely unhappy with their weight and, despite their brush with danger, may well be tempted to turn to extreme weight-loss methods again.

The cases in the last section show how the bodily pressures that are part and parcel of the war on fat can lead vulnerable people—regardless of gender or age—down the slippery slope into an eating disorder. The biobullying Kasey endured in high school was so traumatizing, it left him with lifelong fears about his weight. When he later gained a great deal of weight, he freaked out and, turning to overexercise and self-starvation (methods he had learned as a high school wrestler), developed a full-blown case of anorexia. In Brad's case, the tacit knowledge in his immigrant community about what it takes to be a successful American, combined perhaps with ignorance of the existence of eating disorders in men, have led to the development of an extremely serious and, as of the time the essay was written, unaddressed case of anorexia. In their efforts to be included in the community of good American biocitizens, immigrants such as Brad are unknowingly endangering their health and risking their lives.

Physicians have important responsibilities in the anti-obesity campaign, yet there are hidden dangers to the medical community's extreme preoccupation with weight. Sometimes in their zeal to rid their patients of excess pounds, physicians miss—or even inadvertently help create—other diseases. Nellie's is a case in point. Of course, there were psychological issues at work, too—perhaps the weight-loss campaign became an obsession because it gave Nellie's life the meaning it had lost when her husband died. Still, though, one would expect her doctor to notice the emergence of anorexic symptoms and intervene before it was too late. Taken together, these essays support the emerging view in the eating-disorders community that the intense medical and cultural emphasis on getting rid of obesity is increasing the risk of serious psychiatric disorders.

These findings are notable, but who is noting such things? In four of the five cases of bodily harm, it was a physician who diagnosed the damage. If physicians are seeing many cases of children and teens harming themselves from excessive dieting or exercising or pill use, why aren't such findings part of the larger conversation about eradicating obesity? Why is there so much public information about the dangers of obesity—but so little about the dangers of desperate young people (and older ones, too) driven to take extreme measures to get rid of their fat? Why is there so little public discussion of the possible links between the fight against fat and the development of eating disorders? In the war on fat, the risks of bodily and psychiatric damage seem to be treated like collateral damage, regrettable but secondary costs that are best left unmentioned and uncounted in the interests of winning the larger war against the real threat, which is obesity. Or perhaps such costs are not even seeable and namable because they fall outside the public health crisis frame, beyond the bounds of the dominant narrative about what matters.

In the next chapter we turn to another of the uncharted costs of the war on fat, one that has received even less attention. This is the damage it has done to intimate personal and familial relationships.

8

Families and Relationships Unhinged

I was in a relationship with a guy named Jason for two years; I broke up with him one year ago this month. When we met, Jason was 6'3″and very much in shape. I am 5'3″and weigh about 115 pounds. I am very conscious about my weight. I work out on a weekly basis and am cautious about what I eat. After we had been dating for a while, Jason began to gain a lot of weight. He looked huge compared to me. I used to encourage him to eat better and work out with me, but the weight continued to pile on. Friends began to notice this and some would say things like "It surprises me that you two are together," or "You're so pretty, you can do a lot better." These [superficial compliments] are really rude things to say. For one, they are saying that there must be something wrong with me because it is absolutely shameful to be with someone who is overweight. Two, they are being rude to Jason because they are criticizing his character based on his weight alone. I have always been one to oppose judging others based on their appearance. As much as I tell myself that I broke up with him because his negative qualities were too much for me to handle, there is a tiny part of me way deep inside that knows that part of the reason was that he had gained so much weight and I viewed it as a reflection of myself. I thought that because I take such good care of myself, I deserve someone who does the same.

Laurel, from her Essay "The Effects of Weight in a Relationship"
[SC 261]

In today's weight-obsessed culture, one's value as a person is judged on the basis not only of one's own weight but also of the weight of those one associates with. In *Fat Shame*, Farrell writes about the cultural containment of fat people; although it's fine for them to hang out with each other, once they try to claim a place in mainstream society or to hang out with normals, they are deemed out of line and sanctioned through fat shaming.[1] My students' essays provide ample evidence for such dynamics. As Laurel shamefully admits, fatness is viewed as a "contaminating" factor in relationships; if we associate with fat people it reflects badly on us. The underlying logic seems to be that if we have close ties to fat people, we evidently failed in our duty as a good biocitizen to get others in our world to achieve normal weight. Given the morality attached to weight, people who are fat are viewed as inherently "bad." If we associate with them, others will think we have bad judgment and it (the fatness and the badness) might rub off on us, exposing us to demeaning comments too. In either case, associating with "those fat people" is damaging to "us." These attitudes lead to the kind of social avoidance and rejection of fat people by thin ones that we have seen again and again.

In this chapter we look at the social negotiation and social effects of fatness in two core social domains: families and romantic relationships. Given the polluting quality of fatness, if a family member or partner becomes fat, it is often perceived as destabilizing or threatening to the relationship (or family unit) and becomes a problem to be fixed. The essays we've read include numerous cases of family fights over the weight of a chubby child. They've shed light on the struggles of moms to take pounds off their daughters' bodies and on the special role accorded to male family members (brothers and fathers) in evaluating the desirability of girls' bodies to other males. Think, for example, of April's older brother, who warned that boys would throw things at her if she got fatter, or Tiffany's younger brother who screamed at her "You're FAT!", with an approving nod from their father (see chapter 4). In the world we inhabit, men are supposed to judge girls' bodies, while women must fix them. In this chapter, we read six essays that show with particular clarity how the issue of heaviness is negotiated in familial and romantic relationships, and with what effects. Continuing this section's theme of the uncharted costs of the war on fat, we focus on the damage that can be done to these intimate relationships (rather than to individuals) by the societal emphasis on getting rid of fat at any cost.

In the war on fat, the family is the most important site where the weight of young people is socially negotiated. Based on analyses of the public discourses on obesity (official statements and policies, news articles, and public discussions), feminist scholars have noted the prominent role assigned to mothers in the childhood obesity epidemic and its resolution. Embedding an ideology of intensive or total parenting, in which the mother in particular is supposed to monitor and successfully manage all aspects of her child's life, the obesity discourse tasks mothers with ensuring that all family members—but especially the children, their special responsibility— are good biocitizens who eat right, exercise regularly, and maintain normal weight. Those who fail are deemed unfit, "bad" mothers. Drawing on long-standing cultural discourses of maternal blame, mothers, especially working mothers, and even more so those marginalized by race and class, are seen as the primary cause of childhood obesity, posing threats to the child, the community, and the nation.[2] While the discourse on childhood obesity leaves men invisible and so apparently blameless, women are scapegoated and blamed. Pressing the point, cultural studies scholar April Herndon argues that women (along with fat children) are victims of these discourses and policies pure and simple.[3]

When we distinguish between the written texts, whose discourses these scholars have so carefully dissected, and the broader war on fat playing out in society, we find strong support for their arguments but, at the same time, a more complex picture. Paralleling the silence in the public discourses about obesity and men, my ethnographic research shows that fathers have few if any dedicated roles in the war on fat. They do have a few culturally mandated responsibilities—playing sports with their kids, for example—but, unlike the duties assigned the moms, those associated with dads are poorly defined and fungible, should something more important come up. At the same time, however, we will see that some men play critical roles in the fight against family fat. These need to be brought to light. My research also supports the arguments about mothers while complicating them. Although the public discourses do indeed direct the blame at working mothers, especially those of particular races and classes, the ethnographic research suggest that *all* mothers are under intense pressure to keep their children's weight down. Moreover, the pressures they feel most keenly come not from public discourses such as those examined in existing scholarship; they come from snide comments and dirty looks from people in their social worlds. Not only do cultural authorities such as doctors and teachers expect mothers to successfully fulfill their biocitizen responsibilities to their kids, so too do friends and relatives. Constant media emphasis on the health risks of heaviness and the social value of thinness work to reinforce the already ubiquitous message that being thin and attractive is essential to a girl's career and romantic prospects. Of course, every mom would want that for her daughter. Moms also seek a slender daughter for their own sake, for the mother who fails to control her daughter's weight finds herself criticized for being a bad mother and failing her child. Although each child's genetic makeup reflects the contribution of both parents, the child's, and especially the daughter's, body is often seen as a reflection of the mother's body. Given the shame associated with having a fat daughter, it is no surprise that many moms are deeply invested in efforts to manage their children's weight. Although many of my students complained bitterly about their moms' heavy-handed measures, their essays reveal the extraordinary pressures those moms are under to successfully fulfill their weight-control duties. Those pressures were felt by almost every mom, regardless of working status or ethnic background. Only a few moms who were recent immigrants, and so unfamiliar with American cultural preoccupations, managed to escape the pressure. Ryan's and Kristen's moms are good examples (chapters 4 and 6).

The ethnographic research also suggests the need to consider the science of weight that circulates in popular culture in the form of biomyths. One key biomyth is the notion that a child who is thin is healthy while one with excess pounds is unhealthy. The fear that their heavy child has or will have serious health problems is one of the major drivers of parental concern about weight. Despite the intense pressure on parents, as the mothers in my project discovered it is not at all easy to succeed in controlling a child's weight. Reflecting the ubiquitous biomyth about the controllability of weight, friends and family members (as well as the mothers themselves) invariably assume that mothers are actually *capable* of shaping their children's weight. Although they can influence it to a certain extent—by teaching good nutrition, cooking healthful food, and tracking the food that comes into the household, for example—as any parent knows, there are sharp limits to parents' ability to shape their youngsters' bodies. Not only do genetics and growth spurts interfere, but children eat and play at school and many other places beyond parental control. Children also have many ways to sabotage these efforts. Expected to achieve the unachievable, moms find themselves in an impossible bind. They are asked to do the impossible and then socially punished (by shaming and other forms of critical fat-talk) when they fail. Moms of heavy daughters face a real tactical conundrum. If they rely solely on mild pedagogical fat-talk, it might have no effect. But if they resort to biobullying, the daughter may become resentful or rebellious in ways that could damage the mother-daughter relationship. In the war on childhood fat, mothers have few good options. And the mother-daughter relationship suffers as a result. The ethnographic work thus shows that it is not just mothers who are damaged, although that is bad enough—it is the mother-child relationship, indeed, the stability of the entire family.

In this chapter, we consider four cases of family relationships that are seriously strained by struggles over the weight of a child. In the first three, presented in the first section, we focus on the mother-daughter tie. In the fourth case, we look at the consequences for the whole family. We are interested in how parents deal with an overweight child, how the child responds to parental efforts, and the impact on the mother-daughter tie or the family as a whole. Although the stories are told from the daughters' point of view, we can learn (or can infer) a great deal about the parents—the tactics they try, the frustrations they surely feel—from the descriptions provided by their daughters.

Not coincidentally, three of the accounts are of Asian American families (Filipino, Korean, and Chinese American). But Asian parents are not the only ones who turn to strong-armed tiger mother practices, in Amy Chua's memorable phrase, when their children refuse to lose weight. Dara-Lynn Weiss, the author of a controversial 2012 *Vogue* article (and 2013 book) detailing her no-holds-barred efforts to force her seven-year-old daughter to lose weight, is Caucasian, but she is a tiger mom nonpareil.[4] At the same time, though, it is true, for reasons explained earlier, that in many East and Southeast Asian cultures, heavy-handed parenting techniques are much more generally accepted by parents, children, and the wider (ethnic) community as both appropriate and beneficial to the child and family as a whole. Within these groups, the essays show, parenting essentially means authoritarian parenting. These fine-grained portraits of weight management in Asian American families give us an opportunity to ask whether the praise some have lavished on Asians for being such good, thin, responsible biocitizens is fully warranted.

As Laurel reveals, struggles over weight can also damage intimate relationships. The powerful writing on fat oppression by the sociologist Tracy Royce helps us see the pervasiveness and destructiveness of biobullying, as well as other forms of verbal and emotional violence, in romantic relationships.[5] As she argues, partner abuse is a product of male power on a societal level and a means by which particular men exert power and control over "their" women.[6] Fat shaming in intimate relationships has probably existed since fat became a cultural no-no. What's changed is that fat abuse is now socially sanctioned; indeed, it is seen as deserved and necessary to motivate weight loss. In such an environment, those who are fat-battered by their partners have few ways to defend themselves. Not only is there no commonly accepted language in which they might protest the abuse, there is little social support to bolster such an effort. Fat shaming and other weight struggles can cause terrible damage to intimate relationships and, even more so, to the targeted party as the abuser calls his (or in rarer cases, her) partner demeaning names and the abused, her self-esteem shattered, tries both to defend her dignity and to lose weight in any way possible. For some, Royce suggests, such battering results in symptoms that are indistinguishable from those of posttraumatic stress disorder. In the second section of this chapter, we meet two heterosexual couples in which male fat abuse of the female partner inflicts long-term harm on the victim and ends the relationship.

Frayed Mother-Daughter Relationships

We begin with weight struggles in three mother-daughter relationships. In their desperation to get their daughters to shrink, the moms of all three girls—Destiny, Hillary, and Kelsey—resort to strong-arm, even abusive, tactics that not only do not work but also damage that precious relationship with their daughter. In the first two cases, in which the daughters are not able to talk back and defend themselves, the relational damage appears to be long term; in the third, in which the daughter challenges her mom, the story ends on a happier note.

My Hypercritical, Rude, Nagging, Judgmental, Hypocritical, Clueless Mother: Destiny Airs Her Grievances

In this essay, Destiny, a Filipino American from a middle-class family in San Jose, describes a mother whose weight-badgering is unhelpful in the extreme. The approach taken by Destiny's mom—constant carping, criticism, and invidious comparison—backfires, leaving her twenty-one-year-old daughter angry, depressed, obsessed with her weight, and utterly hostile toward the woman who is making her life miserable.

My Mother, the Weight Cop

When I entered high school, I made it onto the girls' basketball team. [All] athletes needed to have a physical exam before they officially [joined] the team, so I went to see a doctor. A nurse weighed me and checked my height and [informed] my mother that I was overweight. This hurt me so much because I was never really concerned about my weight before. Nobody else had ever brought it up. [Although] my weight was only a couple of pounds [into] the "overweight" category on the BMI charts, the nurse made it seem like such a big deal. It made my mother worry about my weight.

[This new consciousness about my weight deeply] affected me. I [began] working extra hard during practice, not just so I could be better at basketball but so I could sweat more and therefore lose more weight. My mom would watch my games and always criticize me for how slowly I ran because of my weight. She just kept on encouraging me to lose weight, which made me feel fatter than I really was.

I see now how my mother plays a huge role in how I feel about my weight and about myself in general. She's always telling me to watch what I eat. She always criticizes me when I order a soda instead of water, or when I choose white rice over brown. What makes me mad is that when I was a child, she didn't encourage me to eat my vegetables or fruits. She always served me white rice and meat. She never said anything about my eating McDonalds all the time, or drinking soda or whole milk. And now, when I have gotten used to these "bad" eating habits, she judges me. Just because it was easy for her to change her ways of eating doesn't mean that it's easy for me, and I don't think she understands that.

When I am out with mother and we see a bigger person pass by, she always has something to say along the lines of: "See, Destiny, you are going to turn out that way if you don't stop eating junk food." I find this insulting, not only to me but also to the other person. I can't help but think to myself how rude and judg[mental] my mother is and I feel sorry for myself for being her daughter.

Right now I am 130 pounds and 5'0", so my BMI is 25. This is right on the borderline of "normal weight" and "overweight," [yet] my mother thinks I am huge. Every time I go home from college, she tells me that I need to lose weight. She even has the nerve to say multiple times, "When I was your age, I weighed 98 pounds. I was skinny back then." I know she says this to try and encourage me to drop my weight to 98 pounds too. That means that in order to make her happy with the way I look, I need to drop over 30 pounds! When I see her, she brings up my weight more than how I'm doing in school, or what other things I have going on for me. It makes me feel like she cares more about my appearance than how my life is going.

Another thing that irritates me is how she thinks a person should lose weight. She says to quit drinking soda, which I agree is a good start, but she also says to cut out dinner completely. I thought this was ridiculous because, basically, she is asking me to starve myself at night so I can lose weight. [Skipping dinner] is totally unhealthy. This was her method for a while and she dropped some pounds, but eventually she gained them back when she started eating dinner again.

What is funny about this is that she is about the same size as I am, but she thinks she is completely skinnier. I try on her clothes and she asks, with a shocked expression, "You fit *those?*" She has completely no clue how much it hurts me when she criticizes me about my weight. She should approach me differently instead of making me feel horrible about myself.

An Angry, Hurt, Self-Doubting Daughter

Don't get me wrong. I love my mother, but her thoughts and opinions about weight really frustrate me. Sometimes it gets to me. I look in the mirror and I think I'm fat. I've cried many times about my appearance. When I eat "healthy" it is because I am feeling fat, not because I want to be healthy. The same goes with exercising. I hate exercising, and I only do it because I feel fat.

It's really sad that I feel this way about myself. I am a very good person. I am nice, friendly, smart, funny, etc. I know that I am beautiful on the inside and that I have a lot going for me in the future. However, there's that part of me that feels extremely insecure about my weight. I've counted calories, gone on crazy diets that hardly last, made myself throw up, starved myself, and done tons of research just so I can make myself lose weight. I love every part of myself except that insecurity, but this insecurity plays such an important part in my life that it stops me from being the person that I am or want to be. Being pressured to be skinny is stressful and really depressing. I know that one day, I just won't give a crap anymore about what others—especially my mom—think about my weight.

Destiny and Her Mom: A Great Rupture

From the moment her daughter was diagnosed as overweight, Destiny's mom has tried every tactic she can think of to persuade or force her daughter to lose weight. Those tactics reflect two familiar myths: that weight is under individual control and that a daughter should have the same body type and weight as the mom. Yet these beliefs are belied by the facts. Destiny has tried every technique under the sun but nothing has worked. And her body reflects the influence of her father's genes as well as her mother's as well as an environment different from the one faced by the mom when she was growing up. The mom, wanting the best for her daughter but oblivious to these realities, continues to pressure her youngster, creating the conditions for intense conflict over Destiny's weight.

The impact on Destiny has been deep and damaging. Even though she is only on the borderline of overweight, she has come to see herself as fat, and fat is her dominant identity, crowding out the person she wants to be. Like other self-identified fat persons we have met, Destiny is depressed, insecure, and self-doubting. With her constant carping, an evidently caring mother may have unknowingly inflicted enduring emotional damage on her daughter. The high-pressure tactics have also caused grievous harm to the mother-daughter relationship. Mom is unlikely to realize it, but her daughter is full of anger, shame, and disappointment at her treatment of Destiny's weight. How can this bond be repaired? Perhaps time will bring the answer.

Getting Back at my Mother: Hillary's Defiant Story

Hillary is a twenty-one-year-old Korean American from a lower-middle-class family based in Cudahy (in LA County) and then in Los Angeles proper. Deeply hurt by her mother's jabbing comments about her weight, Hillary rebels and tries to hurt her mother right back by doing the opposite of what she urges.

> Ever since I was a little girl, my parents have uprooted my family time and time again. [We moved in] part because of failed business ventures. An even bigger reason was the LA riots of 1992. It was easier to make friends when I was in elementary [school]. It got harder when I got a little older, especially when I moved to a city where I was the only Asian person in a Hispanic-dominated community. I felt out of place and had a hard time approaching other kids in the neighborhood, which led to more time [spent] indoors watching television. I began to gain weight when I was 9 because of the lack of exercise and the fact that I lived next door to Taco Bell and across the street from El Pollo Loco. At the time I was estranged from my older brother, who had moved out on his own. The last time he had seen me I was a skinny little kid. When I met up with him again, the first thing he did was scold me for being so fat. That was the first time I was called that, and all I did was

cry. Before that day, I hadn't thought so badly of myself. I knew that I wasn't as thin as I had been, but I didn't hate myself for it. But then I began to be more conscious of how others viewed me and started wearing baggy clothes to hide my weight.

Abandoned by My Mom

Then junior high came along, and just as I was finally getting comfortable, my parents moved us from South Gate to Koreatown. Now I was in a community that was predominantly Asian and although I looked like I belonged, I still felt out of place. Uncomfortable in my own body, I continued to wear baggy clothes and a sweater, even on hot days. It was at this time that I began having a strained relationship with my mother because she had started making comments about my weight. I felt like I was abandoned by my own mother, who was supposed to be the one to make me feel safe and loved. She began to tell me that I shouldn't eat too much and that I should only eat one meal a day. Although many girls in my position would have developed anorexia or bulimia, I knew about the dangers of such acts and refused to put myself through that. My mother would look me up and down every day with a look of disgust. I probably cried myself to sleep every other night—when[ever] she would say something hurtful.

Going on a diet never crossed my mind. Instead, I began to eat *more* than I could [easily] stomach just to get back at her in my own way. I wanted to show her that I didn't care what she said, as though I could somehow hurt her by showing that her words were insignificant to me. Then I would go off to bed feeling guilty about all the junk I had put into my body because ultimately I didn't want to be overweight. I hated looking in the mirror and seeing a fat version of myself staring back. I couldn't stand to look at my widening face, protruding stomach, thick legs and arms, or double chin. At lunch time I would be ashamed to eat in front of people for fear of being chastised for eating when I needed to go on a diet. So I would get a bag of chips from the student store and have a few of them before sharing [most of the bag] with my group of friends. Then I would go home and raid the fridge.

When my mother began to control what I bought from the market, I began to go buy [treats] myself and hide them in my closet. Sometimes she would find them after I left for school and throw them out. I continued to buy junk food, but now I had it in my mind that I had to finish it all before she got a chance to get rid of it. I never purged on purpose because I hated the feeling, but sometimes I would get sick and throw up from eating too much. This [continued] through high school, when my mother became more adamant about my losing weight. She began to say things like, "No one's going to marry you if you're fat." She even gave me positive feedback when I would tell her that I had nothing to eat that day.

The Look That Says a Million Words

I'm sad to say that I still struggle with issues about my weight because, let's face it, we all want a quick solution and fast results instead of the slow and steady. I [think I] still have a skewed view of myself because I still prefer to wear bigger shirts so as to not accentuate my stomach. I don't know if I will ever be satisfied with my body. Even if I somehow lose the weight, I think that I'll find something else about myself that would bother me because I've basically lived my whole life being judged on how I look. My mother has toned down on the hurtful comments because I informed her that it just makes me binge on junk food even more, but she still says a million words with just one look.

Hurting Herself to Hurt Her Mom: Hillary's Contradictory Body Project

In this troubling story, Hillary's mom, worried about her daughter's weight gain, starts showing concern with gentle comments and weight-control suggestions. But her daughter, feeling deserted by the person who is supposed to love her unconditionally, reacts by fighting back and doing the opposite of whatever her mother urges. The result is an escalating battle in which every weight-loss tactic the mom introduces, from persuasive to more coercive, is met with a countertactic by a daughter so wounded she is determined to hurt her mother at any cost. Even as the mother continues to wage an unwinnable war, the daughter is so blinded by her anger that she stubbornly refuses to adopt even the most basic practices of the good biocitizen. Instead, her project of rebellion calls for embracing the identity of a bad biocitizen by stuffing her face, indulging in junk food, and holding onto the idea that a quick-fix solution will materialize. So intent is she on causing anguish to her mother that she ends up hurting herself, gaining weight that she hates and feeling guilty about it all. Hillary's mom tried every biocitizen tactic available, but they all backfired, leading to weight gain rather than loss and a badly strained relationship.

A Spitting Image: Kelsey as Joan

Finally, we meet Kelsey, a tall, slender twenty-one-year-old white girl whose relationship to her mom is so close—in the photo she shared with me they looked like identical twins!—that, when her mom begins criticizing her weight, it leads to a cataclysmic fight whose end neither could have foreseen.

I grew up in the small town of Murrieta, California, as a white, upper-middle-class girl. I had a better family life than anyone could ask for and a home full of love and encouragement, for the most part. I have the best relationship with my mom, except for one thing: she constantly critiques my weight. Now I know why.

Sisters?

"Are you sisters?" is a common question [people] ask when my mom and I are together. We've even heard, "Are you twins, you two?" And when my mom blushes and responds, "No, I'm her mom, we started young," gasps and shock [follow]. We even sound the same; when the home phone rings, most people ask, "Is this Joan or Kelsey, because I can't tell." My entire life I have been dubbed my mom's twin, Joan's "mini me," her spitting image. I've always liked being like my mom. I genuinely think she is a beautiful person with a kind soul. However, when I ran into some weight issues from the end of my freshman year to the start of my junior year [in college], she mentally destroyed me to the point where I didn't want to visit home.

[It all started when,] at the end of my senior year in high school, my boyfriend of two years woke up one day and decided he no longer wanted to work to have a relationship with me. I was in complete shock. He was everything to me for two years. He was my first kiss and the person I lost my virginity to. After the break-up I was devastated. When college started in September, I had already lost some weight, but not a drastic amount. Then I found out that my ex-boyfriend's [dorm-room] window and my window faced each other (he had followed me to UC Irvine). For the next couple of months, he harassed me by throwing food at my window, bringing girls back to his dorm and engaging in sexual acts right by the window, and pounding on my window at three o'clock in the morning. I didn't realize that, as each month went by, I was losing more and more weight from all the heartache and trauma. By finals week of my first quarter, I was so feeble and sick that I had to be hospitalized. That was when I found out that I was 102 pounds at 5'10" [BMI of 14.6, dangerously low].

I was so sick that I had to be sent home. I was even excused from finals. I stayed between 102 and 105 pounds (size 00) for most of December and January. When I reached around 107 to 110 pounds, my mom told me that I looked beautiful and that 115 to 120 was a good weight to keep. (Throughout high school, I had never weighed more than 120 pounds.) When I started going to therapy and sustaining good health, I was not only able to eat again, but I wanted to eat everything. By the end of my freshman year I weighed in at 137 pounds and stayed between 135 and 138 pounds my sophomore year [BMI of 19.4–19.8, at the low end of "normal"]. Whenever I went home, my mom would tell me that I needed to lose a little bit of weight, and that as my mother—who stood 5'9" and weighed 130 pounds [BMI of 19.2]—"it was her job to tell me when I looked a little overweight and unhealthy" because that's what her mom always did. It didn't bother me much at first, but each visit home got worse, with more nagging and discomfort, especially because no one had ever bothered about my weight [before].

The Biggest Fight of Our Lives

When I went home for Christmas break my sophomore year, my mom and I got into the biggest fight we had ever had. I had just gone to the salon and gotten my hair dyed (from blonde) back to its natural dark brunette color. My mom flipped out, saying I looked "harsh and less radiant." That is when I lost it. I told her that I was tired of constantly being critiqued about how I looked [and] especially about my weight. I told her that it was my body and I thought I did a great job of taking care of it and representing myself well. I told her that it hurt me that she thought I was more beautiful when I was going through the worst period of my life than when I was happy and mentally healthy at 135 pounds. She cried hysterically.

Now I understand why my mom constantly discussed my looks: I am a reflection of her, according to society. When I changed my hair from blonde to brunette, I no longer represented my beautiful blonde mother. I had become more of my own person. When I was heavier than she was, my image became hers because she was "guilty by association." As her spitting image, according to society, I was responsible for being beautiful, slim, and fit for the both of us. What is ironic is that, at 135 pounds, I was still slender for my height, but I wasn't as slender as mom. To society [and] to my family, it was my duty to stay as slender as she.

After I explained the pressures of biocitizenship to my mom, she understood [my feelings of frustration and hurt]. It was intimidating to try to fit into the "Joan mold." She now tells me constantly how lucky she is to have a daughter with a compassionate heart and a good head on her shoulders. [Better that] than to focus on the extra five pounds I have gained or lost since my last visit home. I am now at peace with myself.

A Mother's Concerns Unraveled

In this illuminating essay, Kelsey turns her lens on a momentous episode in her life to uncover the complex underpinnings of her special relationship with her mom. Joan comes across as a caring but relentless biocop who sees it as her duty to chide her daughter to make sure she stays within the "family norms." In what may be common practice in this privileged segment of society, the mom's ideal weight for her daughter was not only below her own BMI but also well into the unhealthy range. (Kelsey does not mention this, accepting that her mom's ideal was in fact "healthy.") Kelsey becomes very upset that her mom is harping on her weight and ignoring her emotional well-being. Unlike the Asian girls we have met, who mostly endure parental bioabuse in silence, Kelsey confronts her mom, claiming ownership of her own body and insisting that her mental health is more important than her weight.

Reflecting on the painful fight that ensues, Kelsey comes to see how, in the biocitizen thinking that shapes these interactions (a term she learned in our class), parents are responsible for ensuring the healthy weight of their children. Then, going beyond what she learned in class, Kelsey explains how kids' bodies become reflections of the older generation's parenting skills, such that a fat kid means a bad parent and a bad biocitizen. Not only are their parenting skills being evaluated, so too are their own bodies, for a daughter's body is seen as a reflection of the mom's. Although the physical resemblance between the two makes this an unusual case, Kelsey's sensitive analysis of her situation helps us comprehend why virtually all the moms we have meet are so deeply invested in their daughters' weight.

Crushed by Male Fat Abuse

In previous chapters, we saw how fat abuse by relatives and peers worked to crush young people's sense of themselves as good, worthy social beings.

Devastating though these effects are, the consequences of fat abuse by an intimate partner, most often male, appear to be even worse. In this section, we witness the effects on two women who have endured sustained and brutal male fat abuse: Leanne, a young Vietnamese American woman who was physically beaten by a boyfriend and a middle-age Mexican American woman who was verbally and emotionally abused by an alcoholic husband. Fat battering in intimate relationships can, of course, occur in couples of any ethnicity. The essays I gathered also include a case of a middle-age Caucasian couple in which the wife was verbally assaulted with epithets like "heifer" for years before being rescued by a sister who removed her from the home and helped her heal [SC 169]. Whether the weight is the "real" reason for the abuse in these cases or just a pretext hardly matters because the effect on the abused person is the same. In both cases presented here (and in that of the Caucasian couple), it was an outsider to the relationship who cared deeply about the victim who told her story.

Scarred for Life: Leanne's Struggles to Survive

In this tender essay, a loving boyfriend tells the story of Leanne, a vulnerable nineteen-year-old Vietnamese girl from a middle-class San Francisco family who was beaten for a year by a former boyfriend who was displeased with her body image. Despite the loving support of her new partner, Leanne suffers from wounds that are likely to take years and years to heal.

Men have [extraordinary] power to influence how women view their bodies. [When violence is involved, it can be even greater.] The subject of my essay is my girlfriend of three months, Leanne. She told me her story about a past abusive relationship and how, as a result of it, she struggles with her weight.

A Violent Ex

Leanne was a senior in high school and dating a guy [who] was a year older and had already graduated. She had been with him for several years, but at the beginning of her senior year he began to beat her. She had been having a hard time with life. Her parents moved to Vietnam for work and she was left to live with her sister. Leanne is a very dependent person and needed her sister's support. She has told me that she would have been a better person if her parents had [stayed in the United States].

Her boyfriend was beating her because they would often get into fights and he would be dissatisfied with her body image. She is very reluctant to share the full story with me, but she has told me she was beaten for about a year. She ran away from home, did drugs, and ditched school to suppress the pain. She was afraid to leave [him] for fear that he would do something even worse. One night he dragged her by the hair from the living room to the bathroom, where he [repeatedly] hit her in the bathtub. She was terrified. She remembers the cold water all over her and [how red it was] from the blood [gushing] out of her nose.

One day in class, her classmate noticed that Leanne had a black eye. The classmate told the counselors, who told the police. The police officers came that day and asked who did that to her. Too afraid to tell them, she made up the excuse that she fell down the stairs. [Again], she feared for her life. She told me that part of the reason he was beating her was that he was dissatisfied with her body weight. She had put on a few pounds and he became abusive over it. He thought that by instilling fear and beating her, she would [gain the willpower to] lose the weight.

Long-Term Fractures

These struggles have proved consequential to her [relationship with her] family. She feels isolated and alone because she is withholding the story from them. It's a huge burden that she cannot get off her chest and move on from. It also has an effect on her love life. It took me a very long time to get her to open up. [Even] today, she still has trust issues and is afraid of being physically touched in any way.

The abuse [she endured] has had a profound effect on how Leanne looks at her body. Leanne is a girl who is easy to manipulate and has a hard time letting things go. At a young age, when she was developing as a woman and growing into her body, she was shaped by this traumatic experience, which has stuck with her. I can tell that she is very self-conscious about her body. She often [refuses to] eat unhealthy food, works out a lot, and eats small meals to make sure she does not gain any weight. I have told her I would love her no matter how she looked. However, she does not believe me and works without telling me to maintain a certain body image and weight. When we go out to dinner, she tends to get the salad rather than the steak. I tell her that her weight is good all the time, but she doesn't believe me. I think she is scarred for life. She often goes on crazy diets to cleanse her body and binge eats [and then purges] to look slim for special events.

Every so often we talk about her experiences. Although I know she is very hesitant to talk about it, it helps her cope when she does. She has told me that she just wants to look good all the time because she is afraid of men judging and hitting her. I told her I would never hit her. Although she believes me, and I have never done so, she is still afraid that it will happen again. I know she lives in fear of seeing him again.

Leanne's story shows that when it comes to our bodies, we are highly sensitive. I try to work on improving Leanne and making her feel loved once again. I really love this girl and just want to give her all the [care] she deserves.

Putting Leanne Back Together Again: A New Boyfriend's Valiant Effort

Leanne's story provides stark testimony to the human damage that can be done when fat abuse becomes physical. The violence left her with emotional scars, relational difficulties, and bodily compulsions that may last a lifetime. Emotionally, Leanne appears fragile in the extreme, indeed, near a point of breaking into pieces. So afraid is she of that violent ex that she won't tell anyone the full story, making it hard for her to move beyond the trauma. Her self-esteem is shattered to the point that she is unable to believe that her new boyfriend loves her or that she is beautiful. Unable to open up to anyone, she is isolated from those who love her the most. She is so emotionally traumatized that she is terrified of being touched and incapable of intimacy. The label posttraumatic stress disorder is not far-fetched in this case. The beating has also left Leanne with a set of extreme and potentially harmful body practices (cleansing diets and purging) that she obsessively pursues in a desperate effort to ensure she does not gain weight. It is no wonder that her new boyfriend fears that Leanne is scarred for life. One can only hope that, with his love and caring, Leanne will be able to slowly heal and put together a new life.

My Mother, My Hero

In this almost unbearably sad ethnography, a daughter recalls a painful childhood in a financially struggling family that was dominated by a raging alcoholic father who viciously berated her mother for her weight and appearance, leading her mother to retreat into silence and self-starvation. The daughter uses her essay to try to come to terms with what happened those many years ago in her OC-based Mexican American family.

I want to write about weight issues and the victimization of people who are vulnerable because society makes it acceptable for people to discriminate against them just because they don't fit conventional [weight] norms. From the many readings we did for class, [the one I found most] touching was the reading about women being abused by their partners for being really fat [an article by Tracy Royce]. I remember crying after reading all the abusive things that [people] say to fat women. I felt so heartbroken because I couldn't understand why fat women were being discriminated against, and by their romantic interest and loved one, no less.

One of the Most Beautiful Women in the World

When I was young I would watch [my mother] get dressed up for outings she and my dad would go on during the weekends. I remember thinking she was the most beautiful woman in the world. I loved the way she fixed her hair and her make-up; [I loved] her beautiful outfits and her shoes. When I was growing up, I never thought my mom had any weight or body issues. My mother was always well put together and she would do the same for my sister and me every morning before we went off to school.

It wasn't until after my second to last brother was born that I noticed she had gained weight. This was all normal, of course, as she had gained weight from being pregnant. I don't remember when it started or how it ended, but there was a point when I remember my father putting my mother down for her weight and appearance. As women we suffer from so many different traumas in our lives. Sometimes instead of seeking help, we deal with our problems by hiding them and only end up [with yet] another problem, often an eating disorder or body issue.

A Drunken, Abusive Father, a Silent, Suffering Mother

After that pregnancy, my mother struggled a lot to take the weight off. [She] would exercise and watch what she ate. She would also make us eat only healthy foods and she made sure we went to the park and played and were active. I don't think she was ever overweight. I think my dad just had some serious problems he was dealing with—[in particular, a serious drinking problem]—but since he didn't know how to deal with them he took them out on my poor mother. He was really abusive toward her, often insulting her looks and putting her down for her weight. She was seriously traumatized by everything my father would yell at her [during] his drunken spells. It's not hard to see why my mom would end up with body issues, since my father would exploit her and put her on the spot when he had been drinking. My father would say that she should watch what she was eating and how much she ate; he would [even] tell her to change [her clothes] if he didn't like what she was wearing. My father was [so very] hurtful.

My mom suffered so much [yet] never said anything or fought back. She suffered [mostly] in silence, never telling anyone what she was feeling or even talking to my dad about how he was hurting her. At one point she let everything my dad was taking out on her affect her to the point that she lost [a huge amount of] weight. With that, she also lost a sense of who she was. For a long time I remember my mother being very emotionally disconnected from us kids. I resented my father for taking my mother's voice away; he made her a silent victim to his demons.

I don't know if [back then] I knew what it all meant, but even if I did know, I think I would have just dismissed it because I figured my dad had a problem: he was an abusive alcoholic who needed help. I [probably] felt the need to sympathize with both of them, and didn't know how much pain all the putdowns caused my mother. I [feel differently] now. I understand that even though my dad had a problem, it in no way made it right to call my mother names for her weight and body image.

Today my mother has found peace and acceptance of who she is. My mother has learned to love herself and I know it's the best thing she could have done because she couldn't keep living life the way she was living. My mother is my hero and she is such a great hard-working person. I'm happy she found God and peace and didn't let my dad's problems bring her down and leave us without a mother. My mother is my best example of believing in yourself and being self-assertive. Even if someone or something is hurting you, you can't let it get you down because you have to [keep believing in yourself].

A Mother and a Family Torn Apart

In this poignant essay, the effects of years of verbal battering and emotional abuse of a wife by an alcoholic husband are seen dimly through the eyes of a sad, sensitive child who could not quite understand why her father was hurting her mother and why her mother emotionally abandoned the family. Unable to talk back, her mom slowly retreated into herself, becoming emotionally withdrawn from her children. Although the details remain sketchy, it seems that the mother developed an eating disorder, losing a huge amount of weight and, with it, her sense of self. Somehow— apparently through religion and an embrace of God—she found peace and self-acceptance.

This essay reveals the damage that intimate-partner fat abuse can do not only to the intended victim but also to the whole family. The children, not wanting to criticize and potentially lose either parent, are put in the middle, forced to look on silently as one parent bashes the other. The victim of the abuse is forced to remain silent, unable to confide even in her own children for fear they would be forced to take sides, which might lead to the breakup of the whole family. The result is that the mom is left alone, and the children, having already lost their father to alcoholism, are left without a functioning mother. The father made not just the mother, but also the whole family, the silent victim to his demons.

Families Pulled Apart

Families can be torn apart not only by destructive fat abuse of one parent by another but also by overzealous biocitizenship efforts directed at a child who is overweight. Stories of parents and siblings "ganging up" on an indolent family member were surprisingly common in the essays, and they were found in virtually every ethnic group. Sometimes, when the pressure is too great and the target is unable or unwilling to comply, the efforts have the tragic effect of wrenching the family apart. One family that met that fate is the Lis.

Good-Bye, Abby

In this ethnography, we meet the Lis, a middle-class Chinese American family from Hacienda Heights in which the parents, and especially the father, are so single-mindedly focused on ridding their middle child of a few extra pounds that they can't see that their harsh techniques are eroding her self-esteem and forcing her out of the family. This essay was penned by her younger sister, who saw the injustice but was powerless to stop it.

My parents have always made it clear to me and my two older sisters that health, exercise, and staying in shape were key in life. My mom's life revolved a lot around her appearance. She always had to do her make-up in the morning, she always wanted to change her hair color to stay trendy, and she always wanted to lose weight. My oldest sister Melanie and I maintain our weight pretty well. We're not involved in a sport nor do we work out often, but we just have a higher metabolism rate than my second sister, Abby.

Remedy for the Chubby Child: Diets, Diet Pills, and Lots of Laps

Ever since we were little, Abby was always a little bit chubby, but not to the point where she would be considered overweight or unhealthy. However, my father frequently stressed that she needed to stop eating so much and lose weight. My mom would constantly give her diet supplements. Melanie and I would always tell my parents that they needed to stop pressuring Abby to lose weight because it was becoming a burden in her life, and if she was comfortable and happy with her body, then my parents should be okay with it as well.

My family has always been very close and we enjoy going out and spending time together, but a lot of times I believe Abby feels left out. Especially when we were little, we would all go to my neighbor's house to swim for fun. Melanie and I would play in the deep end and go on the slide, but my father always made Abby swim laps. So many laps I would start to lose count. When I was younger [I guess] I was too self-absorbed to notice the way my parents were treating my sister. Now that I look back on our childhood, I find myself in disgust with the way my parents would treat Abby. It brings tears to my eyes to remember her being constantly tormented by the people she depended on the most.

Abby hated going swimming or hiking with us. She always made excuses that she had cramps or a lot of homework. My father would just call her lazy and unhealthy, but she was only trying to avoid the torment. She loved hiking and swimming. When we would go to a friend's house she was always the first one in the pool. She was confident in her body, and she didn't have a problem with exercising. Going hiking and swimming started to become less frequent as my sisters and I got older because we always wanted to stand by each other's side. We didn't want to leave Abby alone at home and we didn't want to give our parents the satisfaction of being able to treat Abby differently just because she was a little chubby.

I know my parents never meant to hurt Abby the way they did. They just wanted her to be "healthy." But she was actually very healthy. She was the only one in my family that played a sport in high school. She was involved in badminton and had practice every day. Her team even won the CIF [California Interscholastic Federation] championship in high school, but my parents never seemed to be proud of her because they were too focused on her body. Not only was Abby in a sport, but she always ate less than Melanie and I did. Abby never ate junk food, she only liked fruits, and she always made her own salad after class. [Mean]while Melanie and I would sit in front of the television and stuff our mouths with Oreos and Chip Ahoys.

My parents even took Abby to the doctor's so she could be prescribed diet supplements, but the doctor informed my parents that Abby wasn't overweight but average for her age and height, so they shouldn't worry. However, that didn't stop my parents from trying to get Abby to lose weight. Not even a doctor's opinion [or] knowing she had an average and healthy BMI could change their minds. My parents were basing [their view of her] health fully on [her] appearance.

My parents didn't even know how to put Abby on a diet because she already ate healthy and was in a sport. So my father thought it would be beneficial to take her running every Saturday morning. Abby knew from the beginning that she didn't want to do it, especially not with my father. Every Saturday morning, he would wake her up and try to convince her to go running. Basically, every Saturday morning, Abby woke up to the reminder that her body wasn't good enough, that *she* wasn't good enough.

During Abby's senior year in high school, she was still very much involved in her sport and [in school activities]. She always had straight As on her report card and scored an almost perfect score on her SATs. Compared to Melanie and me, she was the most hardworking one. However, Abby started to gain a little weight during her senior year. I didn't seem to notice but my parents noticed right away. They took her to the doctor again to see if she could get dietary supplements, but the doctors informed my parents again that she was still at an average weight for her height.

Escaping the Torment

I could see over the years that Abby has definitely become the most distant from my parents, and I feel like the main reason is [that] my parents cannot accept her for who she is. Abby is currently attending UC Berkeley and my family is from southern California, but Abby loves it at Berkeley and when she comes home for winter break, I can tell she dreads it. At home she is judged by her own parents, and at Berkeley people could care less [about her weight]. I don't think my parents realize that they have driven a wedge between our family and my sister.

I know that now Abby is slowly recovering and learning to love herself. She doesn't visit home much, and even though I miss her a lot, I think it's the best for her and for my parents. I'm glad she is able to be away from people who bring her down and able to focus on herself and her schoolwork without having to worry about [the constant burden of their disapproval]. My parents will never realize that they did something wrong, but I am glad my sister and I are able to see this happen because we have learned not to treat other individuals like this. Our family may be torn apart, but I know that Abby will continue to feel better about herself and within a couple of years, I hope, our family will be much closer.

Biocitizenship Run Amok: Abby's Parents Force Their Daughter Out

However one defines tiger parenting, this case would fit the definition. Abby's parents single-mindedly pursue a rigidly low standard of desirable weight, even ignoring the professional views of two doctors. Rather than trying to persuade Abby, they use harsh, coercive techniques to get her weight down. By treating Abby as different from the rest of the family, emphasizing her weight above all else, and refusing to praise her for other achievements, the parents have conveyed the loud and consistent message that she is little more than her weight and that she is not good enough for them or the family. Undoubtedly in response, Abby has spent her life as an overachiever—eating exceptionally healthfully, excelling in sports, and getting all As. Yet none of this is good enough for her parents. If her sister is right, the emotional impact on Abby of being reduced to her "chubbiness," excluded from the family, and constantly pressured to be who she is not, has been devastating. In typical Chinese fashion, she has never spoken back to her parents. Instead, she has withdrawn from the family. Although we don't hear her voice, Abby appears to be resilient, leading one to hope that she will eventually overcome the turmoil of her past and, as her sister puts it, come to "love herself." As for tiger parenting by virtuous biocitizens, not only did it erode their daughter's emotional health, it also tore the family apart, leading Abby's sisters to reject their parents' methods and commit to never treating another human being that way. Most ironically, the tiger tactics of these well-meaning but overly zealous biocitizens did not even work to lower her weight (which was at a healthy level in any case). The limits to biocitizenship could hardly be more clearly illustrated.

Who's Counting the Costs to Our Core Relationships?

In a biocitizenship culture that makes parents responsible for nurturing a family of thin, fit citizens, and in which the body size of our intimate partner is held to reflect our own human value, weight becomes a huge and often troubled issue in family and intimate relationships. The ethnographies here provide especially graphic examples, but almost every account in this book suggests the same conclusion. In all three relationships examined here, frustration with a fat child or partner led to use of increasingly harsh, abusive methods to bring their weight under control. In no case did the person targeted actually lose weight. But in every case, both the person targeted and that core relationship were damaged.

Among the three daughters, one found a way to move past the painful conflict with her mom, but it involved rejecting her mom's values. For the other two, who protested and rebelled against their mothers' efforts to shape their weight, the relationship remained fraught for years after the weight issue first surfaced. In the intimate-partner relationships, the fat abuse by the male partner inflicted great emotional and physical trauma on the women and eventually ended the relationship. And in the Li family, the coercive tactics of the parents led to the breakup of a tight-knit family, with one child forced out and the other two left feeling bitter that their sister had been subject to a grievous injustice.

The California ethnographies suggest that the scholarly description of moms as victims of the obesity campaign is fully appropriate. Although working women of color and lower class, the mothers emphasized so far, may receive the brunt of the public blame for the obesity epidemic, virtually all moms are burdened by onerous weight duties. This chapter shines a glaring spotlight on the impossible position in which the war on fat places the nation's mothers: they are made responsible for producing a generation of thin, fit young people, yet the tools available are not capable of doing the job. Although we have heard their voices only indirectly, reading between the lines of the essays, we are left feeling that being a mother today means constantly struggling to accomplish the unaccomplishable and, in the end, feeling like a failure—to oneself, one's children, one's family, and one's community. Moreover, they must endure the reactions of their daughters, who feel betrayed by their moms for not loving them unconditionally, when they (the moms) were just trying to be fulfill their duties.

Yet the language of victim may well be too simplistic. A closer look at the social dynamics of fatness shows that, from the vantage point of some daughters (and, in cases not presented here, also sons), in their efforts to be good biocitizens mothers are also drawn into being (well-intentioned) perpetrators of harsh language and tactics that amount to bioabuse. Further complicating the picture, men too play critical roles in the war on fat. Men may be invisible in the public discourse, but they are anything but invisible in the lives of real people with extra pounds. In the SoCal essays, men appear as both agents and targets of the war on fat. Interestingly, in their role as agents—that is, those trying to get others to change their weight—men rarely appear as biopedagogizers, yet they appear frequently as bioabusers who ridicule, castigate, or coerce others to lose weight.[7] In this capacity, men occupy a full spectrum, from ruthless abusers to sympathizers with those subject to abuse. At one end of the continuum, some, such as the husband of the beautiful mother or Leanne's ex-boyfriend, are vicious fat-abusers. Others, such as Abby's dad, appear to be harsh biocops. At the other end of the continuum are men such as Leanne's new boyfriend, who, in sympathizing with and supporting a traumatized girlfriend, are real life-savers. Beyond their role as agents in the war on fat, many men, including those deemed "too fat" and those labeled "too skinny," are the targets of concerted weight-talk and biocitizen tactics and suffer accordingly. Binh, Jason, and Huy (chapters 4 and 5) are unforgettable examples. The complex role of men and boys in the war on fat needs much more attention.

The war on fat was launched in the name of reducing the health and economic costs of obesity to the nation. As in all in public health campaigns, those costs were calculated in terms of dollars and cents. There has been little discussion of the costs to the nation of the war on fat itself, especially those costs that cannot be converted into monetary values. This and other chapters have made clear that the human costs of the war on fat are huge—both in terms of the emotional and psychosocial costs to individuals who both see themselves and are treated by society as fat subjects and of the relational costs to couples, families, and intrafamilial bonds. Who is "the nation" if not all of us, the sum total of our moms and dads, families and relationships, and individual selves? The real loser is society at large.

These forms of harm to the most fundamental social units of American society deserve a place in the public discussion about the national fight against fat. What price are we as a nation willing to pay to keep waging this battle? What if the battle is not being won, or is not even winnable with the "weapons" now at hand? What if the war on fat is inflicting all this human harm *and* is not working to reduce weight? I return to these questions after considering one final and critical issue: whether the campaign is helping very fat people, who face potentially serious health risks, to lower their weight.

9

DOES BIOCITIZENSHIP HELP THE VERY FAT?

If the public health campaign succeeded in lowering weights, the physical, psychic, and relational damage inadvertently done by the battles over weight might perhaps be worth it. That is, from a societal point of view, we might decide that these costs are acceptable trade-offs for a reduction in obesity. We now turn to that most fundamental question: Does the central dynamic of the larger societal war on fat—virtuous biocitizens, with the help of medical professionals, educating and pressuring people to diet and exercise to achieve normal weight—actually work to get heavy people to shed pounds?

In the essays we've read, we've met a great many overweight young people. Under pressure from their families, doctors, friends, and the wider culture, most undertook diet and/or exercise programs, but few lost weight. Three patterns emerged. In the first and by far most common pattern, the young people dieted and exercised but failed to achieve long-term weight loss. They invariably blamed themselves for "not trying hard enough" and redoubled their efforts, becoming ever more obsessive about their weight-reduction regimens. We might call these *frustrated weight-losers*. The majority of Americans would probably fit this profile. In the second pattern, some did lose substantial amounts of weight but only through excessive dieting and exercising or other risky practices (such as drug use) that posed threats to their health. We can call these *endangered weight-losers*. In the third and least common pattern, a handful of over-weight young people lost weight and kept it off but only by making body management the central focus of their lives. We called these *health freaks*. The California ethnographies suggest that the campaign against fat has not worked all that well for overweight people.

From a public health point of view, the most critical target of the war on fat is the very fat (or, in the language of medicine, "obese") person who, research suggests, faces elevated risks of health problems and perhaps early death. As we saw earlier, public health researchers routinely emphasize that obesity is statistically associated with dozens of medical conditions, many very serious.[1] Some of the strongest evidence for the risks comes from the data on mortality. A major meta-analysis published in 2013 shows that, compared with people of normal weight, obese people face an 18 percent higher risk of death from all causes.[2] All of this increased risk comes from the higher weight classes. People categorized as "severely" and "morbidly obese" (BMIs of 35–40 and 40 and above) have a 29 percent higher risk of mortality from all causes than normal-weight people. Those who are only slightly obese (BMI of 30–35) actually have a 5 percent *lower* risk of early death. Although debate on the protective nature of overweight and mild obesity continues, few doubt that the health consequences of higher levels of obesity are cause for real concern.

Whether biocitizenship works depends in part on why people become and stay very fat. The forces inducing obesity and discouraging weight reduction are numerous indeed. Some of the most promising research today suggests a potentially large role for endocrine-disrupting synthetic chemicals—materials found since the 1950s and 1960s in our air, water, and food systems and in household items—in damaging the normal function of metabolic hormones and stimulating the production and growth of fat cells.[3] The operation of such factors, though, remains invisible in the essays. Here we take a close look at three clusters of obstacles that are important generally and that loom large in the narratives.

The Biology of Heaviness: Genes and Diets

Despite an obesogenic environment, the biologically fortunate—those with what are colloquially called "skinny genes"—have little trouble achieving and maintaining medically normal weights. The majority are not so lucky, however. Research published in 2014 shows that obesity gains a foothold early—before age five, but certainly by age eleven, after which change is rare—suggesting its genetic and, to a lesser extent, environmental roots.[4] Genes act on weight through their influence on food preferences, hunger, fullness after eating, metabolic rate, and many other things, all topics of active research today. Family history is an important risk factor for obesity. It has been shown that similar BMI levels in families are largely due to genetic similarity. Estimates of the heritability of weight are remarkably high, ranging from 47–90 percent in studies of twins to 24–81 percent in family studies.[5] On a population level, some 25–40 percent of the variability in weight can be explained by genes;[6] among children, 30 percent of individual differences in body weight can be genetically explained.[7] Although genetics interacts with the environment, those born with "fat genes" will certainly have a harder time losing weight than those who do not.

One of the most important biological factors underlying fatness is the supposed cure: dieting itself. As we saw earlier, restricting calories produces modest weight loss in the short term, but the vast majority of dieters regain all the weight and many gain back more weight than they lost. What explains this counterintuitive outcome? The science of eating shows that the human body fights weight loss. Dieting induces hormonal and metabolic changes that make the weight-reduced body different from a similar-sized body that has not dieted.[8] Dieting discourages weight loss by, among other things, slowing the rate at which the body burns calories; increasing the body's efficiency at extracting calories from food that is eaten, causing the dieter to digest food faster and get hungrier quicker; causing the dieter to crave high-fat foods; and increasing his or her appetite. The research shows that for at least six years after weight loss, and perhaps much longer, the body defends the old, higher weight. The result, researchers say, is a "coordinated defense mechanism with multiple components all directed toward making us put on weight."[9] No wonder so few of the overweight young people I worked with were able to lose weight and keep it off!

Yo-yo dieting (or weight cycling, that is, repeated loss and regaining of weight), common in dieters but especially in fatter ones, is particularly pernicious. When one diets, the body produces less of the appetite-suppressing hormone leptin. This boosts the appetite and slows the metabolism, leading to weight gain. If one diets enough, it can actually push up one's set-point weight, the weight to which the body reverts when one is not dieting.[10] The science thus says that it is quite possible to diet *up to obesity*. Weight cycling also appears to be associated with increased risk of disease and mortality.[11]

Emotional Eating and Its Corporate Exploitation

In many cases, people put on excess pounds through what is known as "emotional eating"—eating driven by emotional needs and based on external or psychosocial signals rather than internal cues such as feelings of hunger and satiety. As Linda Bacon, author of *Health at Every Size*, explains, many of us seek—and gain—emotional nourishment from food, but our efforts ultimately backfire.[12] Because food cannot fulfill our emotional needs, we eat and eat, never feeling satisfied but often gaining more weight, which then deepens our sense of personal failure. And because we've largely lost the ability to hear our internal biological signals, we become more vulnerable to external messages about food. In an environment saturated with tempting food and food ads, there are few restraints on our appetites. The California essays are full of cases of emotional eating, cases in which young people living stressful lives turn to food—invariably high-fat, high-sugar, and high-salt food—for comfort and end up feeling guilty, compounding the distress and self-hatred. Binh, who ate to calm his nerves (chapter 4), and Sajeda, who soothed her loneliness with hot Cheetos (chapter 3), are prime examples. A more extended description of how it develops and precipitates a downward spiral of weight gain followed by more distress comes from the essay by Vui:

> I started college, and between classes and a bad relationship I ate my way through sadness and stress and disappointment in my life. I always felt hungry when I [got] stressed out or when I was having a bad day. The hunger

would not go away until I ate to the point where I was sleepy. I then just slept it off and woke up to yet another hungry stomach and the cycle continued. Although I knew that my eating habit was unhealthy, I did not care because I felt that I had no other way to make myself happy and to escape the issues in my life. The more I ate the more weight I gained, and the more weight I gained the worse I felt and the more I ate. This caused me to gain more weight, until I became the heaviest I had ever been in my entire life. [SC 2]

Our desire for food to comfort ourselves in times of duress is then exploited by profit-hungry food corporations. Food companies have become exceedingly clever at taste-engineering chips, cookies, and other junk foods to be so emotionally appealing and physiologically irresistible that the average person keeps eating them far beyond the point of caloric satiety. Processed-food companies, in other words, have made junk food addictive.[13] In *The End of Overeating*, David A. Kessler, former FDA commissioner, explains how food corporations, relying on sugar, fat, and salt, strategically create food that is highly palatable—that is, that keeps us coming back for more—and how exposure to such hyperstimulating foods leads some to develop conditioned hypereating that leads to sustained weight gain.[14] Just as emotional drivers often lead people to *undereat* to the point of anorexic self-starvation, emotional forces can lead people to *overeat* to the point of obesity.

The problem of snacking up to metabolic disorder and obesity is not confined to the emotionally needy, however. If J. Eric Oliver, political scientist and author of *Fat Politics*, is right, this style of eating is now part of the American way of life—one that may be particularly persistent because it expresses core American values of individual choice and freedom.[15] The emergence since the 1970s of tasty prepackaged snack foods, he argues, fundamentally changed eating in this country, allowing the individual (rather than the family food preparer) to decide when and how food should be taken and encouraging solitary eating. The rise of snacking has also changed the function of food. With most snack foods containing ingredients that act like opiates on the brain, serving as narcotics, stimulants, and/or tranquilizers, eating is no longer about getting adequate nutrition. Instead, it is a means to satisfy our individual psychological needs, whether they be stress reduction, boredom alleviation, or self-medication. What

Oliver suggests is that it is our very Americanness—our free-market system and our core values of individual liberty—that is making us fat. The problem is deep-rooted indeed.

The Fattening Effects of Poverty

As the statistics make patently clear, living in poverty is a major risk factor for obesity; especially among children and teens, the poor are disproportionately obese.[16] The complex ways in which social and economic disadvantage produces obesity are rooted in the larger political economy of U.S. capitalism, an important topic that falls outside the scope of this book but that others have written about in compelling ways.[17] The research of Paul Ernsberger suggests that the links between poverty and fatness run both ways, with fatness also promoting economic distress as a result of manifold discrimination against fat people.[18] In these essays, which focus primarily on young people, the effects of fat stigma on economic well-being are not yet visible, yet the effects of poverty on weight can be ferreted out.

I've left this topic for last for the simple reason that none of my students chose to write about it. Although the subjects of one in eight of the essays grew up in families that were financially struggling, no one wrote about the role of poverty in their own history of weight struggles. Either they did not see how structural constraints such as unemployment, low incomes, and unsafe neighborhoods shaped their eating and exercise habits, or they were ashamed of their family's circumstances and did not want to stress these factors. Perhaps both were at work.

In suggesting that everyone can be thin if she or he just tries hard enough, the dominant biocitizen narrative remains silent about the role of poverty and class. In reality, however, good biocitizenship is an option only for the middle class and the well to do, who have the time, money, and cultural know-how to eat well, exercise much, and focus on their weight rather than socioeconomic survival. Dara-Lynn Weiss's 2013 memoir of her efforts to get her seven-year-old daughter to lose weight suggests the extraordinary amount of resources required to achieve even a relatively modest weight loss (of 15 pounds, from 93 to 78). In *The Heavy*, Weiss describes an almost a full-time job, entailing preparing special foods, checking food-nutrient levels online, taking the girl to frequent medical appointments, attending meetings at her school, working through the daughter's constant "whining and complaining," and much more.[19] Few are the mothers with the time, financial wherewithal, and unbending determination required to succeed in such a project!

Such class dimensions of biocitizenship, however, are not part of the public story about obesity. Rarely do proud, high-achieving virtuous biocitizens acknowledge the role of their social and economic privilege in their weight and health achievements. Just as the larger biocitizen narrative, by focusing exclusively on individual responsibility, essentially blames the poor for their fatness (they are "lazy, irresponsible," and so forth), so too did my students blame their fatness and failure to follow the practices of a good biocitizen on their own slothfulness and other shortcomings. Overwhelmingly, my students had internalized the culture-wide narrative of personal deficiency, failing to see the role of structural forces in their own plight. Yet there is one account in which the work of cultural, social, and financial deprivation in producing obesity emerges in full force. This is the story of Pedro, and I present it in this chapter.

Biology, emotional eating, and poverty—these factors, often in combination, are some of the most powerful forces keeping the weights of many far above medically normal today. Can the pleas of caring biocitizens overpower these forces and help rid the obese of their fat? In this chapter, we meet six obese or borderline "morbidly obese" young and middle-age people whose weight has been the focus of concerted anti-obesity efforts by the virtuous biocitizens in their lives. We meet two hefty youngsters with supervirtuous biocitizen parents, two heavy middle-age Californians facing a wide array of concerned biocitizens, and two large-bodied young people whom many try to rescue from the fat-inducing environments of Cleveland and Los Angeles.

When Parental Biocitizenship Backfires

In this section we meet two sets of parents of quite chubby children who, in their efforts to ensure their children's health, start early and impose severe biocitizenship regimes on their youngsters. Unfortunately, the efforts backfire. Both Ishtar and Jennifer end up putting on so much weight that they become technically obese.

Rejecting the Biocitizenship Narrative at Last: Ishtar's Story

Ishtar's OC-based parents are part of the large, well-educated, and prosperous Iranian community of SoCal, which has high expectations for its members. Being a good biocitizen is crucial to being a good Iranian American. In plain yet affecting prose, twenty-one-year-old Ishtar, who with her family lives in Huntington Beach, reveals how well-meaning biocop parents who start too early and try too hard appear as tormenters to a young child.

Growing Up Fat with Super-Biocitizen Parents

From a young age I was above average in weight, and this was always a concern to my parents. My parents invested a 100 percent effort in their kids, so it's no surprise that something like weight, which they assume causes tons of problems like diabetes, worried them. My dad is very health conscious. He runs to work every day, runs marathons, and even completed the Iron Man competition. For as long as I can remember, he has been uncomfortable with my weight.

[As early as] elementary school, they had me on some sort of diet. While other kids had chips or cookies along with their sandwich, I had a piece of fruit. I would wish to have a yummy snack in my lunch like the other kids and thought how lucky they were not to have to worry about what they eat. I wondered why they could eat all this junk food and still be skinny. I was even very active at this age. Whether soccer, basketball, or volleyball, I was always playing some sport.

During elementary school I felt different from other kids. I was very shy and found it difficult to make friends. [Although] I was actually in decent shape, weighing about 140 at 5'6", this is the point where I probably felt the fattest. My parents stressed weight loss and rewarded me whenever I lost some weight. They would be so proud when I would eat less and be more healthy.

My mom also was above average in weight and we would do diets together. I tried Weight Watchers and the Atkins Diet. Whatever diet I would do, after a couple of weeks the restrictions would be too hard and I would end up quitting. Any weight I would lose I eventually would gain back—and then some.

A time when I would feel comfortable, I remember, was when we would take a summer trip to Iran, where my parents were born. My two aunts and their two girls were all larger women—even bigger than I was. They were concerned about how little I ate and urged me to eat more. For once, while I was there, I didn't feel out of place.

At one point in middle school, I would have a Slim Fast drink for breakfast and three fruits for lunch and then have some kind of rice and meat dish for dinner. Weight and diet were always on my mind. I did all the sports they offered. I got the MVP [most valuable player] award in volleyball and the Coach's Award in basketball. I got all As throughout all of middle school. [Yet] I never felt very proud of myself. These accomplishments were just what should be expected of me; I didn't feel successful because I was bigger than a lot of girls.

When I look back at pictures of myself at that age, it amazes me to see that I wasn't fat at all. I attributed my difficulty making friends and attracting guys to my weight, when really it was a lack of confidence and shyness.[20] I analyzed everything I said before I said it and often I would decide to just not say it. I wasn't comfortable in my own skin and felt awkward whenever trying to have conversations with people.

New Friends Bring Self-Acceptance

These feelings continued into high school. I had three close friends who could be described as the "nerdy" type. I really wanted to meet new people and in my sophomore year [met a group of new friends who] were different from the old ones—they were outgoing and funny. With these new friends, I started to come out of my shell and grow more comfortable with myself.

I had gained weight from eighth grade until sophomore year. I was around 160 pounds. At one [point] the pressure that came with trying to lose weight was just too much. I decided that I just wasn't going to care anymore. It was so freeing eating whatever I wanted without counting the calories. Without special attention to my weight, though, it just kept going up. My parents tried everything to get me back to dieting. My dad tried a scare tactic and told me that if I didn't lose weight, my friends would leave me, I would find it hard to get a job, and I would never have a boyfriend. This hurt me a lot, but I wasn't as fragile as before, [and] I was not going to go back to being shy and uncomfortable. I was happier at this higher weight than I ever was dieting and keeping my weight under control.

By the end of high school I weighed around 190 and was at my most comfortable and confident. The weight gain continued throughout college and I am around 210 pounds now [BMI of 33.9, edging on "severely obese"]. I do, however, have the most love for myself and [more] confidence than I have ever had in my life. I have plenty of friends, a great social life, and guys who are interested in me. I decided to just accept myself and be comfortable with myself. It is now obvious to me that I do not need to lose weight for social reasons, which was my main concern at one point. I do plan to eat healthier, though, and exercise, and if weight loss comes with it, then great!

Sick of Feeling Bad about Herself: When Concerned Parents Push Too Hard Too Soon

Ishtar's case shows how a bioitizenship program can run aground when it fails to heed basic child psychology. A girl with her mom's large body type (and so facing biological limits to weight loss unacknowledged by her parents), Ishtar watched as her diets not only failed but also led to greater weight gain. Unable to feel like a "good person," she had little self-confidence and no friends. After years of such anguish, all she really wanted was to feel good about herself. So when she finally found a group of supportive friends, she simply gave up on her parent's quest, freeing herself at last of the fat label and the anti-fat regimen.

In the biocitizenship view held by her parents, slenderness is essential to both good health and a rewarding social life. As a child, Ishtar's only concern is social acceptance; she is simply too young to grasp the possible implications of her heavy weight for her health. Once she finds approving friends, she rapidly casts off the "bad person" identity and practices her parents have thrust on her and claims a different identity, that of a self-loving large person with an active social life. In Ishtar's case, the well-intentioned but excessive biocitizenship program imposed by her parents backfired. They ended up producing the very fat child they had worked so hard to avoid.

Yo-Yo-ing up to Obesity: Jennifer's Losing Battle with Weight

Jennifer is a twenty-one-year-old middle-class Filipino Chinese from the Bay Area town of Union City who seems to have arrived in this world heavy. Diagnosed as overweight at age four, Jennifer was put on a medically managed weight-loss program by her mom. She remained on it for the next fifteen years, with results that dismayed everyone.

The Beginning of a Lifelong Struggle

Ever since I can remember, I have been considered "fat." I remember coming home from pre-school and being fed Nissin's Top Ramen, macaroni and cheese, and McDonald's Happy Meals. My mom did not know better than to feed me instant meals because she had just immigrated to the U.S. from the Philippines, where there were maids and nannies to feed the children, and because she didn't really know how to cook. On top of that, she was the stay-at-home mother of four young children. So, I guess I cannot really blame her for what happened next.

I vaguely remember going to a doctor's appointment with my mom one day when I was 3 or 4. I was just going for an [ordinary] check-up. To my mom's surprise, the doctor informed her that I was 4 pounds overweight. Essentially, my weight was medicalized at the [tender] age of 4. From that moment, I have been struggling with my weight. [Following] the doctor's suggestion, my mom began limiting my intake of junk food and sweets. One [time] when I was 6 or 7, I was craving M&Ms. So, I opened the pantry and took the M&Ms upstairs, where we weren't supposed to be eating. Eventually I confessed and I got in trouble. My mom tells me that her limiting my food might have been the reason for my increasing weight gain throughout childhood. She still feels guilty about it today because she believes that if she had not listened to the doctor and had just let me eat sweets when I wanted to, I wouldn't have always wanted what I couldn't have. Thus, I wouldn't have kept indulging and gaining weight.

One (Unsuccessful) Diet after the Other

A few years after that first appointment, I was much more overweight. I wouldn't have considered myself obese, just really chubby. My doctor's weight-loss suggestions weren't working, so she suggested exactly what I should be eating at meals: one-quarter plate protein, one-quarter carbohydrates, one-half vegetables. After hearing something like that I just craved food more. I couldn't stop myself when eating. I was just a little kid—I didn't know better, and my mom couldn't very well keep track of what I was eating all the time because I was already in elementary school and she had started working again. Plus, we hired a nanny who loved to feed me.

When I was 8, my dad felt that he was gaining too much weight so he, along with my chubby nanna and my chubby grandma, went on the vegetable soup diet. (I get my chubby genes from that side of the family.) Essentially, my dad was eating boiled-down, repulsive vegetable soup that was pureed to be disguised as something more edible. He tried to put me on it, but it was so disgusting that I wanted to cry. After my brother called me a cheater for sneaking bacon bits into my soup, the tears came. That's when my parents decided that I shouldn't be dieting like that at such a young age.

Starvation Diets Bring Temporary Success

When I was 9 or 10, I started to have crushes on boys. I had never had a boy "like me back." I was fat, and that's what needed to be fixed about me. So, at the age of 10, I decided to go on a diet. I began the cracker and water diet. I stopped eating breakfast; I would just drink water. By this time, my nanny had moved back to Arizona and my parents were separated, so my mom moved out. There was no one to make lunch for me, really, so I made lunch for myself. My lunch consisted of 6 to 8 crackers. For dinner, I would eat a regular-sized meal so I could hide the fact that I was dieting, so no one could tell me that what I was doing was unhealthy. No one—not my siblings or my dad—noticed.

From November to January, I lost 15 pounds. I can remember the joy I felt when I would step on the scale and [discover I had] shed another pound. By March I had lost another 10 pounds. By that time, people had [begun] noticing the weight loss and complimenting me on it. [By] the spring of 2001, I was a size 2, the skinniest I had ever been. For the first time in my life, I was skinny like my mom and sister. I had always been a good, hardworking student, but I had never felt so proud of myself as when I lost about 30 pounds. The feeling was remarkable, and I gained confidence. At the end of that school year, in fifth grade, I was finally satisfied because boys started to like me. From then until my sophomore year of high school I was thin. It still sickens me, though, that I need to starve my body in order to gain confidence. During those thin years I always watched what I ate for fear of being fat again.

Happiness—and Unwelcome Weight Gain

[In] high school, I started to find a balance between the social and scholarly aspects of my life. I was confident in both areas and I was happy. Toward the end of freshman year and the beginning of sophomore year, I gradually started gaining weight. By junior year, I had gained 15 pounds, going from 130 in my freshman year to 145 in my junior year. That year I started a relationship with my current boyfriend, and he made me happy. He made me feel beautiful, so I didn't have to obsess over my looks and weight. We both love to eat. So, when we got together we went out to eat a lot. I pretty much stopped watching what I ate.

By pre-prom season [of my junior year] I was 150-plus pounds. I went shopping for a prom dress with my mom. We found this beautiful dress that was perfect in every way except that I was a little bit too big for it. Reluctantly, my mom bought the dress and suggested that I go on a liquid-based diet. For 2 or 3 days I basically just drank dietary iced tea, and it made me cranky. I ended up looking great for the prom. [But] then the problems [began to pile up].

I had started eating regularly again, but my body reacted so badly to the starvation I had put it through that I gained tons of weight. From the summer of junior year at 165 pounds to the end of senior year, I gained about 30 pounds. I kept packing the weight on, even though I wasn't necessarily eating excessively all the time. From then until now, my junior year of college, I have yo-yo-ed a bit, bouncing between 185 and 200 pounds.

Right now I'm 195 pounds and 5'4" tall. I would consider myself fat but not obese. According to the BMI scale, I am obese [BMI of 33.5], but I try not to think about myself as fitting into some sort of regulated scale. I have always been big-boned and I can't really help that. I have many things to be proud of, yet I can still honestly say that I am not proud of my body. Whether I am willing to do something about it is the question.

Dieting up to Long-Term Obesity

Jennifer's case illustrates the sharp limits to the current approach to weight loss. Despite her doctor's and parents' concerted efforts over many years to get her body to shed pounds, for Jennifer the standard approach simply has not worked. She can maintain a normal weight only by constantly monitoring her weight and keeping herself on a near-starvation diet. Indeed, the approach actually backfires, for no sooner does she let up on the diet than her weight quickly swells, rising much more rapidly than it would have absent the prior self-starvation. Her body seems to be rebelling against the weight cycling by adapting to the famine phase, processing food more slowly and raising her set-point weight. If this is what has happened, then her long history of off-and-on dieting may have made it impossible for her to now keep the weight off. Put another way, Jennifer appears to have dieted her way up to long-term obesity. Buying into the biomyth that parents can control their kids' weight, her mom feels guilty, telling a psychologizing tale in which depriving a daughter of junk food only increased her craving for it. But any such psychological dynamics, even if true, are largely beside the point. To understand why Jennifer is heavy, one may need look no further than genetics (on her father's side) and the biology of dieting, both neglected by the personal-responsibility model of weight.

On Death's Doorstep: Good Biocitizens
Confront the Dangerously Obese

We now turn to two middle-age individuals, a father and an aunt, who are quite obese and suffer serious obesity-related health problems. It is here, where health problems begin to pile up, that the successful implementation of weight-loss programs becomes critically important. For many who have tried to lose weight and failed again and again, bariatric surgery often seems the only hope. Between 2010 and early 2012, southern California was blanketed with 1–800-GET-THIN billboards (and buswraps and mailbox flyers and radio commercials) announcing the lap-band as the easiest, cheapest, most fail-safe way to lose weight.[21] No warnings were included about medical risks. From the before and after photos and the promises of affordability they made, it is clear that the ads targeted working-class people of color. For those who did not see the exposes in the *LA Times* about the five patients who had died from botched surgeries performed by the clinics behind the ads, the billboards must have made bariatric surgery seem like a simple, low-cost, safe solution to the medical and social problems brought on by obesity. In any case, one of the people we meet in this section, Susanna, hit on weight-loss surgery as the solution to all her life problems.

When Biocitizenship Fails: An Obese Father
Paralyzed by Life's Problems

In this troubling story, we meet a well-to-do OC-based Caucasian businessman in his early forties who binge-eats to cope with life's traumas. Deeply concerned about his growing heft, his family and friends do their best to urge him to take responsibility for his health. Depressed, he cannot hear, instead continuing on his self-destructive path.

Ever since I can remember, my dad has been overweight. When I was in elementary school, even after long days of work, my dad would run around outside and play with me. We would go to the community club to play volleyball or basketball, or go swimming. [But] this was when he was younger, healthier, and in better shape. Upon hitting his late thirties, my dad began to slowly gain more and more weight until he fell under the category of obesity.

One Crisis after the Other

My father is currently the president and owner of a vitamin company; he used to run four health-food stores as well. However, towards the end of my grade school years, his health-food stores began to be in crisis. With the influx of large chain health-food stores my father's stores could no longer meet the competition, and he was forced to close his last store. This put great stress on my father and was most likely the beginning of his weight gain problem. I do not remember too much, but from what my mother tells me my dad would stay up late into the night calculating numbers and figures, trying to keep his business alive. The combination of stress and lack of sleep fostered a desire to binge-eat to cope with the stress. I remember numerous times waking up [and looking forward to] eating my favorite sweet breakfast cereal before school, only to find the once almost-full box empty. I remember saving a piece of birthday cake for my after-dinner dessert and finding it half-eaten at night. Sometimes we would ask my dad if he ate it, but after being denied a response over and over again, my mom, sister, and I would stop asking and just assume it was Dad again.

My dad's eating problem worsened with the onset of a lawsuit over his company and my grandfather's sudden heart attack. A few years after that, his mother began to have serious health problems [requiring hospitalization]. All these [developments] heightened his stress and spurred his desire to eat [as a coping mechanism]. By staying up late, my father was able to eat as much as he wanted of anything he wanted without fear that someone would call him out. Every trip to the hospital he made to see my grandmother, sometimes two or three times a day, again entitled him to another meal. The increase in greasy, fried restaurant food also contributed to my father's weight gain. [Meantime] he was still binging [on] "midnight snacks."

Hiding from All the Concerned Biocitizens

My father fails to acknowledge that he has a "binge-eating disorder" and that he eats too much or is overweight. No one in his family even knows his true weight. He will not even let us look at his driver's license for fear that we will see his weight. He refuses to go to the doctor unless it is absolutely necessary and will not listen to anyone who tells him he has a problem. We all know the doctors tell him he is overweight and is at risk for numerous health problems, and yet he still does not listen. He knows he is a little heavy but [insists] he is completely healthy. His usual response to someone's concern over his weight, other than [to ignore it], is that he runs a nutrition business and takes all the necessary health vitamins and supplements and therefore does not need other help.

As my father's weight has risen, more and more people have come up to him, out of full respect, to confront him about his weight problem. It used to be just my mother (who eventually gave up), his mother (who still persists every day), his father, and his brother. Recently, his non-immediate relatives have begun to confront him, then his close friends and co-workers, my grandmother's friends, our neighbor, and even the waitress at a restaurant he visits frequently. It appears that the more people who confront my father about his weight problem, the [more pressure he feels], and the more he denies the dismal reality staring him in the face. Food has become his sole coping mechanism. By denying the problem, he is refusing to take responsibility for his actions. Rather than turning to help, he is pushing away the ones who love him the most.

Addressing the Wrong Problem: A Father's Needs Misread

In this story we see full-fledged biocitizenship in action, but it did not produce the intended effect. With food the only safety net protecting this father and businessman from falling into an emotional abyss, he hangs onto the binging as though for dear life. Frustrated, some of his earlier supporters, including the author, give up on him and blame him for not taking responsibility and pushing away those who love him. Their attitude seems to be that, if their efforts as good biocitizens do not work, it is the target's fault; he is bad, irresponsible, and essentially irredeemable. They appear not to realize that deep-seated emotional issues may make him incapable of even hearing their pleas.

This father's tragic story highlights some important limits of the biocitizenship approach, which focuses intently on people's weight, even though oftentimes excess weight is but the external manifestation of emotional traumas that people don't know how to, or cannot bear to, address. In times of great stress, people binge-eat because food, especially high-fat and high-sugar food, is biologically and emotionally calming. Most fundamentally, dad has an emotional problem, not a weight problem. If the caring biocitizens in his life had instead showed compassion and helped him address the underlying emotional issues, or encouraged him to see a therapist, the weight issues might eventually have been resolved. Their single-minded focus on this dad's weight was counterproductive, for the greater the pressure on him to lose weight, the more he denies the problem and the greater his social isolation and risk of eventual weight-related disease. In this disturbing case, the biocitizenship approach has backfired, deepening this dad's problems.

A Random Encounter in the Store: How My Aunt Susanna Almost Died

In SoCal, where biocitizenship culture is intense, stranger-to-stranger weight pedagogy is quite common. In some cases, the insensitive remarks of a stranger, coming on top of years of self-loathing and failed attempts to lose weight, can push someone to take drastic action. In this essay, we meet Susanna, the middle-class Mexican American aunt of one of my students, who turned in desperation to bariatric surgery to solve her marital and other life problems.

A Life Spiraling out of Control

In mid-September 2009, my Aunt Susanna checked herself into the emergency room in a hospital near Long Beach for what she could only [describe] as a [terrible] mistake. Four months before that, in May, she had undergone a procedure because she was depressed, overweight, and tired of being tired. She had received a gastric bypass in hopes of living a "normal" life, which was code for saving her marriage, career, and sanity. Her life had spiraled out of control and every mistake she claimed to have made she attributed to the weight she had gained over the previous five years.

[Earlier] that year, she had been approved by her medical insurer to proceed with the gastric bypass surgery with a BMI of 36 because she had a history of hypertension.[22] Her doctors immediately approved her. Her first surgery was scheduled for late May and was described as a "minimally invasive procedure done through microscopy." When my aunt woke up, she complained that she felt as though she had just eaten a large meal and desperately needed to vomit. This feeling would continue for the next four months. By the time she checked herself into the hospital that September, she had lost 100 pounds and was severely dehydrated, malnourished, and hungry. There was no sign of her weight leveling out, either. She told the doctor that she was unable to eat more than a spoonful of soup at every meal; any more would be thrown up.

The heartbreaking part of the story is that my aunt was already losing weight. The previous year, [she] had signed up for an exercise dance class and was slowly losing weight and building [muscle] tone while doing something she loved. [But] one day, while at the store, she was approached by a man whom she described as weighing "at least 500 pounds" who told her she should be buying fat-free milk at her weight. This devastated her. A man who was nearly twice her weight felt entitled to criticize her body and her agency in choosing her food. The following day my aunt made an appointment with a gastric bypass surgeon and later that month she found herself with a smaller stomach.

The Roux En-Y

She received the roux en-Y procedure, which is the most common form of bariatric surgery and the one that is supposed to result in the least amount of nutritional deficiency. The operation was a disaster. Too much of the bowel was removed and her stomach was about 75 percent of what it should have been. When rearranged into the Y-configuration, a small flap of intestine was left inside her stomach, still attached to functioning stomach tissue. This is why she felt full all the time, and the flap of skin was triggering homeostatic processes that eject food from the body. At 5 feet, her starting weight was 240 pounds. By the end of September she weighed 130 pounds.

The second, third, and fourth surgeries were attempts to stretch her stomach to the proper bypass size. All three attempts were failures. She spent the next three months in and out of the hospital. By January 2010, her weight had dropped to 87 pounds. Doctors gave her little chance to live. In February, 2010, the top gastric bypass surgeon in California contacted my aunt offering to fix her stomach. Desperate, she reluctantly agreed, and he was able to fix the issue. I later looked into the training of the doctors who performed these surgeries. The final surgeon my aunt visited was the only one trained to perform microscopy surgeries. All the others went to weekend training sessions. Finally, with her stomach at the proper size, my aunt's weight leveled out at 125. She was at her target weight, but it came at a high price. She suffered and almost died in the pursuit of the perfect weight.

Susanna: Now Thin but Not Healthy

"Severely obese" and suffering from hypertension, Aunt Susanna was a prime candidate for obesity surgery. In her case, the biocitizenship approach worked as it was supposed to—through public shaming—but the effects were not the right ones because surgical complications almost led to her death. Even if she is able to keep her weight down by adhering to the rigid postoperative dietary restrictions she must follow for the rest of her life, Susanna is left with serious nutritional and other health risks, on top of the emotional and relational problems that drove her to the surgery in the first place.

Aunt Susanna's case illuminates problems with other aspects of our culture's orientation to heaviness as well. One is the cultural endorsement of quick-fix solutions. The ubiquitous ads that, at the time, were promoting surgery as a low-cost, simple solution to obesity worked to normalize a decision that in other parts of the country might have seemed extreme. Her story also sheds light on the unappreciated consequences of our tendency to narrate our life problems and their solutions in terms of weight. If, instead of tackling the bodily manifestations of her problems, Susanna had instead addressed the underlying emotional and relational issues, she might be on her way to recovery right now. Finally, our culture so despises obesity that fat people are urged to lose their excess weight at any cost. The risks of surgery are considered nothing compared to the emotional, social, and economic costs of living as a fat person in this society. Susanna's story makes plain that the surgical "cure" can be far worse than the "disease."

No Biocitizens in These 'Hoods: Poor and Fat in Cleveland and Los Angeles

Maps featured on the CDC website show the fifty states of the United States in vivid colors that range from blood red and dark orange (for the fattest states) to gold, dark blue, medium blue, and finally light blue (for the skinniest). With 34.6 percent of its residents obese, Mississippi is the fattest state; Colorado, with 20.5 percent, is the thinnest.[23] California, at 25 percent, is in between but on the skinnier end—more Colorado than Mississippi. Although the U.S. state is not a very meaningful unit for the study of weight because states are made of up diverse regions, such maps convey the important truth that the weight of Americans, far from being a product of individual effort alone, is rooted in larger cultural, economic, and political contexts that influence the ways individuals are able to care for their bodies and health.

While conducting research for this book, I discovered that people in weight-conscious, self-perceived "healthy" regions such as southern California have fantasies of rescuing relatives from other, heavier parts of the country by bringing them to California for a fat-cure. They believe that by lifting them out of their fat-inducing environment and teaching them the weight-wise ways of southern Californians, they can transform them into virtuous biocitizens who will retain their SoCal ways after they return home. Our first essay tells the story of a family who invited a relative from a fat city in a fat state—Cleveland, Ohio (29.2 percent of Ohioans are obese)—to come live with them for the purpose of learning how to get her weight and life under control. The fat-cure worked—for a while. In the second essay, we meet Pedro, who grew up in a poor minority area of Los Angeles. More than any other in this book, Pedro's life story shows how poverty creates the breeding grounds for obesity and how the poor end up blaming not the poverty but themselves for their failures.

For the Sake of Sylvie: The California Cure

Sylvie is an eighteen-year-old African American from a relatively indigent family in Cleveland. At her aunt's urging, and with her mother's consent, she spent almost three years in San Diego with her aunt, who sought to remake her into a proper SoCal biocitizen.

An Unhealthy Upbringing

My cousin Sylvie, [who lives in Cleveland,] has struggled with weight since she was a little girl of about 5. My aunt Cheryl, the sister of Sylvie's mother, Cara, knows better than I do how her social influences, eating habits, and lack of physical activity have affected her life. By her sophomore year in high school, Sylvie had been struggling in school, ditching classes, and not completing homework assignments, to the point that she was no longer on track to graduate. She was very involved in her social circle, however. She would go along with her popular group of friends, participating in underage drinking and a lot of partying.

Weight in the black community in Cleveland is an issue. Every summer when I visit, I notice that a lot of my relatives and others in the community are "obese" or "overweight." The mood in Cleveland is very slow and somber, drastically different from that of the southern California lifestyle that I'm familiar with. In addition, Sylvie's mother, Cara, who also struggles with weight, did not discipline her daughter and, more important, did not notice her tremendous weight gain and unhealthy eating habits. Cara and her husband work long hours and care for their autistic twin sons, who are younger than Sylvie and require much attention and energy. After repeatedly catching wind of Sylvie's extensive social engagements and poor performance in school, my aunt Cheryl and her sister Cara agreed that Sylvie needed a change in environment to set her on the right track for educational and health purposes. In the summer of 2008, when Sylvie was 16, she moved from her parents' home to live with my aunt in San Diego.

The SoCal Cure

My aunt Cheryl lives with muscular dystrophy but is quite active and mobile provided she has the proper [equipment]. However, she knew she could use the extra help at home, and Sylvie desperately needed a change. Being overweight has [lowered] Sylvie's self-esteem. Sometimes I wonder if it causes her to look to others—mainly her friends, new and old—for approval. If her friends want her to go somewhere, or if some activity will boost her popularity, she wants to be part of it.

In the fall of 2009, during a physical my aunt insisted that Sylvie undergo, doctors diagnosed her with non-alcoholic steatohepatitis, or "fatty liver." Doctors stressed that continuance of this condition would result in serious health complications [in the future]. My aunt placed Sylvie on a strict diet to combat the condition. My aunt would prepare baked instead of fried chicken, steamed vegetables, and foods higher in protein and daily fibers and lower in fat, cholesterol, and sodium. Sylvie lost 30 pounds over the course of six months through eating healthy home-cooked meals and performing light nightly exercises. Sometimes she would simply take a walk around the neighborhood; at other times she would lift weights in her bedroom.

Back to Cleveland

In 2010 my aunts Cheryl and Cara agreed to allow Sylvie to return to Cleveland for the summer. This was a reward for her after she had greatly improved her grades and become very active in a positive social environment, her school choir. Sylvie of course was excited. Unfortunately, the visit may not have been the best for her health or social progress. Perhaps because she is an incorrigible teenager, she is highly susceptible to peer influence. Over the summer and then when she returned to San Diego, she neglected her exercise routine and started eating fatty foods, fast food, and unhealthy food. My aunt feared this would happen and unsuccessfully encouraged her to [switch] back to the [diet] plan she had [originally] adopted. Currently (in early 2011) Sylvie is almost 19 and has gained all of the 30 pounds back, plus an additional 15 pounds. Now she weighs almost 280 pounds. She has yet to return to the doctor for a checkup on her fatty liver.

Two months ago, Sylvie received an acceptance letter from Virginia State University. My aunt Cheryl and I know that this would not have been possible without the drastic change in her lifestyle in San Diego. We worry about her health and hope she will revert back to healthy living before it is too late and she begins to fall sick. Yet she is an adult now and will have to make her own health and life decisions [from now on].

A Tale of Two Mothers or a Tale of Two Cities?

In this fascinating essay, Sylvie's SoCal-based cousin tells a classic biocitizenship story that centers on individual and parental responsibility for obesity. In this account, Sylvie is too heavy because her parents are irresponsible. Moreover, her friends are a bad influence. In the cousin's view, the San Diego aunt Cheryl can give Sylvie the SoCal fat-cure and bring her weight down. And sure enough, the San Diego plan works like magic. But no sooner does she return to Cleveland than the SoCal project fizzles; Sylvie gains back what she lost and then some, ending up at 280 pounds and with the fatty liver unattended to.

Beyond the palpable (and predictable) moralism in this story (the bad parents, the good aunt, and the bad visitor who gets what she deserves), what is interesting is how the author, with her insistent focus on individual responsibility for health behaviors and outcomes, fails to recognize how Aunt Cara's "bad parenting" and Sylvie's "irresponsibility" might be a product of larger forces that are beyond their control. Census statistics paint a powerful portrait of two different worlds inhabited by Cara and Cheryl, one of poverty and one of privilege. In 2010, in one city, Cleveland, the median household income was $27,349; in the other, San Diego, it was $62,480. In Cleveland, a mere 13.1 percent of adults had a bachelors or higher degree; in San Diego, 40.8 percent were so fortunate. Cleveland was predominantly African American (53.3 percent black, 37.3 percent white), while San Diego was majority white (58.9 percent white, 6.7 percent black).[24] Although the myriad ways in which social and economic deprivation begets heavy, diseased bodies remain out of sight here, if we could track those forces, this story of the irresponsible aunt Cara would certainly turn out to be a story about two places: Cleveland, where lack of access to education and good jobs breeds obesity, and San Diego, where social and economic privilege provides the conditions for people to become good biocitizens—and brag about it. The author's story is right as far as it goes, but by neglecting larger structural forces, it blames the poor for their plight and leaves us without an understanding of the kinds of reforms that are necessary to help people like Sylvie avoid ending up very heavy and at risk of chronic disease.

Anything but Lazy: Pedro's Struggles to Control His Weight

Pedro is a twenty-three-year-old Nicaraguan American who grew up in a part of LA where two-thirds of the residents are Latino and one-third live below the poverty line. Pedro's story reveals the kinds of economic pressures and cultural disadvantages that can pile up, one on top of the other, to turn poor kids into fat kids and fat kids into fat adults and parents. This essay is adapted from an interview with Pedro, which I taped, transcribed, and reorganized into a chronological narrative.

"El Gordo"

I was born in Willowbrook, an unincorporated area of LA [and] then at age 12 moved to nearby Downey. Yeah, it was the 'hood. A lot of Latinos there. My mom is from Nicaragua, my dad from Armenia. Since high school, I've been living on campus because my dad lives in a one-bedroom apartment with my sister. My mom has been in jail for the last ten years; she was framed for something. So, basically, I'm on my own. My girlfriend and infant son live with me.

When I was little I was overweight. I was like really big. I was like 160 in fourth grade. When my mom used to take my sister and me to the doctor, he would say, "You're fat, you know." Almost literally, he said in Spanish, *gordo.* [Responding to a prompt] No, he didn't tell me my BMI. I was a child, and I don't think my mom would have understood. My mom spoke broken English. The pediatrician was Egyptian and he spoke very bad Spanish. Our weight was a big part of what we always talked about. We would check blood sugar and all that stuff. To check for diabetes or pre-diabetes, I guess, because it runs in my family or something.

Being heavy didn't bother me that much at the time. In middle school, in PE every week you had to run the half mile in a set period of time. I was a big guy so I couldn't really finish in time. Most of my exercise came during the summer [when] I would ride my bike everywhere. I was good coming out of middle school and going into high school. I didn't do sports in high school [because] I have asthma. But I didn't really want to do sports anyway. I like my guitar and music. And my dad didn't like my staying after school. They wanted me home whenever possible.

Four Hot Dogs a Day

During my fittest time in high school, I would come home every day and eat four hot dogs because that was the easiest thing to make. And I was fine. I didn't really eat healthy per se; I think it's the fact that I ate very little, though, after or before that. During the day, lunch was always small at school. Everyone [else] would buy stuff [i.e., other food], but I didn't really have any money so I would stick to what the school gave me.

I was average when I came to college. I gained a little weight the summer before because I worked at Starbucks and every day I would drink and eat Starbucks or Taco Bell, which was on the way to work. Coming in here, I weighed like 190, which is still good in my opinion. And then, you know, by the end of my second year I weighed like 230. [At 5'6", Pedro had a BMI of 37.1, "severely obese."] It's hard to eat healthy here. You have to learn to cook yourself, and you're lazy and don't have time. So [I] just make a hot pocket or something. And then my third year I was not eating too well—I'd eat a bowl of rice and one Subway sub every day—so in a few months I went down to 200. I felt really good and tried to maintain that weight. I have pictures if you want to see them. I have so many pictures of me, it's ridiculous. I took them for a reason. And I show people these pictures. I have them here [in my phone] because I need to see them for inspiration; I need to know what I can look like—my potential. Because if [I don't have the photos], I'm just like, I feel bad a lot of the time.

My weight has fluctuated so much in the past year and a half; I've gained 70 pounds [to a BMI of 43.6]. I had knee surgery to repair a meniscus that I tore at the gym. That set me back a lot. I had the surgery like six months later because I didn't have the insurance. I was in bed and depressed because I couldn't work out. And then I messed up my knee again, less than a year ago, and had another surgery. I'm having trouble just starting to jog. And I was so used to like running everywhere—that was my thing. So I've [had to] put the whole working-out thing on the backburner for now. I hate it, you know, because I've seen what I can do. I've tried—I try eating healthy, I try eating small portions. I'm seeing a therapist and that's one of the things we talk about.

No Money for Fruit or a Nutritionist

The week my son was born, my girlfriend and I had Jack in the Box three times a day for a week! There was no time to cook at all. [Responding to prompt] Of course, in middle school and high school health ed classes, there was always someone to tell you what a nutritious diet is. But you hear it and hear it; I heard it often enough that I was like, "Eh, I know what it is." Everyone knows that fruits and veggies are good for you. But you don't always have fruits [available to eat]. We don't buy fruits a lot because they expire and we forget about them. Or it's hard to buy enough fruit for every day because it's not that cheap. We're getting food stamps—actually, free food from WIC[25]—right now, and it's a limited amount.

People tell me I'm fine the way I am, but I know I can look better. It's so easy to be, like, "Oh, those toy story cookies look good, let's buy a box." I would eat one or two a day, which felt alright because four were 140 calories. And then just last week I was like, "Those cookies look good," and I ate 16 of them in one sitting. I felt so bad about that. It didn't help that this past weekend, my girlfriend's mom brought fried chicken over. I ate so much. It felt so greasy. I feel like I took five steps back from wherever I was the week before. So it's things like that, you know. I made an effort; it's not that I'm lazy. That's a misconception a lot of people have—that overweight people are just lazy. But they're not. I've tried, you know, I've been from 200 to 230. I've been 70 pounds lighter, and I've lost weight. And I have other things to do [like study and tend to a newborn]. But then you have other people who have the same stuff to do, but they weigh less.

You think, you know, that something's wrong with you. You think you're not—I don't know—I think I'm doing something wrong. I think when I diet alone, I can control my weight at least to a more reasonable level. Like maybe 220 or 230, instead of [my current] 270 or 260 [BMI of 42–43.6]. But it's hard; I just don't know how to do it. I've recently thought of seeing a nutritionist, you know, but there's a small co-pay. In my situation, every ten dollars adds up.

It's hard to go on a regular diet because my girlfriend and I don't have a lot of money, so when we buy groceries it has to be stuff we both like to eat. We buy hot pockets, we buy orange chicken, and every time we make it, we make the whole package, so it's like, oh, extra food, we'll just eat it all. My girlfriend's always saying, "I want to lose weight, I feel fat." I tell her, let's do something about it. But when it comes down to cooking, we make the food and we eat it and we forget that we're supposed to be watching our weight. For us, food is just so good; we forget we're supposed to be counting calories.

A Sisyphean Task

Nowhere are the effects of socioeconomic disadvantage on weight more starkly evident than in this story of Pedro's battle to keep his weight down. He has been the object of efforts of virtuous biocitizens his whole life (doctors and teachers, although not parents), but their encouragements and blandishments have proved powerless in the face of entrenched poverty. Pedro grew up in a poor community with parents who were unable to foster good eating and exercise habits and seem to have passed on genetic proclivities to heaviness and diabetes. As a young adult, Pedro knows what foods are good for him, but he can't afford them and, even if he could, he has no time to prepare them. Instead, he lives on the kind of high-fat, high-sugar, high-salt diet that packs on pounds and undermines health. He dreams of consulting a nutritionist but cannot afford the modest co-pay. He wants to exercise, but his asthma and two surgeries have kept him inactive. Meantime, much to his distress and confusion, Pedro's weight just keeps on rising, reaching morbid obesity.

As if being fat and facing the associated health risks were not punishment enough, he suffers a huge dose of shame and guilt. Although pushing back on the equating of fat with lazy, Pedro internalizes the narrative that he is to blame for his weight and that he is bad person because he overindulges in bad food. Like the fat people we met earlier, Pedro suffers from the sense that there is something fundamentally wrong with him, but he doesn't quite understand what it is. He also suffers feelings of deep inadequacy, feelings he can ease only by gazing at photos of his thinner self. If Pedro's case is typical of those living on the margins—and much evidence suggests that it is—then the message of biocitizenship has reached the truly poor, but it does not and cannot work because becoming a thin, fit citizen takes time and money, and the poor have neither.

The Limits to Individual and Societal Responsibility for Weight

The accounts we've just read tell a troubling story about the ability of the biocitizenship approach to help those at greatest health risk. No matter how many well-intentioned family members and friends stepped up to educate, urge, and/or cajole these heavy people to lose weight, the effort never succeeded. To the contrary, in virtually every case the program backfired, doing more damage than good. Sorting out why everyone's efforts went awry will help us see some of the real-life limits to our current approach to reducing fat.

The ethnographies of Jennifer and Ishtar reveal how biology can conspire with psychology to undermine the efforts of earnest biocitizen parents and doctors to induce weight loss through scolding and imposing diet and exercise rules. With both girls apparently inheriting "heavy genes" from a parent, biology alone may have made the quest for normality an impossible dream. Psychological dynamics also played a role, though. The biocitizen program involves imposing an identity of "fat and bad" on the heavy target. When that identity is forced onto a very young child, it can have unexpected and devastating effects. In one case, the daughter found the identity and the restrictions so intolerable that, as soon as she found friends who valued her as she was, she relabeled herself "fat and good," and gave up the effort to shrink down. In the other case, a girl given that degrading identity undertook dangerous diets in an effort to shed it. As she began to crave the foods that were forbidden, she found devious ways of getting them and, in turn, packed on the pounds. After years of on-and-off dieting, both ended up gaining more weight than they had ever lost.

In the stories of the middle-age relatives, the efforts of concerned biocitizens also proved counterproductive. In the case of the father who coped with life's problems by binge-eating, caring biocitizens emerged as one would hope, but all their weight-talk seems to have deepened the dad's resistance. The more they confronted him the more he withdrew, putting himself in danger of losing his family and perhaps losing his life. In the case of the aunt, the "helpful" suggestion of a stranger precipitated a drastic weight-loss strategy that almost ended in her death. In both of these lives, biocitizenship failed because it was unable to address the fundamental causes of their weight gain: life's numerous stresses and the emotional problems accompanying them. As with so many instances when social ills become framed as medical problems, the biomedical "cure" does not fit the real "disease." And so, of course, it does not work.

In the ethnographies about Sylvie and Pedro, the biocitizen program did not and could not work because it failed to address the ways that the food insecurity, economic insecurity, and social marginalization that plague poor neighborhoods make it impossible for their residents to pursue the health-focused lifestyle demanded of the virtuous biocitizen. In the case of the Cleveland cousin, the biocitizenship project of a SoCal aunt worked wonders for a while, but it was not transportable back to the home environment. As for Pedro, the efforts of teachers and doctors in his early life were simply overwhelmed by the realities of extreme cultural, social, and economic deprivation. Although the achievement of a thin, fit body is really possible only for the middle and upper classes (especially for those with the right genetic endowments), the dominant narrative about obesity remains silent about the brutal realities of class. Instead, it preaches individual responsibility and blames the poor for their heavy weight and ill health. We are able to hear Sylvie's voice only indirectly, so we do not know how much she was bothered by these attributions of blame. Raised in health-obsessed SoCal, Pedro, however, takes them as yet another sign that he has failed in life and deserves his exclusion from the community of the deserving. On top of the injuries of obesity and the health risks it entails, he must endure the insults of blame and self-blame.

If the biocitizenship approach to weight control does not work when it matters most—when aimed at fat people facing potentially serious health risks—isn't it time to step back and rethink the war on fat?

Part 4

What Now?

10

Social Justice and the End of the War on Fat

We now live in a society in which one [mean] comment can destroy a child's life. This book must be a call to action.

Courtney, Cambridge, Massachusetts, and San Diego, California, April 2014

For some fifteen years now, Americans have heard the official obesity story again and again—the one about the threatening national epidemic and how we must all join in a massive campaign to fight fat. Rather than challenging that narrative, in these pages I've set it aside to tell a different, more human story about how the war on fat has played out in society and with what effects. The essays have put faces on the complex struggles that are obscured by the simple, seemingly transparent statistics of public health. In these final pages, I draw together the main findings that have emerged from the essays and analyses and then suggest some things we can do to begin ushering in a new, postwar-on-fat future.

The Societal War on Fat: Biocitizenship and Its Unintended Consequences

My story began with a narrative about the recent history of the anti-obesity campaign—how it took root and flourished in an entrenched culture of thin worship and fat hatred, and then, as it gathered steam, absorbed some of the meanest strands in that culture: an almost visceral hatred of corpulence and a deeply rooted moralism that equates fat with bad and thin with good. The anti-fat campaign not only built on that antipathy toward largeness, it also deepened it. As it began recruiting more and more sectors of society to fight fat, the public health campaign quickly transformed into a sprawling multisectoral war on fat. At this point, the historical narrative winds down, and my students' essays about their lives start shaping the story line.

From their ethnographies, it is clear that these young people grew up in a world full of earnest biocitizens all trying to mold them into successful thin, fit Americans. In the private spaces of their homes and family gatherings, in the public spaces of the schools and malls, in social media sites and on the Internet, almost everywhere they turned, they encountered a barrage of fat-talk in which everyone was judging everyone, including them, by their bodies. When a youngster began to put on excess pounds, well-intentioned biocitizens sprang into action, starting with informative fat-talk—the tips on diet and exercise, and the compliments or veiled insults telling people how heavy they were. Much concern has focused on the harmful effects of those put-downs, and that is warranted, but the essays suggest that the compliments deserve just as much attention, for comments such as "you lost weight, you look great!"—which are so commonplace as to go unnoticed—were just as powerful in encouraging weight-consciousness and weight-loss efforts as the slights. When the pedagogy didn't work, worried caregivers turned to more abusive fat-talk, stigmatizing and shaming people to motivate healthful change. The bioabuse documented in the ethnographies was shocking—from derogatory labels like "slut," "fat, ugly piece of shit," and "bloated lump of fat" to hateful behaviors like throwing trash at the fat girl or faking a heart attack to stress the dangers of excess pounds.

These ways of treating the overweight and obese are mean-spirited and cruel, to be sure, but what this book newly reveals is that they are also culturally legitimate. Southern Californians seem to feel that, given that there is a national epidemic of obesity and everyone is responsible for maintaining a normal BMI, the irresponsible, selfish people who refuse to do so, and so harm the rest of us, fully deserve the derision, condemnation, and censure they get. The (apparent) scientific authority behind the discourse seems to encourage the bullies to feel even more justified and self-righteous in using any means necessary to bring the noncompliant into line. Although female confidantes sometimes comforted the target of the attacks in private, remarkably, in public there was no push-back, no one who came to the defense of those targeted for abuse. Instead, the victims were left to suffer on their own. As Binh lamented, "my damn relatives just let me take it." Not only is such abuse considered deserved, it is deemed beneficial to the target, who is expected to see the light at last and change his or her ways. The essays make strikingly clear that biobullying is a pervasive, widely condoned, and actively encouraged feature of our culture today.

Few Pounds Lost, but Many Untoward Consequences

Despite the monumental efforts and massive resources of so many social forces, the biocitizenship approach of making the self and society primarily responsible for weight is not achieving the campaign's primary goal. A tiny handful of our subjects did shed pounds and keep them off, at least for the time covered in the essay, but they were the exceptions. Among the many overweight people we met, the vast majority were frustrated weight-losers who, despite failed efforts to lose pounds, kept on trying. A small number were endangered weight-losers who succeeded in shedding pounds—but only by engaging in extreme practices that posed threats to their health. The smallest number were self-proclaimed health freaks who achieved normal weights but only by making bodywork the center of their existence. Even those at greatest health risk—the very fat—failed to lose weight and, in some cases, added pounds despite the concerted efforts of the virtuous biocitizens in their lives. Why did biocitizenship fail? Because the heavy weights stemmed not from individual laziness or laxity but from a complex of deeply rooted emotional, biological, and economic problems that all the coaxing and badgering of earnest biocitizens could not address.

Previous chapters uncovered some of the troubling if unintended consequences of the way obesity has been tackled in the war on fat. My students' heartfelt essays reveal that that war has turned virtually everyone with any extra body fat into diet-, exercise-, and weight-obsessed fat subjects—people who often were only slightly overweight, but who saw themselves as fat, took fatness as a core identity and became obsessed with relieving themselves of that stigmatized identity. Notably, it was not so much a desire to be thin and attractive as it was a desperate need to restore "health" and to avoid social condemnation that motivated change. Rejected as socially contaminating and undeserving of friends, fat people ended up socially isolated. And fatness brought emotional trauma wrought by years of verbal abuse about being lazy, ugly, irresponsible, and unfit for participation in American society. Having so many people feel so bad about themselves may be good for American capitalism, but it is not good for the health and happiness of American society.

It was not only heavy people who came to feel fat and to take fatness as their core identity. Young people who had medically normal and socially acceptable weights but were subject to ubiquitous fat-talk came to see themselves as at risk of gaining weight. As the fear of fat came to inhabit their consciousness, they became potential fat subjects and reorganized their lives around avoiding that dreaded fate. Of all those we met, the ultra-thin were some of the most tormented by weight worries. Subject to constant comments about their "weakness," "freakiness," and "anorexia," these extremely thin people came to view themselves as unhealthily underweight—defective, socially unacceptable skinny persons—and did everything in their power to change that. Thick or thin, the essays suggest, almost everyone was a fat subject of some sort.

The ethnographies also reveal a larger society preoccupied with, even obsessed by, weight, a society of individuals who take health as a super-ordinate value and devote much of their lives to micro-managing their diets and exercise patterns in hopes of achieving thin, fit bodies. They live, in short, in a healthist society, and the war on fat has intensified that trend. Yet as the stories of Jade and Sarah, the self-identified health freaks, make patently clear, healthism is not necessarily good for our health. Assuming there exists an "optimal" or "perfect" health—what one critic calls the "chimera of health"—healthists blindly pursue it at any cost, subjecting their lives to rigid discipline and taking bodily practices to extremes that could endanger their health.[1] Healthism today relies heavily on the popular science of diet, nutrition, and exercise found on the Internet, attributing objectivity and beneficence to "experts" who may possess neither of these things. Thinking they are creating scientifically managed lives, healthists may be remaking their lives according to the advice of self-proclaimed experts who are peddling their own prejudices—and often their own commercial products, some of them dangerous—in the name of science. Perils abound. Moreover, healthism crowds out other life goals. What is lost are other identities, other notions of what it means to be a good American. Jade and Sarah are extreme cases, but most of the young people we met lived by healthist values to some degree. The transformation of so many into weight-obsessed people diminished them as human beings by keeping them focused on fighting fat rather than studying, advancing their careers, helping their families, or trying to do good in the world.

Michelle, Meet Pedro: The Unseen Dangers of Targeting Children and Teens

The public face of the anti-obesity campaign today is Michelle Obama, whose Let's Move! campaign has generated great enthusiasm. With its appealing images of kids playing basketball and planting gardens with the first lady, her message is that we should focus our energies on children, teaching them healthful habits that will last a lifetime and giving their moms or other caregivers the information and tools they need to buy and prepare healthful meals and to get their kids to become active.

Following the standard public health approach, Let's Move! focuses on the high obesity rates in the black and Hispanic communities and promotes the biomyths that young people and their parents can control the weight of the young and that it is their ignorance of healthy practices and failure to take responsibility that are the problem.[2] As Obama put it in a 2013 speech to the nation's largest Latino advocacy group, "We need to step up [and] own this as a serious problem in our communities. We need to . . . start questioning the behaviors and beliefs that are making our kids sick."[3] The Let's Move! campaign seems to assume that minority children (and their moms) are underexposed to health-promotion messages and information; once properly educated they will eat well and exercise much. There could be areas of the country where that is the case, but, given the ubiquity of such messages—in the schools, in doctor's offices, and in the popular culture found on TV and the World Wide Web—I am hard pressed to imagine where they are. In California, children are, if anything, *overexposed* to these health messages. Yet this knowledge does not necessarily translate into health. Perhaps the first lady could meet Pedro, who as a child heard the fruit-and-veggie messages again and again but has not, either then or now when he is a young parent, been able to eat as well or exercise as much as he'd like to because of the force of economic duress. The SoCal data provide virtually no support for the notion that ignorance and laziness are at the heart of the childhood obesity problem.

The evidence from southern California suggests the need for concern— if not alarm—about targeting children. What the essays in this book say is that our young people, supposedly the major beneficiaries of the war on fat, may actually be its biggest victims. Children and teens suffer some of the greatest damage because their minds and bodies are not yet fully formed. Children are highly susceptible to social judgment, especially from the authorities in their lives charged with their upbringing and care. Children are also highly sensitive to the norms and judgments of their peers because their greatest desire is simply to fit in and be "normal, like everyone else." The ethnographies suggest that children are particularly vulnerable because the emotional wounds from being labeled "fat" at a tender age can last a lifetime. So much trauma accumulates around the fat person identity that, even after losing the bodily fatness, the fear of looking fat or of getting fat again haunts them. Having grown up with the war on fat, today's youth have been raised to believe that obesity is a major national problem, that it is their duty to be thin and fit, and that they are bad people and bad Americans if they fail. The young people we have met are members of the first war-on-fat generation—the targets of anxious efforts by parents to raise healthy, socially valued youngsters; of doctors to diagnose and preempt weight-based "disease"; and of schools to create weight-loss-promoting environments. The young people have been molded into fat subjects by the constant fat-talk of their caregivers, their peers, and the wider culture; this identity has come to inhabit their consciousness, making it hard for them to imagine any other way of measuring their human value and of living their lives.

Although subject to such anti-fat pressures their whole lives, these young people have had no public voice in any of it—either in their designation as the main target or in the ways the war on fat has shaped their selves and lives. Hence the value of the auto-ethnographies I have gathered, which permit us to hear some of their voices. Some of the stories my students relayed are distressing in the extreme. Who can forget Annemarie, the star basketball player who felt powerful and in charge of her life until that day in seventh grade when a school nurse declared her overweight, turning her into nothing more than another fat girl anxious about her body? Or Jason, the third grader who could beat the fifth graders at handball but was forced to give up his game because he could not bear all the bullying about his skinniness? Or the ultra-thin Linh, whose family believed she was too mentally and physically weak to take on the rigors of graduate school, forcing her to curtail her life ambitions? So many young lives and dreams have been cut short—the stories are endless. All this human trauma has been imposed on these children and teens—and to what end? Of course, the promise was health. In most cases, though, the teasing and interventions did not improve physical health (few if any of the youngsters lost weight) but, instead, harmed the young people's mental or emotional health. For those whose bodies did not match the culturally and medically mandated body size, the war on fat punctured their dreams and diminished their lives. Instead of playing with their friends, they were online looking up weight-loss techniques, dieting, and exercising in an endless battle against their own bodies. This excessive weight worry needs to be part of the conversation about obesity today.

Concrete Bodily and Psychiatric Harm

Not only is the war on fat not lowering weights, it is actually harming people—and not just fat people but all people who are the "wrong" (that is, abnormal) weight and are trying to rectify it, a category that included most of the people I worked with. The harm took many forms. It included the bodily harm from starvation diets, excessive exercise, and diet drugs. It also included psychiatric peril, namely, the disturbing possibility that the relentless dieting so energetically encouraged by the wider culture, by coaches of certain sports, and by many doctors was causing people to slip noiselessly into full-blown eating disorders. Such risks to Americans' physical and mental health are built into our approach to eradicating obesity. By encouraging the badgering of people to lose weight, offering no effective methods, and stigmatizing them for failing, that approach drives them to take their body projects to dangerous extremes.

The young people I worked with were completely unaware of the risks they were taking. Told repeatedly that dieting, exercising, losing weight, and being thin are good for their health, and hearing no warnings about limits on or dangers of these practices, they energetically undertook them, believing they were doing healthy things for their body. To most of my subjects, disordered eating and excessive exercise were normal behaviors, just their and their friends' way of life. By unintentionally fostering and normalizing disordered eating, and focusing laser-like on anti-fat messages, the war on fat may be worsening the problem of eating disorders among the young.

The war on fat is also tearing the fabric of our society. Struggles over weight too often damaged mother-daughter bonds, leaving daughters of nagging moms feeling angry, wounded, and abandoned by the person who was supposed to love them unconditionally. And in families where the parents imposed rigid bodily standards on all and insisted they be met, battles over weight sometimes broke up the family by forcing members who could not make the grade to leave. "Good-bye Abby," the story of the Li family, is a sad reminder of this rare but painful possibility. Fat abuse in romantic relationships—which remains unmeasured but certainly is quite common—can destroy its victims and end relationships, especially in cases of extreme and prolonged abuse, such as the two we read.

The war on fat is particularly unkind to the nation's mothers. Moms, already responsible for so much, have been given a set of onerous new tasks they must accomplish to be a "good mother." Existing critiques have drawn this conclusion from studies of the discourse promoted by the war on fat. This book adds a vital ethnographic perspective. Although we have heard moms' voices only indirectly, their kids' essays make clear that the war on fat has put mothers in an impossible bind. They are charged with nurturing a whole family of thin, fit biocitizens when there are no tools with which to successfully do so. And then they are criticized and shamed and blamed for failing to do so—not only by faceless government officials and the kids' doctors and teachers but also by friends and relatives. And these are not just working mothers of lower-income and ethnic minority status, the groups on which others have mostly focused. The California research suggests that all mothers are subject to these expectations and criticisms. On top of these pressures concerning their children, mothers

have their own bodily unhappinesses and struggles to deal with. As the
advocacy group Families Empowered and Supporting Treatment of Eating Disorders (FEAST) insists, parents and especially moms are not the
problem in the development of eating disorders or of disordered eating;
instead, they are caught in a vise, with no way out.[4]

The ethnographies were relatively silent about fathers (except as part of
"team parents"), embodying the widespread assumption that fathers bear
little responsibility for their children's body size. This is of course patently
untrue: fathers affect their children's weight through their genetic contribution, their role in creating the home environment, their comments about
what it takes to be successful in life, and so on. Even where the contribution
of the father was glaring, the dad's role was scarcely mentioned. Striking
cases were those of Seth and Jason, who got so much grief for being skinny
although their fathers had also been skinny at their age. Those fathers quietly shared their experiences with their suffering sons, but neither spoke
out to the critical mother or family friends in defense of his son's skinniness. It is as though the fathers' knowledge and experiences had little legitimacy, as though weight were a mothers' matter only. Fathers did have
one dedicated role. While moms were invariably in charge of diet, some
dads took charge of creating and enforcing rules on exercise. This was not
so much a cultural expectation, because there was little evidence that men
who failed to promote exercise were sanctioned, as it was a project that
some men took on probably to feel proud that they were doing their part
in making their child healthy and to gain social approval for being a "good
father." Overall, though, the fathers' role was distinctly secondary to that
of the mothers, reinforcing the assumption that mothers should and can
successfully control the children's weight.

Recalculating the Balance Sheet?

The dominant narrative stresses the costs of obesity to the nation's health
and economics. The emotional, social, bodily, and relational harm inflicted
on individual Americans in the name of fighting fat is not counted. Indeed,
such costs are not even measured and, thus, remain invisible to the public
and policymakers alike. The 45 essays presented here and the other nearly
190 accounts that I gathered provide stark evidence that the approach we

have now is doing real, measurable damage to our selves, our psyches, our relationships, our families, and especially our young people. The sheer amount of human suffering that individuals and families are enduring in the name of fighting fat is staggering. What if these costs could be measured and tallied up? Would we find them acceptable? What if the war on fat imposed all these costs and made little dent in the obesity problem? What would we say then?

The Social Fabric of Body Weight: More Reasons
Gender, Ethnicity, and Class Matter Now

The ethnographies also suggest the need for a reset in our conversations about gender, ethnicity, class, and weight.

Sheryl, Meet Sajeda

Fat used to be a feminist issue, as the psychologist Susie Orbach put it in her 1978 book, but the official discourse of today's anti-obesity campaign is remarkably silent about gender, treating fatness as an equal-opportunity "disease." Among young people, levels of overweight and obesity are at rough parity today, with boys slightly more overweight than girls (15.3 compared to 14.4 percent), and slightly less obese than girls (16.7 versus 17.2 percent; data for 2011–2012).[5] What the statistical data cannot tell us, however, is what that means to boys—whether being heavy invades their sensibilities the way it generally does among girls. The California ethnographies allow fairly strong conclusions about gender. They say that, statistical parity notwithstanding, fat still is—or should be—a feminist issue. Although boys were subject to vicious fat abuse too, and they suffered emotionally on account of it, in every case the boys were able to rise above the taunts and resist taking on the global identity of fat boy. Because boys' worth is evaluated primarily on the basis of their achievements and because boys rely much less on others' views for their sense of self, boys such as Binh managed to escape the feeling of being a devalued "fat person." These findings are consistent with those of Lee F. Monaghan from the United Kingdom, where heavy men have a variety of discursive strategies they can mobilize to construct socially acceptable masculine identities for themselves.[6] In California, girls subject to similar kinds and amounts of abuse invariably took on the fat-girl identity and felt bad about themselves as persons. Regardless of all the advances girls have made in education, sports, and other domains, their worth is still ultimately tied to their appearance. As Sajeda and many others wrote, despite all their accomplishments they could not feel good about themselves because their bodies were too big. By so insistently and publicly stressing thinness as essential to health and civic belonging, the war on fat is undermining girls' self-esteem. Twenty years ago, Naomi Wolf underscored this reality in her book *The Beauty Myth*.[7] Today feminist gurus such as Sheryl Sandberg, who tell young women they can be successful by just "leaning in," simply do not get it about body size.[8]

Yet, before we declare boys relatively free of weight worry, we must recall the plight of the underweight, which has been worsened by the war on fat's constant drumbeat about weight. Being relentlessly skinny posed agonizing problems for everyone we met, but the problems were especially severe for men, for to be a "real man" (and to be a good biocitizen) requires being big and buff. To escape the constant comments and feelings of falling short as a person, virtually all the ultra-thin men tried everything they could to bulk up. They had no lasting success—indeed, some actually lost weight—leading to extraordinary personal suffering, which they could not openly express for fear of being called a sissy. Although skinny men are a distinct minority, being concentrated among one broad ethnic group, their problems deserve more attention.

Good and Bad Ethnicities? Undoing Inaccurate and Harmful Stereotypes

What about the stereotype of the "good Asian," who is supposedly helping the nation solve its obesity problem by staying thin? The aggregate statistics on weight and ethnicity support this image, but the ethnographies tell a different story. In comparison with families of other ethnic groups, the Asian families were distinctive in sharing elements of a traditional parenting style rooted in values of respect for authority, hard work, and parental discipline. Among themselves, the Asian families differed in the degree to which they incorporated more "American" parenting methods into the mix. Especially in families living in Asian-majority communities, parents had highly demanding body ideals for their children, often imposing standards that were even more strict (read: skinny) than the cultural standards of mainstream society established by well-known celebrities. In Chinese, Vietnamese, and Korean cultures, in particular, the norm for women was to be rail thin. Such extreme ideals may have reflected both Asian beliefs in the ability of hard work to overcome any obstacle and the conviction that Asians needed to try harder and do better than Caucasians to get ahead in American society. In the tight-knit, ethnically homogeneous Asian communities that dot the southern California landscape, the achievement of such norms was a critical measure of social success for individual and family alike. In these communities, comparison and competition between families for the best-bodied children was intense. So too was the fat shaming directed at parents with heavy kids. These dynamics help explain why Asian parents, especially those in largely Asian communities, were hypervigilant virtuous biocitizens, so obsessed with raising thin kids (the "fit" part was less emphasized) that their treatment of the weight issue very often bordered on abusive. Asian parents used the most heavy-handed and authoritarian weight-control methods of any group. By spreading fat hatred, the war on fat playing out in the wider society added fuel to this cultural fire, both legitimizing minority parents' efforts to shame their kids into losing weight and providing new cultural discourses with which to do so.

Although many of the Asians looked thin by the standards of the dominant culture—hence, the stereotype—they were too thick by the standards of their own cultures and so became subject to insistent parental efforts to get them to become even thinner. In many families, body size became another source of intergenerational strain. Little did the Asian parents know how much trauma their well-meaning efforts inadvertently inflicted on their sons and daughters. Their youngsters' responses varied—from quietly compliant to sullenly cooperative to defiantly hostile to, in the rare case, openly resistant. The overall result of all this pressure, however, was extraordinary levels of emotional duress in the younger generation, many of whom, for reasons of genetics or biology or fat-dense environments, simply could not meet their parents' goals. Bringing loss of face to their parents as well as themselves, the young people of Asian descent experienced the most weight-based distress documented in the essays. Four of the six cases of relational harm were in Asian families. My students' essays thus support the notion introduced earlier that harsh, tiger-type parenting tends to produce not compliant and successful children but resentful, hostile, and emotionally damaged ones.[9]

If the stereotype of the thin happy Asian overlooks the extreme pressures many young Asians are under to become even thinner, it also misses the reality that not all Asian Americans are pleasingly skinny. Strikingly, five of the six cases of "obese" young people were East and Southeast Asian (the other was South Asian).[10] And some were unpleasantly skinny. In the essays, there appeared to be a biological tendency among many Asians to have shorter, thinner frames than the young people of other ethnic backgrounds. Not one Hispanic, Middle Eastern, African American, or Caucasian male was skinny, but a great many Asians were. Moreover, thin bodies were not necessarily healthy ones, for Asian bodies seem to have more fat and more risky patterns of fat deposition (that is, abdominal fat) than do other bodies.[11] All in all, the image of the "good Asian" received little support in these SoCal ethnographies. Like the stereotype of the hypersuccessful "model minority," the stereotype of the superhealthy "thin Asian" conceals more than it reveals and sets up a false image of perfection that almost no one can live up to.

There were not enough cases of African Americans and Latinos to draw conclusions about the stereotypes of the "bad black" and the "bad Hispanic." Certainly, there was no evidence of any kind of ignorance of the health consequences of obesity or laziness about dieting and exercising.[12] One intriguing pattern did emerge, though. In almost all the families we encountered, the parents were relatively relaxed about their children's weight and, when they encouraged weight loss, they used supportive methods such as promoting participation in sports or slow, steady weight loss through sensible dieting. In several cases not featured here, Latina mothers helped protect their daughters from the trauma of weight abuse that many Caucasian and Asian kids suffered by telling them they were beautiful at any weight and refusing to accept a doctor's label of overweight because they "did not want to make their daughters suffer more than they have to" [SC 162, 163, 190, 219]. The essays suggest that, far from being ignorant, such cautious, measured responses to a child's weight gain are *more sensible* than the agitated reactions of some other parents, which led to emotional and, in cases, even bodily harm in their youngsters.

The Hidden Injuries—and Privileges—of Class

One of the most powerful findings to emerge from the essays is the close connection between poverty and, more generally, class or socioeconomic security, and weight. The dismaying story of Pedro (and, to a lesser extent, Sylvie) shows especially clearly how social marginalization and economic disadvantage breed overweight in one generation, which gets reproduced in the next. The essays make very clear that everyone, rich and poor alike, hears the warnings of the war on fat—they are ubiquitous and inescapable—and that virtually everyone wants to be thin and fit but only some are able to achieve this. Pedro, poor and member of a minority, is precisely the kind of person the anti-obesity campaign is supposed to help, but because it only lectures people like him to "eat better and exercise more," neglecting the very real economic and structural constraints on his ability to do so, it could not help him lose weight. Instead, it left him feeling like a bad person, a failure to himself, his family, and his country.

Meantime, the offspring of the middle class, who formed the vast majority of subjects in this book, took for granted their ability to buy the things that go into good biocitizenship. Their complaints centered on lack of willpower, stress in their lives, or biologically obtuse bodies. For their part, the truly rich faced a problem of a different kind—body ideals so exacting that only loads of time and money could produce them. Not recognizing their own privilege, some of the middle- and upper-income young people prided themselves on their own bodily virtue while scorning others who were unable to reach that standard. Such is the power of class in America—remaining invisible even as it creates great social, bodily, and moral divides.

Medicine and Its Social Reach

So far I've said little about the role of public health and medicine, but health professionals have had a big hand in how things have turned out. It was experts in these fields (which for simplicity I call simply "medicine") who first created the national crisis of obesity and then declared a national war on fat. To this end, medicine has insistently pathologized heaviness, labeling overweight and obese people defective and diseased and, in the process, defining these conditions—their understanding, definition, and treatment—as belonging within the sphere of medicine itself.

Bull's-Eye on Children

Yet medicine had no safe, effective, long-term treatment for these conditions. And so the onus was put on children, with the goal now being to prevent obesity in the next generation.[13] But medicine had few proven techniques to apply to this problem either. When the clinical guidelines for managing the childhood obesity epidemic were developed, the expert group in charge had to rely on best-guess medicine—essentially reduced calorie diets and greater exercise—in hopes that effective measures would soon be discovered. With few options and much hope, medicine encouraged the biomyths that people can control their weight and that parents can successfully manage their children's weight. It promoted the use of the BMI because it was easy to calculate. And, because children's health practices are shaped by many institutions beyond the family, health officials outlined a campaign in which virtually every sector of society played a role.

Questions of Social Justice

All this seemed reasonable at the time and, after all, public health campaigns are always launched on the basis of partial knowledge and optimistic best guesses. Yet fifteen years have passed, new data are available, and it is time to take stock of the results. When we pay close attention to these accounts of how children and teens have been personally affected by the war on fat, questions of social justice come to the fore. With its many tales of tortured selves, of emotional and bodily harm unintentionally inflicted by medicine itself, and of damage done to relationships and families, this book suggests that the war on fat has perpetrated a grave injustice. It is unjust to classify one-third of children and teens—to say nothing of two-thirds of adults—as "biologically abnormal" and "diseased" when the field of medicine has no safe, reliable means to enable them to lose the weight and keep it off, and so become "well" and "normal." The ethnographies suggest that the diagnosing of so many as "diseased" when medicine has no way to successfully "treat" them consigns perhaps the majority of young Americans to feelings of being damaged and defective; to being excluded from the community of good, valued Americans; and to the anxious pursuit of the near-impossible quest of becoming thin. This life-diminishing labeling without effective treatment is all the more unjust when one considers that most people are heavy in good part because of weight-prone biologies, genetics, and/or environments—forces that lie beyond their own *and* medicine's grasp.

Clinical Medicine Challenged Too

Many sectors of public health and medicine have reaped benefits from the war on fat. But the war on fat has probably not been so good for the nation's roughly 900,000 clinicians,[14] especially those in primary care or family medicine, who are on the front lines of an ongoing, almost unwinnable battle with their heavy patients. Given the difficulty of achieving weight loss and the intensity of the emotions surrounding it, for them fighting the war on fat has mostly been an exercise in frustration. Indeed, many surveys show that primary care doctors feel ill equipped to treat obese patients and believe that their efforts are ineffective, futile, and unrewarding.[15] One of the most striking findings of this research is the extraordinary negativity many patients felt toward medicine and its treatment of their weight. In California, many children have come to dread going to the doctor for an ordinary check-up, fearing that he or she will calculate their BMI and deliver a moralizing lecture or, worse yet, declare the child overweight and unhealthy, precipitating a series of unpleasant changes in how the child is treated by doctor and parents alike. Many fat adults, treated in demeaning ways by their caregivers, simply stop going to the doctor;[16] heavy children rarely have that option. How can a doctor form a good working relationship with a young patient who so fears the F-talk that he or she does not even want to visit the doctor?

The essays reveal the BMI, that handy but flawed tool, to be a source of countless problems in the clinic. To be sure, a few doctors that we met used the chart judiciously, giving more weight to their own judgments of the child's overall health than to an elevated BMI number. But this cautious approach to BMI scores was relatively rare. Whether through obesity-fighting zeal or through ignorance, most doctors they described appear to have followed recommended practice, diagnosed children with high BMIs as "unhealthy," and initiated treatment. The results were rarely good. In

this book, we met many young people whose identities were spoiled, childhoods stolen, and lives damaged by the rigid application of that problematic scale.

There is another injustice here, for medicine (rightly) encourages young
people to participate in sports but then sometimes (wrongly) diagnoses
them as "overweight and unhealthy" when they develop strong, muscular
bodies. Muscular athletes, such as Ryan, who were misdiagnosed as "unhealthily overweight" developed an abiding distrust of "the man in the
white coat," whom they saw as an illegitimate teller of bodily truths. Under
the Hippocratic oath, medicine is supposed to "first, do no harm," but in
the cases of misdiagnosed athletes, the label of unhealthy and overweight
caused iatrogenic injury, resulting in strong, healthy youngsters such as
Alexis ending up with anxiety disorders caused by body anxieties rooted
in their BMI-based diagnosis. In Annemarie's case, the diagnosis left her
deeply confused about her actual health and undermined her confidence in
her ability to know her own body.

For these young patients, encounters with their doctors were disempowering and de-skilling, in the end undermining their ability to manage
their own health. Perhaps because underweight is not as stigmatizing as
overweight, one young person (Seth) who was misdiagnosed as "unhealthily underweight" and possibly "anorexic" was able to step outside his diagnosis to see the flaws in the label he had been given—though not until his
identity had been tarnished. Physicians lose trust, credibility, and authority
when the diagnostic tool they use produces so many faulty diagnoses. Few
young people we met were indifferent about their physicians. Those with
negative experiences of any sort were wary at best and hostile at worst.
Such guardedness and suspicion hurt medicine and hurt patients' health.

School Fitness Tests at Fault

Reforms in the schools are a critical part of the anti-obesity campaign and
schools around the country have taken them up with vigor. Although only
a few of the essays alluded to changes in lunch menus or vending policies,
an extraordinary number mentioned the school fitness tests and the trauma
they inflicted on ten- and twelve-year-olds who were informed that they
had a "bad BMI"—a measure they had never heard of before—and were
"unhealthy." In every case, the BMI was the only measure of fatness used,

and the verdict was delivered by a medically trained figure imbued by children and parents with the authority of science. The BMI testing worked to compare and rank children, establishing a new, authoritative, and "scientific" hierarchy of good and bad students, proper and not proper Americans. Bad BMIs robbed youngsters of their sense of themselves as normal, healthy kids. The red numbers made them feel different from and inferior to their peers, marked them for sure-to-be unwelcome changes that would take away their childhood pleasures, and induced a body consciousness that lasted their entire young lives. Are such costs to young children worth the benefit to schools of being able to measure and track students' BMIs? Do the schools really need this information, given the uncertain relation between the BMI and health? Do school administrators even know that bad BMIs cause so much anguish and that they can shatter a child's happy life in an instant?

If One Comment Can Destroy a Child's Life, What Should We Do Now?

In the story I have untangled, the human costs of the war on fat are the consequence of the all-out offensive against heavy bodies and persons now being waged in our society. A concern with social suffering and social justice calls for ending that war. Academics such as myself are generally reluctant to draw real-world policy conclusions from their social analyses, but every reader of this book in draft demanded to know: Now what? How can we change things? As Courtney, a student at Harvard who grew up in southern California and so understood every word, urged, this book must become a call to action. So now, shifting register, I share some thoughts.

People in many quarters are now pushing back against entrenched ways of treating the obesity issue. This book has described some of the pushback coming from professionals in the fields of fat studies, eating disorders, cardiology, and epidemiology/health statistics. Changes are bubbling up in the culture as well. Television is featuring women with some meat on their bodies, such as Lena Dunham, star of the HBO series "Girls," and Mindy Kaling, star of Fox TV's "The Mindy Project." Fat-positive and fat-pride photos and postings abound on such sites as Pinterest, Jezebel, and the Huffington Post. Fat fashion is becoming more mainstream, with

2014 bringing Full Figured or Plus Size Fashion Weeks in New York, London, and Paris. The bear community is openly celebrating the bigness (and hairiness) of large gay men as physically and sexually attractive. And there are thousands more points of light.

These are all promising developments, but much more is needed. While scientific research on obesity is critically important and should continue, the larger war on fat that is playing out in society and especially the maltreatment of heavy people need to be brought to an end. Why is such fundamental change required? I offer eight reasons, listed in bullet-point form. The first three are discussed at length in this book, but they are also well-established points that have been made by others on the basis of extensive data and/or analysis. The war on fat is:

- Based on science that, despite enormous progress, is far from resolving the most fundamental questions of cause, consequence, and effective treatment for obesity. As leading specialist Richard L. Atkinson stated at a major obesity conference in late 2014, "We have an encyclopedic ignorance of obesity."[17] The scientists need more time.
- Not working to reduce obesity in adults or prevent it in children.
- Worsening discrimination and social inequalities along lines of gender, class, race/ethnicity, and weight.

The findings in this book show that the war on fat also is:

- Causing injury to selves, psyches, relationships, families, and society as a whole.
- Putting everyone—fat, thin, and in between—at risk of emotional, social, and bodily harm.
- Imposing human costs likely to exceed its possible benefits.
- Creating a meaner culture.
- Posing ethical challenges for the field of medicine.

Clearly, ramping down the war of fat is a huge and vastly complicated project. It is hard to know even where to begin. But there are positive steps that we can take. These steps should certainly include a renegotiation of the social contract with corporations promising to help us fight fat. Because my work did not deal with corporate America, however, I must leave that discussion to others.[18] The steps I am more equipped to discuss include changing the culture to challenge the sexism, racism, and classism that infuse the war on fat. Others entail changes in medicine's treatment of obesity, in particular, deemphasizing obesity in favor of more direct measures of health. Here I offer six more concrete suggestions aimed at mitigating some of the main problems that I have identified in this book. I offer these not as firm proposals but as open-ended suggestions that I hope will provoke discussion and debate.

- Tell the public the truth about the biomyths.

Most of the trauma documented in this book has stemmed from people's unquestioned belief that the biomyths are scientific truth. Let's publicly acknowledge the limitations of these convenient shorthands. Let's educate the public about the importance of genetics and the environment in obesity, the limits of dieting, and so on. And let's mobilize the science press and the bloggers to get out the word.

- Ban the use of the BMI except for surveillance, screening, and study.

Everyone knows the BMI is badly flawed, but everyone keeps using it, and for things for which it was not designed. Let's restrict its use to what it was created for. Where it still must be used, let's remember its limitations. In doctors' offices, let's use it only in conjunction with other measures of obesity and encourage prioritizing assessments of patients' overall health over BMI scores.

- Ensure that BMI testing respects children's right to privacy.

BMI tests in schools may still be needed to track population-level changes, but let's ensure they are conducted in ways that guarantee children's right to privacy and freedom from shaming. They should be conducted in private, and the results should not be sent home in BMI "report cards."

- Create fat-talk-free zones.

Following the model of summer camps that have "no body talk" rules,[19] let's establish fat-talk-free (FTF) zones where not just insults but also compliments about weight are forbidden. Such spaces could help foster wider cultural change by raising awareness of the extent of weight preoccupation in our society and by giving people a chance to try out new ways of relating to themselves and each other.

- Launch a nationwide campaign against fat bullying.

This book should put to rest the persistent calls from some quarters to use stigma and shaming as tools to induce weight loss. This book presents overwhelming evidence that these techniques not only don't work but are harmful, causing lifelong trauma to many victims. Instead of being encouraged, the shamers should be shamed! Let's establish a human right to be free from weight bullying and launch a nationwide campaign to fight fat shaming and bullying everywhere.

- Give "Let's Move!" a makeover.

Let's take this popular campaign and make it over to focus on child health, fitness, and overall well-being. Let's continue to emphasize good food and fun exercise but also use it to fight fat bullying, to teach kids that weight is not so all-important, and to foster a kinder culture in which kids have empathy for those with different-size bodies. Let's address this movement to all ethnic groups, not just African Americans and Hispanics, and let's encourage dads as well as moms to be involved. If the generation born in the 1990s is the first war-on-fat generation, a group whose lives have been dominated and all too often diminished by this all-out battle against extra pounds, then, with the help of Let's Move!, the young people born in the 2010s could be the first postwar-on-fat generation, a group in which weight is no longer the measure of health and human value, a group that, while working to adopt healthful practices, understands that bodies come in all sizes, each beautiful in its own way.

Appendix

**Personal Essay Prompt: Weight, Diet, and
BMI in Everyday Life (2 points)**

Students wishing to earn 2 points extra credit may write a personal essay on
how the issues surrounding weight that we're discussing in class play out in
their lives or in the lives of people they know well (family members, close
friends). You could write about any of the things we've talked about in class.
The aim here is to illuminate how these issues shape our lives. The way to
approach this is to think of a person whose life has been deeply affected by
one of these issues and then describe how. Alternatively, you could take a
particular incident in someone's life and write about that. The aim is to provide a richly detailed account: describe how the person felt, what she or he
said and did, how it affected others, what struggles erupted in his or her family, what meaning these struggles had in his or her life, and so on. The more
of this kind of personal detail you can include, the richer your story will be.

Your essay can deal with any issue around diet, weight, fatness, skinniness, the medicalization of obesity, bariatric surgery, weight loss programs,

BMI, and so on. Of special interest are essays about the BMI—how it's affected someone's life and sense of who s/he is. Also of particular interest are essays on how these issues affect the lives of guys.

I want to encourage you to write one of these essays because this class deals with stuff that affects all of us personally. I'd like there to be a space where you can reflect on what these things mean in the lives of those you know best. These essays will be turned in to the professor and kept completely confidential. No one else will have access to them without your explicit permission.

The essays should be 3–5 pages, doubled spaced. (It's fine to write more if you wish.) The first page should include your name; student ID; email address; and, for the subject of your essay, the person's ethnicity and the name of the city where s/he grew up and lived during the events described in the essay. Please give your essay a title. Giving something a title often helps us organize and focus our thoughts about the topic. The essay can be turned in any time, but it is due by Thursday, March 3 at the latest. Please turn them in to the instructor.

Producing Virtuous Biocitizens: Survey Results

TABLE A.1 Weight Worries (%)

A. How often do you think (or worry) about your weight?	Women	Men
Almost all the time	17.2	6.8
Much of the time	39.8	23.1
Occasionally	37.0	40.2
Rarely	6.0	29.9
Total	100.0	100.0

B. Do you think you are:	Women	Men
Way too heavy	7.9	3.4
Somewhat too heavy	43.8	28.2
Just about right	42.3	47.9
Somewhat too thin	5.1	16.2
Way too thin	0.4	4.4
N.A.	0.4	0.0
Total	99.9	100.1

Notes: Data from 2010 and 2011 beginning-of-term surveys (470 women and 117 men; excludes 14 gender not specified). N.A., not available.

TABLE A.2 Body Mass Index Awareness (%)

A. When did you first learn your BMI?

Elementary school (ages 4–10)	4.5
Middle school (ages 11–13)	38.6
High school (ages 14–17)	36.3
College (ages 18+)	13.0
N.A.	7.7
Total	100.1

B. Who first brought your BMI to your attention?

Doctor	18.3
Parent, relative	4.0
Instructor	52.4
Self[a]	8.3
Friend	5.2
Two or more people	2.5
Other	2.0
N.A.	7.3
Total	100.0

Notes: Data from 2010 and 2011 beginning-of-term surveys (601 students). N.A., not available.
[a] Those who answered "Self" discovered their BMI scores on the Internet, in magazines, on television, and so forth.

TABLE A.3 Physician Concern about Body Mass Index (%)

Has a doctor ever told you that your weight or your BMI was something to worry about and work on?

	Women	Men	All
Yes	19.8	14.8	19.1
No	70.7	77.1	71.6
N.A.; not sure	9.5	8.2	9.4
Total	100.0	100.1	100.1

Notes: Data from beginning-of-term survey (341 students total, including 273 women, 61 men, and 7 with gender not indicated). N.A., not available.

TABLE A.4 Parental Concern about Weight (%)

A. Have your parents ever criticized or scolded you about being the wrong weight?

	Women	Men	All[a]
Yes	62.3	37.7	57.5
No	37.4	62.3	41.9
N.A.	0.4	0.0	0.6
Total	100.1	100.0	100.0

B. When you were growing up, were your parents very concerned about their weight?

	Moms	Dads
Yes, much of the time	24.8	5.9
Yes, some of the time	43.2	25.4
No, not much at all	31.4	66.7
N.A.	0.7	2.0
Total	100.1	100.0

Notes: Data in Panel A from 2011 beginning-of-term survey (341 students, including 273 women, 61 men, and 7 with gender not indicated); Data in Panel B from 2011 end-of-term survey (303 students of both genders). N.A., not available.
[a] Figures are skewed due to the large number of women relative to men.

TABLE A.5 Diets (%)

A. Last fall, were you on a diet; if so, what kind?

	Women	Men	All
Yes, restricting	16.5	13.1	15.5
Yes, counting calories	6.2	1.6	5.3
Yes, skipping some meals	5.9	1.6	5.0
Yes, other kind of diet	2.6	4.9	2.9
Yes, two or more kinds	8.1	6.6	7.6
No, no diet	58.6	70.5	61.3
Not sure; N.A.	2.2	1.6	2.3
Total	100.1	99.9	99.9

B. Have you ever been on a diet of any kind?

	Women	Men	All
Yes	67.4	44.3	63.0
No	32.6	55.7	37.0
Total	100.0	100.0	100.0

Notes: Data from beginning-of-term survey, 2011 (341 students, including 273 women, 61 men, and 79 with gender not indicated). N.A., not available.

TABLE A.6 Exercise (%)

Last fall, how many times a week did you exercise?

	Women	Men	All
3 times or more	22.7	39.3	25.8
2 times	20.5	8.2	18.2
1 time	9.9	18.0	11.4
No regular exercise program	46.2	31.2	43.4
Other	0.7	3.3	1.2
Total	100.0	100.0	100.0

Notes: Data from beginning-of-term survey, 2011 (341 students, including 273 women, 61 men, and 7 with gender not indicated).

TABLE A.7 Beliefs in Core Tenets of Biocitizenship Culture (%)

A. Weight can be safely and effectively controlled by virtually everyone; achieving normal weight is a matter of personal willpower.

	Women	Men	All
Agree	53.5	62.3	54.8
Not sure	17.6	9.8	16.7
Disagree	28.9	27.9	28.5
Total	100.0	100.0	100.0

B. The BMI is a reliable, scientifically sound measure of body fat that applies to everyone, regardless of body shape, ethnicity, and so on.

	Women	Men	All
Agree	25.6	34.4	27.3
Not sure	27.8	39.3	30.5
Disagree	46.5	26.2	42.3
Total	99.9	99.9	100.1

C. If family members or friends are overweight, it is our responsibility to let them know we've noticed, and to provide suggestions for diet, exercise, and other techniques they can use to lose the extra pounds.

	Women	Men	All
Agree	41.8	50.8	43.4
Not sure	33.7	24.6	24.6
Disagree	24.5	24.6	32.0
Total	100.0	100.0	100.0

Notes: Data from 2011 beginning-of-term survey (341 students, including 273 women, 61 men, and 7 with gender not indicated).

Notes

1. A Biocitizenship Society to Fight Fat

1. Nationally representative data from the National Health and Nutrition Examination Survey (NHANES), the gold standard for evidence on Americans' weight, indicate that in 2011–2012, 34.9 percent of adults ages 20 or above were obese and that 33.6 percent were overweight. Among children and adolescents ages 2 to 19, 16.9 percent were obese and another 14.9 percent were overweight (Ogden et al. 2014). Some evidence suggests a renewed rise in adult obesity in 2014 (United Health Foundation 2014).

2. For this narrative, see, for example, Office of the Surgeon General 2001; Carmona 2003; Brownell and Horgen 2004.

3. Office of the Surgeon General 2001.

4. See White House 2010, www.letsmove.gov/ and www.whitehouse.gov/.

5. Loar 1995.

6. The medicalization of excess weight began around World War II but has intensified in the last two decades with the concern about risks to public health (Sobal 1995; Jutel 2006; Boero 2007; on medicalization generally, Conrad 2007; Clarke et al. 2010). Obesity has been classified as a disease by the World Health Organization, the Institute of Medicine, and the Food and Drug Administration, among others. A PubMed search of studies with the term *obesity* in the title or abstract showed a rapid rise of studies beginning in the mid-1990s, followed by an exponential increase during 2000–2010 (Saguy 2013, 108–9). On the earlier history, see Farrell 2011; Stearns 2002.

7. Saguy 2013.

8. Boero 2007.

9. Boero 2012.

10. Based on a search for articles with the term *obesity* in the heading or lead paragraph in Lexis-Nexis U.S. News Sources. Between 2004 and 2010, the media attention to obesity remained high but stopped rising (Saguy 2013, 108–9).

11. Chapman 2009; Perez-Pena 2011; Zernike and Santora 2013.

12. Rae 2010. For deeper insight into these trends, see Jutel 2009.

13. American preoccupation with thinness has been explored by many authors, including historians, Schwartz 1986 and Brumberg 1997, and journalists, Fraser 1998 and Wolf 1991.

14. Shape Up America! 1997.

15. Quoted in Balko 2004.

16. Marilyn Wann, a fat-rights activist, explains, "Calling people 'obese' medicalizes human diversity. Medicalizing diversity inspires a misplaced search for a 'cure' for naturally occurring difference" (2009, xiii).

17. World Health Organization 2011.

18. Centers for Disease Control (CDC) analyses of NHANES data show no significant change in the prevalence of obesity among youth and adults between 2003–2004 and 2011–2012. During the same period, obesity rose in women ages 60 and older, from 31.5 to 38 percent. In the first significant decline found in any group, obesity among preschool children (ages 2–5) decreased from 14 to just over 8 percent (a 43 percent decline), a finding that attracted widespread attention in the media and some controversy in scientific circles when it was announced in early 2014. Among middle and high school–age youth, there was no significant change. Other data show significant declines in obesity between 2008 and 2011 among low-income preschool-age children participating in federal nutrition programs in eighteen states. For the details, see Ogden et al. 2014, and for some media discussion, see Tavernise 2014.

19. Power and Schulkin 2009, 324. The slowdown could also be due to environmental change unrelated to the war on fat.

20. The video went viral, provoking a ferocious backlash online. For more on the campaign, see http://www.strong4life.com/en/pages/LearnAssess/RewindtheFuture/ArticleDetails.aspx?articleid=RewindtheFuture&sectionid=Overview.

21. In early 2011, the weight limits for lap-band surgery were lowered so that adults in the lowest level of obesity (BMI 30+) with one obesity-related condition were approved for surgery. These procedures cost $20,000–$35,000, a sum that doubles when one adds nutritional counseling, personal training, and cosmetic surgery to remove sagging and excess skin (www.webmd.com, accessed July 25, 2013).

22. Pollack 2012a, 2012b; http://www.fda.gov/NewsEvents/Newsroom/PressAnnouncements/ucm413896.htm

23. "It's Hard Enough to Be a Fat Kid without the Government Telling You You're an Epidemic," Jezebel, n.d., http://jezebel.com (accessed July 25, 2013).

24. Associated Press, "Wisconsin News Anchor Strikes Back after Being Called 'Fat,'" *Chicago Sun-Times*, October 4, 2012, www.suntimes.com (accessed July 25, 2013).

25. Rothblum and Solovay present a wide-ranging survey of FAM arguments is *The Fat Studies Reader* (2009). Also noteworthy are Marilyn Wann's irreverent *Fat! So?* (1998) and the website of the National Association to Advance Fat Acceptance (www.naafa.org/).

26. In a major review of the literature on weight stigma, Fikkan and Rothblum (2012) find that fat women are treated more poorly than thinner women and than men of all weight classes, with harmful effects that are wide ranging.

27. Bacon 2008.

28. See Rothblum and Solovay 2009, part IV. On the "smash the scale" campaign, see Bahadur 2013.

29. Members of the FAM were very active in the critique of the "Stop Sugarcoating It, Georgia" campaign.

30. Saguy (2013, esp. 29–36) suggests that thin women and tall, muscular men are accorded more credibility in the debates over obesity. The views of fat-rights activists who are fat themselves are often dismissed because the speakers are seen as having an axe to grind or as trying to rationalize their own weight.

31. Farrell 2011, esp. 6–8.

32. The groundbreaking work is Rothblum and Solovay 2009. The new journal *Fat Studies: An Interdisciplinary Journal of Body Weight and Society* (from 2012), edited by Esther D. Rothblum, is a key locus for discussions in this rapidly growing field.

33. See esp. Saguy 2013; Boero 2012.

34. Boero 2012, esp. 3, 59–93.

35. Reed-Danahay 1997 provides a useful entree into the use of auto-ethnography in anthropology.

36. Farrell 2011, esp. 25–81.

37. Rose 1999; Rose and Novas 2005.

38. Others (Halse 2009; Guthman 2011) use the term *biocitizen* to describe the weight-conscious denizens of today's world. My use differs in its emphasis on the demand that the biocitizen be fit as well as thin. I build on their theoretical projects while also using the term to illuminate how the war on fat operates on the ground and with what effects in real people's lives.

39. Rosenblatt 2001.

40. Crawford 1980.

41. Crawford 2006. Using different terms, Metzl and Kirkland (2010) also argue that health has been transformed into "the new morality."

42. Crawford 1980, 2006.

43. Guthman 2011, 52–56.

44. Crawford 2006, 415–19.

45. Lupton 1995. Foucault's phrase was "the importance of health: at once the duty of each and the objective of all" (1984, 277).

46. Halse (2009) calls the discourse of the BMI a "virtue discourse" to draw attention to its inherent moralism.

47. For a women's studies perspective, see Fikkan and Rothblum 2012. In the rapidly growing literature on weight stigma in public health, see esp. Puhl and Heuer 2009, 2010; Puhl and Latner 2007; Puhl, Peterson, and Luedicke 2013.

48. Puhl and Heuer 2010.

49. "Organizational Chart of Governmental and Non-Governmental Agencies Addressing Food Policy and Obesity," May 2010, yaleruddcenter.org/resources/ (accessed July 25, 2013).

50. Office of the Surgeon General 2001.

51. For the latest inventions, see Weintraub 2014.

52. Halse 2009.

53. Nichter 2000.

54. Christakis and Fowler 2007.

55. Hruschka et al. 2011. Some also challenge the findings on methodological grounds (Lyons 2011).

56. Power and Schulkin 2009, 134–35.

57. This understanding of discourse is influenced by the writings of Foucault, especially his work on scientific-medical discourses of the clinic (1975) and of sexuality (1978).

58. Stearns 2002; Vigarello 2013.

59. Barlow and the Expert Committee 2007.

60. Ibid.; National Institutes of Health (NIH) and the National Heart, Lung, and Blood Institute (NHLBI) 1998.

61. Kuczmarski et al. 1994, 211.

62. Carmona (2003); White House (2010).

63. Mann et al. 2007. On bariatric surgery, see Puzziferri et al. 2014.

64. Pfeifer 2011.

65. On Bloomberg's health initiatives, see Gratzer 2012.

66. Brownell and Horgen 2004; see also www.yaleruddcenter.org. In 2013, Brownell left Yale for Duke. In 2015, the Rudd Center moved to the University of Connecticut.

67. Among childhood programs, school-based prevention programs have produced modest results. The Institute of Medicine sees the U.S. as lagging in evaluating obesity prevention efforts. See AHRQ 2013; IOM 2013.

68. Barlow and Dietz 1998.

69. Barlow and the Expert Committee 2007.

70. Office of the Surgeon General 2001.

71. Key contributions of critical obesity researchers include Gaesser 2002; Campos 2004; Gard and Wright 2005; Oliver 2006; Campos et al. 2006. Critiques of the science can also be found occasionally in mainstream medical and public health journals.

72. In his work on patient organizations encouraging the development of the sciences of their diseases, Novas (2006) coined this term to refer to a faith in the powers of science and technology to find solutions, a faith with political and economic materiality.

73. Ross 2005, 92.

74. Lavie and Loberg (2014, 54–63) provide a useful overview of the relative advantages of peripheral (rather than visceral or abdominal) fat in the risk of co-morbid diseases.

75. Pollack 2013.

76. Lavie and Loberg 2014, 22.

77. Lavie and Loberg 2014; Power and Schulkin 2009.

78. Lavie and Loberg 2014, 156.

79. Power and Schulkin 2009. This suggestion is supported by a study that compared metabolically healthy obese and normal-weight individuals and showed increased risk for adverse long-term health outcomes among the obese, despite their metabolic health (Kramer et al. 2013). This is far from the last word on this subject, though.

80. Lavie and Loberg 2014.

81. Lazar 2013, cited in ibid., 115–16.

82. See note 71.

83. Flegal et al. 2013.

84. Belluck 2013.

85. Miller 2013.

86. Swidley 2013.

87. See, for example, Lavie and Loberg (2014, esp. 92–117) on disputes over weight and mortality and Boero (2012, 16–39) on struggles over the designation of obesity as a leading health indicator. The most systematic analysis is Saguy's (2013) on the credibility struggles over the framing of obesity as a problem.

88. Butler 1990; Bordo 1993.

89. The term *biopedagogy* was introduced by Evans et al. 2008.

90. The term *fat abuse* comes from Royce 2009. *Biobullying*, my term, emerged from a conversation with Alma Gottlieb of the University of Illinois, Urbana-Champaign.

91. Lumeng et al. 2010; Taylor 2011.

92. Puhl and Latner 2007; Puhl 2011; Puhl, Peterson, and Luedicke 2013.

93. The public health literature suggests that stigma not only does not work but may actually worsen obesity by causing people to cope by eating more food and refusing to diet. See, for example, Puhl and Latner 2007.

2. Creating Thin, Fit Bodies: The View from SoCal

1. For this book, the southern California region includes ten counties: the coastal counties of Los Angeles, Orange, San Diego, Ventura, Santa Barbara, and San Luis Obispo and the inland counties of Kern, San Bernardino, Riverside, and Imperial. The 2012 population estimates come from the U.S. Census Bureau, http://quickfacts.census.gov/qfd/states/06/06059.html (accessed July 29, 2013).

2. The quotations in this section come from the 2011 end-of-term survey, which I describe in the next section.

3. Computed from U.S. Census Bureau data, http://quickfacts.census.gov (accessed July 29, 2013).

4. Founded in 1999, CDC's Division of Nutrition, Physical Activity, and Obesity (DNPAO) funds anti-obesity programs in selected states. California received funding in 2000–2002 and then began a new five-year agreement in 2008. From Centers for Disease Control, State-Based Programs, http://cdc.gov (accessed January 18, 2011, and July 29, 2013).

5. California Department of Health Services (CDHS) 2006, 4.

6. Ibid., 1–3.

7. Ibid., 5.

8. Ibid., 8.

9. Schools are required by law to include PFT results in the School Accountability Report Card and to provide students with their individual results (California Department of Education n.d.).

10. This discussion of the BMI is based in part on the Summit Honor Roll, which praises many organizations for spreading BMI consciousness (CDHS 2006, 16–23).

11. Ibid., 9–12.

12. The state instituted the toughest school nutrition reforms in the nation, was the first to require fast-food and large chain restaurants to post nutritional information on their menus, and adopted the first-ever physical education standards in schools (Office of the Governor 2010).

13. Ibid.

14. In a controversial article in *JAMA*, two researchers at the Harvard School of Public Health advocated removing obese kids from their parents' homes, a practice that has been used in some states (Murtagh and Ludwig 2011).

15. Twenty-two percent of the students wrote about eating disorders, which were not part of the assignment. Rather than doing what I asked, which was to choose a central figure and write about his or her experiences, one-quarter of the students wrote rambling reflections on weight culture or general descriptions of a category of people (such as wrestlers). Such evidence supports my belief that the prompt did not overdetermine the essay content.

16. After realizing that I had more than enough essays to analyze, I decided to not contact about twenty-five of the students who had written essays in 2011.

17. The essays featured here do not represent the extremes from the pool. There were much more disturbing accounts, especially of eating disorders, that I was not able to include.

18. Frey 2011.

19. Ibid., app. B. In the other SoCal metro areas, the proportion of nonwhite children in 2010 ranged from 64 to 76 percent.

20. Yen 2012.

21. The ethnic breakdown of the students in my classes was similar to those for the UC Irvine campus as a whole. At UC Irvine in 2012, 18 percent of undergraduates were white, 18 percent Hispanic, 47 percent Asian, 6 percent foreign, and 4 percent of two or more races/ethnicities (University of California, Irvine 2012).

22. In 2011–2012, obesity levels among adults were 47.8 percent among (non-Hispanic) blacks, 42.5 percent among Hispanics, and 32.6 percent among (non-Hispanic) whites. Among children, the corresponding percentages were 20.2, 22.4, and 14.1 (Ogden et al. 2014).

23. Centers for Disease Control and Prevention (CDC) n.d.

24. Carney 2015. See Greenhalgh and Carney 2014 for a refutation of the stereotype of "the ignorant Latino."

25. Bell, NcNaughton, and Salmon 2009; Boero 2012, 52–55.

26. Saguy and Gruys 2010, 245–46.

27. Data are from the U.S. Census Bureau, http://quickfacts.census.gov.

28. Among Asian adults, obesity prevalence in 2011–2012 was 10.8 percent, one-third the level for all adults (34.9 percent) (Ogden et al. 2014; Aoki et al. 2014). I am grateful to Cynthia Ogden for illuminating discussions of these issues.

29. Deurenberg, Deurenberg-Yap, and Guricci 2002; Despres 2012.

30. Nichter 2000; Molinary 2007.

31. Zhou 2009. See also Kibria 1995; Lee and Zhou 2004.

32. Zhou 2009, 187–201.

33. Chua 2011.

34. Juang, Qin, and Park 2013; Kim et al. 2013; Lau and Fung 2013.

35. Calculated from U.S. Census Bureau data, http://quickfacts.census.gov.

36. Income data are for 2007–2011 (ibid.). The median household income in the United States as a whole was $52,762; in California it was $61,632.

37. The cult of the slender body is the subject of a long history of feminist scholarship that includes Ohrbach 1978; Chernin 1981; Wolf 1991; Fraser 1998; Hesse-Biber 2007. Most of that research was conducted before today's war on fat was launched.

38. Dworkin and Wachs 2009.

39. The authors argue that, in response to competition from women in education and the workforce, men are increasingly preoccupied with their appearance, seeking to create big, strong muscled forms that mark them as different from and superior to women. That's the "body panic" of their book's title.

40. Nichter 2000, 45–67.

41. Nichter 2000; Taylor 2011.

42. At UC Irvine, 93 percent of undergraduates hail from California. Another 1 percent are from other U.S. states, and 6 percent come from abroad (University of California, Irvine 2012).

43. Martin 2007. For a more academic treatment, see Counihan 1999.

44. University of California, Irvine 2012.

3. "Obese"

1. A few scholars have studied the development of the fat self among young women (Rice 2007) and men (Monaghan 2007, 2008: Monaghan and Malson 2013). I know of no work investigating the development of "normal selfhood" or "skinny identity," however.

2. Fat people are also less likely to gain admission to college (Fikkan and Rothblum 2011). I thank Esther Rothblum for discussions of these important points.

4. "Overweight"

1. For the numbers, see chapter 1, note 1.

2. In the group of the essays dealing with everyday weight struggles (57 percent of the total), it was hard to classify people as "overweight" or "normal" because many informants frequently added and shed pounds, shifting their BMI category. My rough estimate is that three-fifths of those, or one-third of all the essays, focused on technically overweight people.

5. "Underweight"

1. Age-adjusted figures for adults ages eighteen and older, from National Center for Health Statistics 2012, 106 (table 31).

2. Age-adjusted figures for adults ages eighteen and older, from Barnes, Adams, and Powell-Griner 2008, 11 (table 2).

7. Physical and Mental Health at Risk

1. Austin 2011.
2. See, for example, Sánchez-Carracedo, Neumark-Sztainer, and López-Guimerà 2012; Schwartz and Henderson 2009; Puhl et al. 2014. I am grateful to Anne Becker for illuminating discussions of these issues.
3. Neumark-Sztainer et al. 2012. In 2010, some 50 percent of females and 38 percent of males in a Minneapolis–St. Paul sample engaged in unhealthy weight-control behaviors; 7 percent of females and 4 percent of males engaged in extreme weight control behaviors associated with anorexia and bulimia; and 10 percent of females and 6 percent of males resorted to binge eating.
4. Neumark-Sztainer et al. 2010.
5. Wagerson 2012.
6. This second figure is based on surveys done in four years between 2001 and 2011, with a total of 663 students.
7. This discussion of the hazards of extreme dieting and exercising has been distilled from a variety of websites, including those maintained by eating-disorder specialists. The discussion here mentions only some of the main dangers; it is not meant to be comprehensive.
8. Battaglia 2008.
9. Tendonosis is a degeneration of the tendon's collagen due to chronic overuse unaccompanied by rest. Although therapy can improve function, the cellular damage is unlikely to ever be completely reversed.
10. Many youngsters developed eating disorders as a way to cope with sexual or emotional abuse (five cases) or parental breakup (five cases). In a handful of cases, young people were preparing for careers in fields where slender bodies were de rigueur (music theater and modeling). There is no obvious connection to the war on fat in these situations.
11. Because the FDA regulates prescription drugs and monitors the safely of all drug products on the market, more information is available to the public on the dangers of weight-loss drugs. Prescription weight-loss drugs have a notorious history of safety problems, ably described by others (e.g., Fraser 1998; Mundy 2001). The FDA also maintains lists of dangerous or potentially dangerous over-the-counter products. For more see Food and Drug Administration (FDA) 2011, 2013a, 2013b. For the larger context, see Pollack 2012a, 2012b.
12. At the National Institutes for Health (NIH) website, a search for "dangerous weight loss practices" turned up 259,000 hits. Most items turned out to be about such things as weight-loss guidelines for clinical practice, the efficacy of weight-loss methods, or even the dangers of inactivity and not dieting. I found almost nothing about safety issues. There was even less information on the CDC website, whose webpage on "Obesity and Overweight" was focused entirely on strategies to combat obesity. Searches conducted July 4, 2013.
13. Zelman 2011.

8. Families and Relationships Unhinged

1. Farrell 2011, 7.
2. Bell, McNaughton, and Salmon 2009; Boero 2009; Maher, Fraser, and Wright 2009; Saguy 2013; Herndon 2014.
3. Herndon 2014.
4. Weiss 2012, 2013.
5. Royce 2009.
6. Ibid., 152.

7. The warnings of April's brother—that boys would throw things at her if she did not lose weight (chapter 4)—might be construed as informative biopedagogy, though such statements are somewhat abusive too.

9. Does Biocitizenship Help the Very Fat?

1. Such information can conveniently be found on the CDC website, cdc.gov/obesity/adult/causes/index.html. See chapter 1 for details.

2. Flegal et al. 2013. The findings are from representative U.S. cohorts.

3. A useful nontechnical discussion of this research can be found in Guthman 2011, 100–115. Tang-Peronard et al. 2011 provide an entre into the scientific literature.

4. Cunningham, Kramer, and Narayan 2014.

5. Llewellyn et al. 2013.

6. Brownell and Horgen 2004, 23–24.

7. Llewellyn et al. 2013.

8. Sumithran et al. 2011.

9. Ibid. A longer, more popular account of the research and its context is Parker-Pope 2012. The quotation, from Joseph Proietto, one of the researchers, can be found in Parker-Pope's article.

10. For an accessible description of these dynamics, see Bacon 2008, 47–50.

11. Bacon and Aphramor (2011) report that weight fluctuation worsens disease risk by increasing inflammation, hypertension, insulin resistance, and dyslipidemia; weight cycling is also associated with worse cardiovascular outcomes.

12. Bacon 2008, 31–42.

13. Moss 2013.

14. Kessler 2009.

15. Oliver 2006, 143–58.

16. Low-income adolescents and children are more likely to be obese than other children, but the relationship is not consistent across racial/ethnic groups; it is strongest among non-Hispanic whites and weakest among Mexican Americans (Ogden et al. 2010b). Among adults, the relationship is weaker, holding for women but not men, and again varying by racial/ethnic group (Ogden et al. 2010a).

17. Compelling analyses of the role of American capitalism, government policies, and political culture in the making of the obesity epidemic can be found in Oliver 2006; Guthman 2011, 163–84. A more global take on the role of capitalism in producing hunger and obesity is Albritton 2009.

18. Ernsberger 2009.

19. Weiss 2013.

20. In truth, the heaviness and the lack of self-confidence are closely related.

21. For the history, see Hiltzik 2013.

22. Later in the essay, the author reports his aunt's initial weight as 240 pounds. At 5′ tall, she would have a BMI of 46.9. Although the nephew seems to have gotten one number wrong, that does not affect the narrative.

23. Data for 2011. They come from the Centers for Disease Control and Prevention, www.cdc.gov/obesity/data/adult.html (accessed July 15, 2014).

24. The data are from the U.S. Census Bureau, http://quickfacts.census.gov (accessed August 5, 2013).

25. Special supplemental nutrition program for Women, Infants, and Children, run by the U.S. Department of Agriculture.

10. Social Justice and the End of the War on Fat

1. Skrabanek 1994.

2. See www.letsmove.gov (accessed July 26, 2014).

3. Quoted in Satchfield 2013.

4. See http://members.feast-ed.org (accessed July 26, 2014).

5. Ogden et al. 2014

6. Monaghan 2007; Monaghan and Malson 2013.

7. Wolf 1991.

8. Sandberg 2013.

9. Kim et al. 2013.

10. This was not a result of the way I selected the cases for inclusion in the book. The same ethnic pattern appears in the full collection of essays.

11. Deurenberg, Deurenberg-Yap, and Guricci 2002; Despres 2012.

12. For a fuller treatment of these issues, see Greenhalgh and Carney 2014.

13. In his 2001 *Call to Action*, Surgeon General Satcher outlined strategies for reducing obesity among Americans of all ages (Office of the Surgeon General 2001). By 2003, Surgeon General Carmona in his statements before Congress had shifted the focus to "the growing epidemic of childhood obesity" (Carmona 2003, 2004).

14. This was the number of licensed physicians in the United States in 2010 (Young et al. 2013).

15. Puhl and Heuer 2009.

16. Fikkan and Rothblum 2011.

17. Atkinson 2014.

18. Helpful entrees into this literature are Simon 2006; Nestle 2007; Guthman 2011.

19. Krueger 2014.

REFERENCES

AHRQ. 2013. "Childhood Obesity Prevention Programs: Comparative Effectiveness." AHRQ Pub. No. 13-EHCO81-3. www.effectivehealthcare.ahrq.gov/child-obesity-prevention.cfm.

Albritton, Robert. 2009. *Let Them Eat Junk: How Capitalism Creates Hunger and Obesity*. London: Pluto.

Aoki, Yutaka, Sung Sug Yoon, Yinong Chong, and Margaret D. Carroll. 2014. "Hypertension, Abnormal Cholesterol, and High Body Mass Index among Non-Hispanic Asian Adults: United States, 2011–12." NCHS Data Brief 140. NCHS, Centers for Disease Control, Hyattsville, MD. Available at http://www.cdc.gov/nchs/data/databriefs/db140.htm.

Atkinson, Richard L. 2014. "Labeling Obesity as a Disease—Does This Label Help or Hurt the Cause?" Presentation at Obesity Week 2014, Boston, Massachusetts, November 6.

Austin, S. Bryn. 2011. "The Blind Spot in the Drive for Childhood Obesity Prevention: Bringing Eating Disorders Prevention into Focus as a Public Health Priority." *American Journal of Public Health* 101(6): e1–4.

Bacon, Linda. 2008. *Health at Every Size: The Surprising Truth about Your Weight*. Dallas, TX: Benbella Books.

Bacon, Linda, and Lucy Aphramor. 2011. "Weight Science: Evaluating the Evidence for a Paradigm Shift." *Nutrition Journal* 10(9): 13 pp.

Bahadur, Nina. 2013. "PHOTOS: 'Smash the Scale' Is the New Year's 'Revolution' You Need to Know About." Available at http://www.huffingtonpost.com/2013/12/13/smash-the-scale-new-years-resolution-rev (accessed July 1, 2014).

Balko, Radley. 2004. "'As Threatening to Us as the Terrorist Threat'?" Ideas in Action. June 3. Available at http://www.ideasinactiontv.com (accessed December 20, 2012).

Barlow, Sarah E., and William H. Dietz. 1998. "Obesity Evaluation and Treatment: Expert Committee Recommendations." Part 1 of 2. *Pediatrics* 102(3): e29.

Barlow, Sarah E., and the Expert Committee. 2007. "Expert Committee Recommendations Regarding the Prevention, Assessment, and Treatment of Child and Adolescent Overweight and Obesity: Summary Report." *Pediatrics* 120(Suppl. 4): S164–92.

Barnes, Patricia M., Patricia F. Adams, and Eve Powell-Griner. 2008. "Health Characteristics of the Asian Adult Population: United States, 2004–2006." Advance Data for Vital and Health Statistics No. 394, January 22. Washington, DC: U.S. DHHS, CDC, National Center for Health Statistics. Available at http://www.cdc.gov/nchs/data/ad/ad394.pdf (accessed August 2, 2013).

Battaglia, Emily. 2008. "4 Dangerous Weight-Loss Methods." October 3. Available at http://www.lifescript.com (accessed July 4, 2013).

Bell, Kirsten, Darlene McNaughton, and Amy Salmon. 2009. "Medicine, Morality, and Mothering: Public Health Discourses on Feetal Alcohol Exposure, Smoking around Children and Childhood Overnutrition." *Critical Public Health* 19(2): 155–70.

Belluck, Pam. 2013. "Study Suggests Lower Mortality Risk for People Deemed to Be Overweight." *New York Times*, January 1. Available at www.nytimes.com (accessed July 27, 2013).

Boero, Natalie. 2007. "All the News That's Fat to Print: The American 'Obesity Epidemic' and the Media." *Qualitative Sociology* 30(1): 41–60.

———. 2009. "Fat Kids, Working Moms, and the 'Obesity Epidemic.'" In *The Fat Studies Reader*, edited by Esther Rothblum and Sondra Solovay, 113–19. New York: NYU Press.

———. 2012. *Killer Fat: Media, Medicine, and Morals in the American "Obesity Epidemic."* New Brunswick: Rutgers University Press.

Bordo, Susan. 1993. *Unbearable Weight: Feminism, Western Culture, and the Body*. Berkeley: University of California Press.

Brownell, Kelly D., and Katherine Battle Horgen. 2004. *Food Fight: The Inside Story of the Food Industry, America's Obesity Crisis, and What We Can Do about It*. Chicago: Contemporary.

Brumberg, Joan Jacobs. 1997. *The Body Project: An Intimate History of American Girls*. New York: Random House.

Butler, Judith. 1990. *Gender Trouble: Feminism and the Subversion of Identity*. New York: Routledge.

California Department of Education. n.d. "Program Overview: Overview of the California Physical Fitness Test (PFT)." Available at http://www.cde.ca/gov (accessed November 8, 2012).

California Department of Health Services (CDHS). 2006. *California Obesity Prevention Plan: A Vision for Tomorrow, Strategic Actions for Today (COPP)*. Sacramento: CDHS.

Campos, Paul. 2004. *The Obesity Myth: Why America's Obsession with Weight Is Hazardous to Your Health*. New York: Gotham.

Campos, Paul, Abigail Saguy, Paul Ernsberger, Eric Oliver, and Glenn Gaesser. 2006. "The Epidemiology of Overweight and Obesity: Public Health Crisis or Moral Panic?" *International Journal of Epidemiology* 35(1): 55–60.

Carmona, Richard H. 2003. "The Obesity Crisis in America," Testimony before the Subcommittee on Education Reform, Committee on Education and the Workforce, U.S. House of Representatives, July 16. Available at www.surgeongeneral.gov (accessed January 18, 2011).

——. 2004. "The Growing Epidemic of Childhood Obesity." Statement of Richard H. Carmona, March 2. Testimony before the Subcommittee on Competition, Infrastructure, and Foreign Commerce, Committee on Commerce, Science, and Transportation, U.S. Senate. Available at www.surgeongeneral.gov (accessed December 20, 2012).

Carney, Megan A. 2015. *The Unending Hunger: Tracing Women and Food Insecurity across Borders*. Berkeley: University of California Press.

Centers for Disease Control and Prevention (CDC). n.d. "Compared with Whites, Blacks Had 51% Higher and Hispanics Had 21% Higher Obesity Rates." CDC feature. Available at www.cdc.gov (accessed July 28, 2013).

Chapman, Steve. 2009. "A Big, Fat Political Mistake: Why Jon Corzine Should Have Left Obesity Out of the New Jersey Governor's Race." November 2. Available at http://reason.com (accessed May 2, 2011).

Chernin, Kim. 1981. *The Obsession: Reflections on the Tyranny of Slenderness*. New York: Harper and Row.

Christakis, Nicholas A., and James H. Fowler. 2007. "The Spread of Obesity in a Large Social Network over 32 Years." *New England Journal of Medicine* 357(4): 370–79.

Chua, Amy. 2011. *Battle Hymn of the Tiger Mother*. New York: Penguin.

Clarke, Adele E., Laura Mamo, Jennifer Fosket, Jennifer R. Fishman, and Janet K. Shim, eds. 2010. *Biomedicalization: Technoscience, Health, and Illness in the U.S.* Durham, NC: Duke University Press.

Conrad, Peter. 2007. *The Medicalization of Society: On the Transformation of Human Conditions into Treatable Disorders*. Baltimore: Johns Hopkins University Press.

Counihan, Carole M. 1999. *The Anthropology of Food and Body: Gender, Meaning, and Power*. New York: Routledge.

Crawford, Robert. 1980. "Healthism and the Medicalization of Everyday Life." *International Journal of Health Services* 10(3): 365–88.

——. 2006. "Health as a Meaningful Social Practice." *Health* 10(4): 401–20.

Cunningham, Solveig A., Michael R. Kramer, and K. M. Venkat Narayan. 2014. "Incidence of Childhood Obesity in the United States." *New England Journal of Medicine* 370(5): 403–11.

Depres, Jean-Pierre. 2012. "Body Fat Distribution and Risk of Cardiovascular Disease: An Update." *Circulation* 126(10): 1301–13.

Deurenberg, Paul, Mabel Deurenberg-Yap, and Syafri Guricci. 2002. "Asians Are Different from Caucasians and from Each Other in Their Body Mass Index/Body Fat Per Cent Relationship." *Obesity Reviews* 3(3): 141–46.

Dworkin, Shari L., and Faye Linda Wachs. 2009. *Body Panic: Gender, Health, and the Selling of Fitness*. New York: NYU Press.

Ernsberger, Paul. 2009. "Does Social Class Explain the Connection between Weight and Health?" In *The Fat Studies Reader*, edited by Esther Rothblum and Sondra Solovay, 25–36. New York: NYU Press.

Evans, John, Emma Rich, Brian Davies, and Rachel Allwood, eds. 2008. *Education, Disordered Eating and Obesity Discourse: Fat Fabrications*. London: Routledge.

Farrell, Amy Erdman. 2011. *Fat Shame: Stigma and the Fat Body in American Culture*. New York: NYU Press.

Fikkan, Janna L., and Esther D. Rothblum. 2011. "Is Fat a Feminist Issue: Exploring the Gendered Nature of Weight Bias." *Sex Roles: A Journal of Research* 66(9): 575–92.

Flegal, Katherine M., Brian K. Kit, Heather Orpana, and Barry I. Graubard. 2013. "Association of All-Cause Mortality with Overweight and Obesity Using Standard Body Mass Index Categories: A Systematic Review and Meta-Analysis." *Journal of the American Medical Association* 309(1): 71–82.

Food and Drug Administration (FDA). 2011. "Questions and Answers about FDA's Initiative against Contaminated Weight Loss Products." January 27. Available at http://www.fda.gov (accessed July 4, 2013).

——. 2013a. "Beware of Fraudulent Weight-Loss 'Dietary Supplements.'" June 5. Available at http://www.fda.gov (accessed July 4, 2013).

——. 2013b. "Medications Target Long-Term Weight Control." April 12. Available at http://www.fda.gov (accessed August 4, 2013).

Foucault, Michel. 1975. *The Birth of the Clinic: An Archaeology of Medical Perception*. New York: Vintage.

——. 1978. *The History of Sexuality, Vol. 1: An Introduction*. New York: Random House.

——. 1984. "The Politics of Health in the 18th Century." In *The Foucault Reader*, edited by Paul Rabinow, 273–89. New York: Pantheon.

Fraser, Laura. 1998. *Losing It: False Hopes and Fat Profits in the Diet Industry*. New York: Penguin.

Frey, William H. 2011. "America's Diverse Future: Initial Glimpses at the U.S. Child Population from the 2010 Census." State of Metropolitan America No. 29. Brookings Institute, Washington, DC.

Gaesser, Glenn A. 2002. *Big Fat Lies: The Truth about Your Weight and Your Health*. Rev. ed. Carlsbad, CA: Gurze Books.

Gard, Michael, and Jan Wright. 2005. *The Obesity Epidemic: Science, Morality and Ideology*. London: Routledge.

Gratzer, David. 2012. "The Bloomberg Diet." *National Affairs* 13(fall). Available at www.nationalaffairs.com (accessed July 25, 2013).

Greenhalgh, Susan, and Megan A. Carney. 2014. "Bad Biocitizens? Latinos in the U.S. 'Obesity Epidemic.'" *Human Organization* 73(3): 267–76.

Grinberg, Emanuella. 2012. "Georgia's Child Obesity Ads Aim to Create Movement out of Controversy." February 7. Available at http://www.cnn.com (accessed July 26, 2013).

Guthman, Julie. 2011. *Weighing In: Obesity, Food Justice, and the Limits of Capitalism*. Berkeley: University of California Press.

Halse, Christine. 2009. "Bio-Citizenship: Virtue Discourses and the Birth of the Bio-Citizen." In *Biopolitics and the "Obesity Epidemic,"* edited by Jan Wright and Valerie Harwood, 45–59. New York: Routledge.

Herndon, April. 2014. *Fat Blame: How the War on Obesity Victimizes Women and Children*. Lawrence: University of Kansas Press.

Hesse-Biber, Sharlene Nagy. 2007. *The Cult of Thinness*. 2nd ed. New York: Oxford University Press.

Hiltzik, Michael. 2013. "What California Should Learn from the 1–800-GET-THIN Saga." *Los Angeles Times*. April 19. Available at http://www.latimes.com (accessed August 6, 2013).

Hruschka, Daniel J., Alexandra A. Brewis, Amber Wutich, and Benjamin Morin. 2011. "Shared Norms and Their Explanation for the Social Clustering of Obesity." *American Journal of Public Health* 101(Suppl. 1): S295–300.

IOM (Inst. of Medicine). 2013. "Evaluating Obesity Prevention Efforts: A Plan for Measuring Progress." www.iom.edu (accessed February 3, 2015).

Juang, Linda P., Desiree Baolin Qin, and Irene J.K. Park. 2013. "Deconstructing the Myth of the 'Tiger Mother': An Introduction to the Special Issue on Tiger Parenting, Asian-Heritage Families, and Child/Adolescent Well-Being." *Asian American Journal of Psychology* 4(1): 1–6.

Jutel, Annemarie. 2006. "The Emergence of Overweight as a Disease Entity: Measuring Up Normality." *Social Science and Medicine* 63(9): 2268–76.

———. 2009. "Doctor's Orders: Diagnosis, Medical Authority, and the Exploitation of the Fat Body." In *Biopolitics and the "Obesity Epidemic,"* edited by Jan Wright and Valerie Harwood, 60–77. New York: Routledge.

Kessler, David A. 2009. *The End of Overeating: Taking Control of the Insatiable American Appetite*. New York: Rodale.

Kibria, Nazli. 1995. *Family Tightrope: The Changing Lives of Vietnamese-Americans*. Princeton: Princeton University Press.

Kim, Su Yeong, Yijie Wang, Diana Orozco-Lapray, Yishan Shen, and Mohammed Murtuza. 2013. "Does 'Tiger Parenting' Exist? Parenting Profiles of Chinese Americans and Adolescent Development." *Asian American Journal of Psychology* 4(1): 7–18.

Kramer, Caroline K., Bernard Zinman, and Ravi Retnakaran. 2013. "Are Metabolically Healthy Overweight and Obesity Benign Conditions? A Systematic Review and Meta-Analysis." *Annals of Internal Medicine* 159(11): 758–69.

Krueger, Alyson. 2014. "'No Body Talk' Summer Camps." *New York Times*. June 18. Available at http://www.newyorktimes.com/2014/06/09 (accessed July 27, 2014).

Kuczmarski, Robert J., Katherine M. Flegal, Stephen M. Campbell, and Clifford L. Johnson. 1994. "Increasing Prevalence of Overweight among U.S. Adults." *Journal of the American Medical Association* 272(3): 205–11.

Lau, Anna S., and Joey Fung. 2013. "On Better Footing to Understand Parenting and Family Process in Asian American Families." *Asian American Journal of Psychology* 4(1): 71–75.

Lavie, Carl J., and Kristin Loberg. 2014. *The Obesity Paradox: When Thinner Means Sicker and Heavier Means Healthier*. New York: Hudson Street Press.

Lee, Jennifer, and Min Zhou, eds. 2004. *Asian American Youth: Culture, Identity, and Ethnicity*. New York: Routledge.

Llewellyn, Clare H., Maciej Trzaskowski, Robert Plomin, and Jane Wardle. 2013. "Finding the Missing Heritability in Pediatric Obesity: The Contribution of Genome-Wide Complex Trait Analysis." *International Journal of Obesity* 37(11): 1506–9.

Loar, Russ. 1995. "Doctor's Orders: Ex-Surgeon General Koop Calls for War against Obesity." *Los Angeles Times*. March 18. Available at http://articles.latimes.com (accessed December 20, 2012).

Lumeng, Julie C., Patrick Forrest, Danielle P. Appugliese, Niko Kaciroti, Robert F. Corwyn, and Robert H. Bradley. 2010. "Weight Status as a Predictor of Being Bullied in Third through Sixth Grades." *Pediatrics* 125(6): 1301–07.

Lupton, Deborah. 1995. *The Imperative of Health: Public Health and the Regulated Body*. London: Sage.

Lyons, Russell. 2011. "The Spread of Evidence-Poor Medicine via Flawed Social-Network Analysis." *Statistics, Politics, and Policy* 2(1). Available at https://www.bepress.com/spp/vol2/iss1/2 (accessed July 3, 2014).

Maher, JaneMaree, Suzanne Fraser, and Jan Wright. 2009. "Framing the Mother: Childhood Obesity, Maternal Responsibility and Care." *Journal of Gender Studies* 19(3): 233–47.

Mann, Traci, A. Janet Tomiyama, Erika Westling, Ann-Marie Lew, Barbra Samuels, and Jason Chatman. 2007. "Medicare's Search for Effective Obesity Treatments: Diets Are Not the Answer." *American Psychologist* 62(3): 220–33.

Martin, Courtney E. 2007. *Perfect Girls, Starving Daughters: How the Quest for Perfection Is Harming Young Women*. New York: Penguin.

Metzl, Jonathan M., and Anna Kirkland, eds. 2010. *Against Health: How Health Became the New Morality*. New York: New York University Press.

Miller, Jake. 2013. "Weight and Mortality: Harvard Researchers Challenge Results of Obesity Analysis." *Harvard Gazette*. February 23. Available at http://news.harvard.edu/gazette/story (accessed July 27, 2013).

Molinary, Rosie. 2007. *Hijas Americanas: Beauty, Body Image, and Growing Up Latina*. Emeryville, CA: Seal Press.

Monaghan, Lee F. 2007. "Body Mass Index, Masculinities and Moral Worth: Men's Critical Understandings of 'Appropriate' Weight-for-Height." *Sociology of Health and Illness* 29(4): 584–609.

———. 2008. *Men and the War on Obesity: A Sociological Study*. Abingdon, UK: Routledge.

Monaghan, Lee F., and Helen Malson 2013 "'It's Worse for Women and Girls': Negotiating Embodied Masculinities through Weight-Related Talk." *Critical Public Health* 23(3): 304–19.

Moss, Michael. 2013. "The Extraordinary Science of Addictive Junk Food." *New York Times Magazine*. February 20. Available at http://www.nytimes.com (accessed August 6, 2013).

Mundy, Alicia. 2001. *Dispensing with the Truth: The Victims, the Drug Companies, and the Dramatic Story behind the Battle over Fen-Phen*. New York: St. Martin's.

Murtagh, Lindsey, and David S. Ludwig. 2011. "State Intervention in Life-Threatening Childhood Obesity." *Journal of the American Medical Association* 306(2): 206–7.

National Center for Health Statistics. 2012. *Summary Health Statistics for U.S. Adults: National Health Interview Survey 2010*. Vital and Health Statistics, Series 10, No. 252, January. Washington, DC: U.S. DHHS, CDC. Available at http://www.cdc.gov.nchs/data/series/sr_10/sr10_252.pdf (accessed August 2, 2013).

National Institutes of Health (NIH) and the National Heart, Lung, and Blood Institute (NHLBI). 1998. "Clinical Guidelines on the Identification, Evaluation, and

Treatment of Overweight and Obesity in Adults—the Evidence Report." *Obesity Research* 6(2): 1S–209S.

Nestle, Marion. 2007. *Food Politics: How the Food Industry Influences Nutrition and Health*. Rev. ed. Berkeley: University of California Press.

Neumark-Sztainer, Dianne, Katherine W. Bauer, Sarah Friend, Peter J. Hannan, Mary Story, and Jerica M. Berge. 2010. "Family Weight Talk and Dieting: How Much Do They Matter for Body Dissatisfaction and Disordered Eating Behaviors in Adolescent Girls?" *Journal of Adolescent Health* 47(3): 270–76.

Neumark-Sztainer, Dianne, Melanie Wall, Mary Story, and Amber R. Standish. 2012. "Dieting and Unhealthy Weight Control Behaviors during Adolescence: Associations with 10-Year Changes in Body Mass Index." *Journal of Adolescent Health* 50(1): 80–86.

Nichter, Mimi. 2000. *Fat Talk: What Girls and Their Parents Say about Dieting*. Cambridge, MA: Harvard University Press.

Novas, Carlos. 2006. "The Political Economy of Hope: Patients' Organizations, Science and Biovalue." *Biosocieties* 1(3): 289–305.

Office of the Governor [of California]. 2010. "Gov. Schwarzenegger Convenes 2010 Summit on Health, Nutrition and Obesity: Actions for Healthy Living." Press release. February 24. Available at http://gov.ca/gov/ (accessed April 14, 2010).

Office of the Surgeon General. 2001. *The Surgeon General's Call to Action to Prevent and Decrease Overweight and Obesity, 2001*. Rockville, MD: U.S. DHHS.

Ogden, Cynthia L., Margaret D. Carroll, Brian K. Kit, and Katherine M. Flegal. 2014. "Prevalence of Childhood and Adult Obesity in the United States, 2011–2012." *Journal of the American Medical Association* 311(8): 806–14.

Ogden, Cynthia L., Molly M. Lamb, Margaret D. Carroll, and Katherine M. Flegal. 2010a. "Obesity and Socioeconomic Status in Adults: United States, 2005–2008." NCHS Data Brief, no. 50. National Center for Health Statistics, Washington, DC.

———. 2010b. "Obesity and Socioeconomic Status in Children and Adolescents: United States, 2005–2008." NCHS Data Brief, no. 51. National Center for Health Statistics, Washington, DC.

Orbach, Susie. 1978. *Fat Is a Feminist Issue: The Anti-Diet Guide to Permanent Weight Loss*. New York: Paddington Press.

Oliver, J. Eric. 2006. *Fat Politics: The Real Story behind America's Obesity Epidemic*. Oxford: Oxford University Press.

Parker-Pope, Tara. 2012. "The Fat Trap." *New York Times Magazine*, January 1, 22–49.

Perez-Pena, Richard. 2011. "Skip the Sundae? Christie Is on the First Lady's Side." *New York Times*, February 28, A17.

Pfeifer, Stuart. 2011. "Lap-Band Has Poor Outcomes, Study Finds." *Los Angeles Times*, March 22, B4.

Pollack, Andrew. 2012a. "After 13-Year Drought, the FDA Approves a Second Drug for Weight Loss." *New York Times*, July 18, B3.

———. 2012b. "Diet Drug Is Approved by FDA." *New York Times*, June 28, B1–2.

———. 2013. "AMA Recognizes Obesity as a Disease." *New York Times*. June 18. Available at www.nytimes.com (accessed July 22, 2013).

Power, Michael L., and Jay Schulkin. 2009. *The Evolution of Obesity*. Baltimore: Johns Hopkins University Press.

Puhl, Rebecca M. 2011. "Weight Stigma toward Youth: A Significant Problem in Need of Societal Solutions." *Childhood Obesity* 7(5): 359–63.

Puhl, Rebecca M., and Chelsea A. Heuer. 2009. "The Stigma of Obesity: A Review and Update." *Obesity* 17(5): 941–64.

———. 2010. "Obesity Stigma: Important Considerations for Public Health." *American Journal of Public Health* 100(6): 1019–28.

Puhl, Rebecca M., and Janet D. Latner. 2007. "Stigma, Obesity, and the Health of the Nation's Children." *Psychological Bulletin* 133(4): 557–80.

Puhl, Rebecca M., Dianne Neumark-Sztainer, S. Bryn Austin, Joerg Luedicke, and Kelly M. King. 2014. "Setting Policy Priorities to Address Eating Disorders and Weight Stigma: Views from the Field of Eating Disorders and the US General Public." *BMC Public Health* 14: 1–18.

Puhl, Rebecca M., Jamie Lee Peterson, and Joerg Luedicke. 2013. "Weight-Based Victimization: Bullying Experiences of Weight Loss Treatment-Seeking Youth." *Pediatrics* 131(1): e1–9.

Puzziferri, Nancy, Thomas B. Roshek III, Helen G. Mayo, Ryan Gallagher, Steven H. Belle, and Edward H. Livingston. 2014. "Long-term Follow-up after Bariatric Surgery." *Journal of the American Medical Association* 312(9): 934–42.

Rae, Jessica. 2010. "It's the Year of the Value Diet." June 18. Available at www.cnbd.com (accessed May 1, 2011).

Reed-Danahay, Deborah E. 1997. *Auto/Ethnography: Rewriting the Self and the Social.* Oxford: Berg.

Rice, Carla. 2007. "Becoming 'The Fat Girl': Acquisition of an Unfit Identity." *Women's Studies International Forum* 30(2): 158–74.

Rose, Nicholas. 1999. *Powers of Freedom: Reframing Political Thought.* Cambridge, UK: Cambridge University Press.

Rose, Nicholas, and Carlos Novas. 2005. "Biological Citizenship." In *Global Assemblages: Technology, Politics, and Ethics as Anthropological Problems*, edited by Aihwa Ong and Stephen J. Collier, 439–63. Malden, MA: Blackwell.

Rosenblatt, Robert A. 2001. "Surgeon General Takes Stern Stance on Obesity." *Los Angeles Times.* December 14. Available at http://articles.latimes.com (accessed July 23, 2013).

Ross, Bruce. 2005. "Fat or Fiction: Weighing the 'Obesity Epidemic.'" In *The Obesity Epidemic: Science, Morality and Ideology*, edited by Michael Gard and Jan Wright, 86–106. London: Routledge.

Rothblum, Esther, and Sondra Solovay, eds. 2009. *The Fat Studies Reader.* New York: NYU Press.

Royce, Tracy. 2009. "The Shape of Abuse: Fat Oppression as a Form of Violence against Women." In *The Fat Studies Reader*, edited by Esther Rothblum and Sondra Solovay, 151–57. New York: NYU Press.

Saguy, Abigail C. 2013. *What's Wrong with Fat?* Oxford: Oxford University Press.

Saguy, Abigail C., and Rene Almeling. 2008. "Fat in the Fire? Science, the News Media, and the 'Obesity Epidemic.'" *Sociological Forum* 23(1): 53–83.

Saguy, Abigail C., and Kjerstin Gruys. 2010. "Morality and Health: News Media Constructions of Overweight and Eating Disorders." *Social Problems* 57(2): 231–50.

Sánchez-Carracedo, David, Dianne Neumark-Sztainer, and Gemma López-Guimerà. 2012. "Integrated Prevention of Obesity and Eating Disorders: Barriers, Developments and Opportunities." *Public Health Nutrition* 15(12): 2295–309.

Sandberg, Sheryl. 2013. *Lean In: Women, Work, and the Will to Lead.* New York: Knopf.

Satchfield, Scott. 2013. "Michelle Obama Speaks Out about Childhood Obesity during N.O. Visit." Fox News. July 30. Available at www.fox8live.com (accessed August 26, 2013).

Schwartz, Hillel. 1986. *Never Satisfied: A Cultural History of Diets, Fantasies and Fat.* New York: Doubleday.

Schwartz, Marlene B., and Kathryn E. Henderson. 2009. "Does Obesity Prevention Cause Eating Disorders?" *Journal of the American Academy of Child and Adolescent Psychiatry* 48(8): 784–86.

Shape Up America! 1997. "In Spite of Diet Drug Withdrawal, the War on Obesity Must Continue Says Dr. C. Everett Koop." Press release. September 19. Available at www.shapeup.org (accessed December 20, 2012).

Simon, Michele. 2006. *Appetite for Profit: How the Food Industry Undermines Our Health and How to Fight Back.* New York: Nation.

Skrabanek, Peter. 1994. *Death of Humane Medicine and the Rise of Coercive Healthism.* Edmonds, UK: Social Affairs Unit.

Sobal, Jeffery. 1995. "The Medicalization and Demedicalization of Obesity." In *Eating Agendas*, edited by Jeffrey Sobal and Donna Maurer, 67–90. New York: Aldine de Gruyter.

Stearns, Peter. 2002. *Fat History: Bodies and Beauty in the Modern West.* 2nd ed. New York: NYU Press.

Sumithran, Priya, Luke A. Prendergast, Elizabeth Delbridge, Katrina Purcell, Arthur Shulkes, Adamandia Kriketos, and Joseph Proietto. 2011. "Long-Term Persistence of Hormonal Adaptations to Weight Loss." *New England Journal of Medicine* 365(17): 1597–604.

Swidey, Neil. 2013. "The Food Fighter." *Boston Globe Magazine*, July 28, 17–21.

Tang-Peronard, Jeanett L., Helle R. Andersen, Tina K. Jensen, and Berit L. Heitmann. 2011. "Endocrine-Disrupting Chemicals and Obesity Development in Humans: A Review." *Obesity Reviews* 12(8): 622–36.

Tavernise, Sabrina. 2014. "Obesity Rate for Young Children Plummets 43% in a Decade." *New York Times*, February 25.

Taylor, Nicole L. 2011. " 'Guys, She's Humongous!' Gender and Weight-based Teasing in Adolescence." *Journal of Adolescent Research* 26(2): 178–99.

University of California, Irvine. 2012. "UCIrvine." Statistical portrait. November 1. Available at http://www.oir.uci.edu/portrait (accessed July 29, 2013).

United Health Foundation. 2014. *2014 Annual Report.* www.americashealthrankings.org/reports/Annual (accessed February 3, 2015).

Vigarello, Georges. 2013. *The Metamorphoses of Fat: A History of Obesity.* Translated by C. Jon Delogu. New York: Columbia University Press.

Wagerson, Margarita. 2012. "School Obesity Programs May Promote Worrisome Eating Behaviors, Physical Activity." *University Record Online.* University of Michigan.

January 30. Available at http://ur.umich.edu/1112/Jan30_12/3108-school-obesity-programs (accessed March 16, 2014).

Wann, Marilyn. 1998. *Fat! So? Because You Don't Have to Apologize for Your Size!* Berkeley: Ten Speed Press.

———. 2009. "Foreword: Fat Studies—An Invitation to Revolution." In *The Fat Studies Reader*, edited by Esther Rothblum and Sondra Solovay, xi–xxv. New York: NYU Press.

Weintraub, Karen. 2014. "New Allies in War on Weight." *Boston Globe*, June 30, B5–B6.

Weiss, Dara-Lynn. 2012. "Weight Watcher" *Vogue* magazine. April. Available at http://www.vogue.com (accessed August 5, 2013).

———. 2013. *The Heavy: A Mother, a Daughter, a Diet—a Memoir*. New York: Ballantine.

White House. 2010. "First Lady Michelle Obama Launches Let's Move: America's Move to Raise a Healthier Generation of Kids." Press release. Available at www.whitehouse.gov (accessed July 24, 2013).

Wolf, Naomi. 1991. *The Beauty Myth: How Images of Beauty Are Used against Women*. New York: Doubleday.

World Health Organization (WHO). 2011. "Obesity and Overweight: Fact Sheet." Updated March. Available at www.who.int (accessed May 2, 2011).

Yen, Hope. 2012. "White Population to Lose Majority Status in 2032." *Boston Globe*, December 13, A2.

Young, Aaron, Humayun J. Chaudhry, Janelle Rhyne, and Michael Dugan. 2013. "A Census of Actively Licensed Physicians in the United States, 2010." *Journal of Medical Regulation* 96(4): 10–20.

Zelman, Kathleen M. 2011. "6 Things Never to Do to Lose Weight." Edited June 16. Available at http://www.webmd.com (accessed July 4, 2013).

Zernike, Kate, and Marc Santora. 2013. "Weight Led Governor to Surgery." *New York Times*. May 7. Available at http://www.nytimes.com (accessed August 16, 2013).

Zhou, Min. 2009. *Contemporary Chinese America: Immigration, Ethnicity, and Community Transformation*. Philadelphia: Temple University Press.

Index